Oxford Medical Publications

Adverse Syndromes and Psychiatric Drugs

D0861341

Adverse Syndromes and Psychiatric Drugs
A clinical guide

Edited by

Peter M. Haddad
Cromwell House Community Mental Health Centre
Bolton, Salford and Trafford Mental Health NHS Trust

Serdar Dursun
Neuroscience and Psychiatry Unit, University of Manchester

and

Bill Deakin
Neuroscience and Psychiatry Unit, University of Manchester

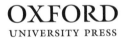

OXFORD
UNIVERSITY PRESS

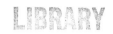
OXFORD
UNIVERSITY PRESS

Great Clarendon Street, Oxford OX2 6DP

Oxford University Press is a department of the University of Oxford.
It furthers the University's objective of excellence in research, scholarship,
and education by publishing worldwide in

Oxford New York

Auckland Bangkok Buenos Aires Cape Town Chennai
Dar es Salaam Delhi Hong Kong Istanbul Karachi Kolkata
Kuala Lumpur Madrid Melbourne Mexico City Mumbai Nairobi
São Paulo Shanghai Taipei Tokyo Toronto

Oxford is a registered trade mark of Oxford University Press
in the UK and in certain other countries

Published in the United States
by Oxford University Press Inc., New York

A catalogue record for this title is available from the British Library

ISBN 0 19 852748 9 (Pbk)

10 9 8 7 6 5 4 3 2 1

Typeset by Newgen Imaging Systems (P) Ltd., Chennai, India
Printed in Great Britain
on acid-free paper by
Biddles Ltd., King's Lynn

Foreword

Psychiatric drugs are far from "clean". They cross the blood-brain barrier and affect the delicate balance of neural mechanisms, as well as producing an extraordinary range of systemic unwanted effects. The authors in their preface tell us that adverse syndromes associated with psychiatric medication have been neglected. This book fills a gap in the medical literature in an original and comprehensive way. One glance at the contents list of this volume will show the great care that has gone into choosing the topics covered in order to provide a helpful and instructive book. It is about clinical practice, while providing the background knowledge to inform that practice. This is the kind of book that everyone will want to keep at hand in order to deal with difficult cases and be prepared for the discussions that inevitably accompany them.

The wide range of chapter headings shows the thought and expertise that has been applied. It is invidious to select topics for mention, but I hope I may be permitted to comment on a few chapters. Neuroleptic malignant syndrome is presented as a distinct clinical entity with a range of apparently related but clinically distinguishable differential diagnoses. Matters such as QTc prolongation are a source of differing reports and opinions. It is helpful here to have the main research data clearly laid out in the chapter on torsade de pointes. It is also worth noting that the topical and important issue of diabetes has been included. At the same time, well-known but complicated topics such as the adverse effects of lithium are authoritatively covered.

The book is user-friendly and lives up to its title. The use of a structured layout for each syndrome means that specific issues can be accessed with ease. The boxed summary at the end of each chapter should prove equally useful for both the busy practising doctor and the revising examination candidate.

As will be seen, many of the adverse effects of psychiatric drugs reside uneasily on the borderline between psychiatry and other disciplines. My own experience as a clinical pharmacologist and emergency physician has shown me that these syndromes can present in unexpected and often life-threatening ways. The editors and authors are to be congratulated on producing this book, and I recommend it to psychiatrists, physicians, and all healthcare workers who are likely to encounter these challenging syndromes.

John A Henry
Professor of Accident and Emergency Medicine
Imperial College, London   April 2004

Preface

The editors' aim is that this book be an easily accessible text that will help psychiatrists, GPs, pharmacists and nurses prevent, recognize and manage common adverse syndromes associated with psychiatric drugs. In addition we hope that it will stimulate interest in psychopharmacology. The book is not intended to be a reference book listing every side effect of psychiatric drugs; other texts cover this adequately e.g. *Compendium of Data Sheets* and *Summary of Product Characteristics*. Instead it concentrates on syndromes. There are several reasons for this.

First, adverse syndromes associated with psychiatric medication have been neglected. Most general psychiatry textbooks deal with adverse syndromes of medication in a cursory manner and some common syndromes are not mentioned at all. This is despite the fact that pharmacotherapy is an important aspect of the treatment of most major psychiatric disorders. Second, many syndromes are common. For example it would not be unusual for a clinician to encounter at least one adverse syndrome, or potential syndrome, in every outpatient clinic or ward round e.g. an extrapyramidal syndrome associated with an antipsychotic, an antidepressant withdrawal syndrome or the possibility of teratogenesis in a woman who is planning to get pregnant and is prescribed an anticonvulsant or lithium as a mood stabilizer. Finally, in contrast to drug side-effects, syndromes have clinical utility i.e. since a syndrome usually has a specific cause and underlying mechanism, its diagnosis will lead to a specific treatment and prognosis. In contrast, since a symptom can have umpteen causes, one cannot make any firm conclusions about cause, treatment or prognosis.

Of course the separation of symptoms from syndromes is not fixed and requires an arbitrary cut-off. For example although the term 'serotonin syndrome' is widely used, in reality there is a spectrum of serotonin toxicity. This argument applies to many of the syndromes discussed on this book. Nevertheless the concept of a syndrome is clinically useful as long as readers bear the spectrum concept in mind. Exactly the same issue applies to most psychiatric diagnoses which are syndrome based and require an arbitary cut-off in terms of number of symptoms, severity and duration. Patients with troublesome adverse symptoms, which fall short of the criteria for an adverse syndrome, still require diagnosis and treatment!

All the syndromes covered in this book include sections on:

- Clinical features
- Pharmacological basis
- Differential diagnosis
- Management
- Risk factors and prevention.

In addition each chapter ends with a boxed summary, complete with eight fixed headings, for each syndrome that has been discussed. We hope that this will provide a quick reference source.

We are grateful to all the authors who have contributed and shared their expertise. Special thanks are also due to Oxford University Press.

Peter M Haddad,
Serdar Dursun,
and Bill Deakin

Neuroscience and Psychiatry Unit
University of Manchester

Contents

List of contributors

Ian Anderson
Senior Lecturer in Psychiatry
Neuroscience and Psychiatry Unit
University of Manchester
Manchester
UK

Heather Ashton
Professor of Clinical
Psychopharmacology
University of Newcastle upon Tyne
Newcastle upon Tyne
UK

Glen B Baker
Professor of Psychiatry
University of Alberta
Alberta
Canada

David S Baldwin
Senior Lecturer in Psychiatry
University of Southampton
Southampton
UK

Thomas R E Barnes
Professor of Psychiatry
Imperial College School of Medicine
London
UK

Hyun-Sang Cho
Postdoctoral Fellow
Department of Psychiatry
Yale University School of Medicine
USA

Deepak Cyril D'Souza
Associate Professor
Department of Psychiatry

Yale University School of Medicine
USA

Bill Deakin
Professor of Psychiatry
Neuroscience and Psychiatry Unit
University of Manchester
Manchester
UK

Serdar Dursun
Senior Lecturer in Psychiatry
Neuroscience and Psychiatry Unit
University of Manchester
Manchester
UK

Nicol Ferrier
Professor of Psychiatry
University of Newcastle upon Tyne
Newcastle upon Tyne
UK

Ken Gillman
Consultant Psychiatrist and Director
Department of Clinical
Neuropharmacology
Pioneer Valley Private Hospital
Queensland
Australia

Peter M Haddad
Lead Consultant in Community
Psychiatry
Cromwell House Community
Mental Health Centre
Bolton, Salford and Trafford Mental
Health NHS Trust
Salford
UK

Salman Karim
Lecturer in Psychiatry
University of Manchester
Manchester
UK

Dora Kohen
Professor of Psychiatry
University of Central Lancashire
Preston
UK

John H Krystal
Professor of Psychiatry
Department of Psychiatry
Yale University School of Medicine
USA

Anna Lambert
Research Assistant
University of Southampton
Southampton
UK

Suzy N Leech
Senior Registrar in Dermatology
Royal Victoria Infirmary
Newcastle upon Tyne
UK

Shôn Lewis
Professor of Psychiatry
University of Manchester
Manchester
UK

Karine A N Macritchie
Specialist Registrar in Psychiatry
Newcastle upon Tyne
UK

Andrew G Mayers
Research Psychologist
University of Southampton
Southampton
UK

R Hamish McAllister-Williams
Senior Lecturer in Psychiatry
University of Newcastle upon Tyne
Newcastle upon Tyne
UK

Trevor I Prior
Assistant Professor of Psychiatry
Department of Psychiatry
University of Alberta
Alberta
Canada

Jerrold Rosenbaum
Chief of Psychiatry
Massachusetts General Hospital
Massachusetts
USA

Paul Strickland
Consultant Psychiatrist
Bolton, Salford and Trafford Mental
Health NHS Trust
Salford
UK

David M Taylor
Chief Pharmacist
Pharmacy Department
Maudsley Hospital
Denmark Hill
London
UK

Ian M Whyte
Professor and Director of Clinical
Toxicology and Pharmacology
New Castle Mater Misericordiae
Hospital
New South Wales
Australia

Angelika Wieck
Consultant in Perinatal Psychiatry
Manchester Mental Health and Social
Care Trust
Manchester
UK

Allan H Young
Professor of Psychiatry
University of Newcastle upon
Tyne
Newcastle upon Tyne
UK

Chapter 1

Extrapyramidal syndromes

Serdar Dursun, Peter M Haddad, and
Thomas R E Barnes

Introduction

Extrapyramidal syndromes (EPS) were recognized soon after antipsychotic drugs entered clinical practice. The first formal report is generally attributed to Steck (1954). Four key syndromes are recognized: acute dystonia; akathisia; parkinsonism; and tardive dyskinesia. Patients may suffer concurrently from more than one syndrome. Akathisia and acute dystonia generally emerge in the first week after starting treatment with an antipsychotic drug, parkinsonism during the first two months of treatment and tardive dyskinesia after at least six months of treatment. Dystonia can also occur late in treatment (tardive dystonia) either in isolation or as part of tardive dyskinesia (TD). Drug-induced EPS need to be differentiated from abnormal involuntary movements, particularly orofacial dyskinesia, which can occur in people with schizophrenia who have not received antipsychotic treatment, and represent a neuromotor component of the illness (Gervin *et al.* 1998; Puri *et al.* 1999).

EPS are important clinical phenomena for several reasons. Both the motor and mental manifestations of EPS can be unpleasant for patients. The movements of tardive dyskinesia, for example, may cause functional impairment and can also be stigmatizing, unfavourably affecting social acceptability (Boumans *et al.* 1994). It is likely that EPS contribute to poor adherence with antipsychotic medication and so play a role in relapse. However studies investigating this area have produced conflicting results (Hummer and Fleischhacker 1996). This may be partly because the rating scales used to assess parkinsonism tend to concentrate on the objective phenomena and it may be the adverse subjective experience of EPS that is more relevant to adherence (Barnes *et al.* 2000). Dystonia (Newton-John 1988; Stones *et al.* 1990) and tardive dyskinesia (Youssef and Waddington 1987) may be associated with increased mortality.

EPS can occur with psychotropic drugs other than antipsychotics, but this is uncommon. For example, akathisia, dystonia, parkinsonism and TD have occasionally been reported with SSRIs (Leo 1996; Lane 1998), with akathisia being the the most common problem. There have also been sporadic reports of EPS with tricyclic antidepressants and monoamine oxidase inhibitors (Gill *et al.* 1997). Although there are not enough data for a definitive statement, it appears that SSRIs are more likely to be associated with EPS than other antidepressants (Schillevoort *et al.* 2002). EPS have been reported with lithium monotherapy (Tyrer *et al.* 1980), and lithium can also worsen antipsychotic-induced EPS (Addonizio *et al.* 1988). Non-psychotropic drugs occasionally reported to cause EPS include the contraceptive pill and anti-dopaminergic anti-emetics such as metoclopramide. For the most part, this chapter will limit itself to EPS associated with antipsychotics.

It has been suggested that risk of EPS could be markedly reduced if conventional antipsychotics were prescribed more judiciously. This argument has been linked to the idea that psychiatrists have tended to prescribe relatively high doses of conventional antipsychotics. Although this is probably true, the argument is simplistic. First, positron emission tomographic (PET) studies show that the threshold level of dopamine D_2 receptor blockade in the striatum associated with therapeutic efficacy is only a little below that associated with the appearance of EPS, such that it would generally be difficult to produce clinical benefit without some risk of EPS (Kapur *et al.* 2000). Second, some patients will exhibit movement disorder despite receiving relatively modest doses of antipsychotic medication. Finally, in the acute setting clinicians may employ higher dosages to harness the sedative effects of a drug rather than its antipsychotic properties. Although benzodiazepines can be used for this purpose, the approach is not without its problems; benzodiazepines may cause behavioural disinhibition and are associated with dependence (Pato *et al.* 1989; Wolkowitz and Pickar 1991).

The newer, so-called atypical antipsychotics have a lower liability for acute EPS than conventional antipsychotics (Caroff *et al.* 2002). This has been demonstrated in individual trials involving amisulpride (e.g. Coukell *et al.* 1996), aripiprazole (Marder *et al.* 2003), clozapine (e.g. Gerlach and Peacock 1995; Kurz *et al.* 1995), risperidone (e.g. Claus *et al.* 1992; Peuskens 1995), olanzapine (e.g. Beasley *et al.* 1996), and quetiapine (e.g. Arvanitis *et al.* 1997; Small *et al.* 1997) as well as in a meta-analysis (Geddes *et al.* 2000). This difference in EPS liability is the main reason that in the UK the National Institute for Clinical Excellence (NICE) appraisal of atypical antipsychotics recommended that atypical antipsychotics are considered as first line agents in the treatment of first onset schizophrenia (NICE 2002*a*). However, this should not obscure the fact that individual atypical antipsychotics differ in their propensity to cause EPS (Tarsy *et al.* 2002). Across their full dose range, clozapine and quetiapine do not differ from placebo in their EPS liability. In contrast, EPS are seen with some other atypicals, as dose-related phenomena. Overall, despite the widespread use of atypical antipsychotic drugs, acute and chronic EPS remain a significant problem in clinical practice (Modestin *et al.* 2000; Halliday *et al.* 2002).

Acute EPS are predictive of an increased subsequent risk of TD (Umbricht and Kane 1996*a*). This suggests that atypical antipsychotics may be associated with a lower incidence of TD. Experience with clozapine tends to support this view (Umbricht and Kane 1996*b*) but, despite some promising results (for example, Dolder and Jeste 2003), the published data on the long term use of other atypicals are probably insufficient for a firm statement to be made on their individual liability to cause TD.

Acute dystonia

Clinical features

A dystonia is an involuntary contraction of a muscle to its maximum degree. The contraction can be sustained, usually resulting in postural distortion (myostatic dystonia) or it can be transient and repetitive (kinetic dystonia) producing an appearance of constant movement. Psychiatric drugs tend to produce myostatic dystonias and these can affect virtually any part of the body including the head, neck, trunk and limbs. In this section we are concerned with acute dystonias. These usually occur early on in drug treatment, are short lived and respond to treatment with anticholinergic drugs. In contrast, tardive dystonias occur late on in treatment, are persistent and unresponsive to anti-cholinergic treatment. They are discussed further in the section on TD.

The neck is the most common site to be effected by an acute dystonia. In one large retrospective study (Swett 1975) neck dystonia accounted for approximately one-third of such reactions. The neck can be twisted in any direction. The jaw and tongue constitute the next most commonly involved area (15–17 per cent; Swett 1975). The tongue may be protruded, retracted or deviated to one side. Patients will often complain that their tongue is 'swollen', although it is actually of normal size; their description is an attempt to explain the unpleasant subjective feeling associated with contraction of the tongue muscles. The mouth may be forced closed (trismus) or open, or the jaw may be deviated to one side. Oculogyric crisis is a dystonia of the extra-occular muscles leading to upward deviation of the eyes so that only the sclera are visible. Strictly it should be referred to as 'oculogyric spasm', as 'oculogyris crisis' is a more complex disorder where spasm is associated with other features (Owens 1990). Although the condition is well known to doctors, it is relatively rare in clinical practice, and accounted for only 6 per cent of the dystonic reactions observed in the study by Swett (1975).

Bilateral contraction of the truncal muscles can lead to arching of the back (opisthotonos), while asymmetric involvement of the truncal muscles can cause the person to lean to one side with one shoulder rotated forward (Pisa syndrome). Dystonia of the limbs can cause particularly bizarre postures. For example, in the lower limbs, patients can exhibit extension of the hips and knees combined with plantar flexion at the ankles so that they appear to walk on tiptoe like a ballet dancer. Sometimes this is combined with adductor spasm causing the legs to be forced together or crossed at rest. On attempting to walk the patient will put one foot across the path of the other with each step ('scissors' gait).

Dystonias can have serious consequences and are occasionally fatal. Lingual dystonias can cause trauma to the tongue. Dystonias of the laryngeal musculature can lead to respiratory distress, stridor and asphyxiation while involvement of the pharyngeal musculature can cause difficulty swallowing and death by choking (Stones *et al.* 1990; Newton-John 1988; Flaherty and Laymeyer 1978).

A key feature of dystonias is the associated subjective distress, with fear and anxiety. This is partly an understandable emotional reaction to a distressing event during which the patient will often not understand what is happening to their body. In addition it has been suggested that distress is a core part of the dystonic syndrome (Cunningham Owens 1999), in the same way that anxiety is an integral part of akathisia.

Acute dystonia has a relatively rapid onset. Subjective symptoms are the first to appear; the patient may complain of stiffness or aching. This is rapidly followed by full muscle contraction. The time to onset of the full syndrome ranges from a few minutes to an hour. Without treatment the natural history can take three forms; (i) the symptoms may be sustained over hours or days, (ii) the symptoms may fluctuate in severity without totally remitting, or (iii) the symptoms may totally resolve but reappear after a short time, producing an episodic picture.

Most dystonias occur within the first 5 days of initiating antipsychotic treatment (Ayd 1961; Singh *et al.* 1990) though the syndrome can occur during chronic antipsychotic treatment and as an acute consequence of abrupt drug discontinuation. Figures for incidence vary widely. The transient nature of dystonias and the lack of a specific rating scale mean that the phenomenon has not been assessed as systematically as other EPS in clinical trials. The results of two prospective studies suggest an incidence of approximately 33 per cent over several weeks in patients treated with fluphenazine (Singh *et al.* 1990; Chakos *et al.* 1992). A study comparing intramuscular haloperidol and olanzapine for rapid tranquillization revealed a 7 per cent incidence of dystonia within 24 hours of receiving im haloperidol and 0 per cent after receiving im olanzapine (Wright *et al.* 2001).

Pharmacological basis

The pathophysiology is unclear. It has been suggested that dystonias reflect excess dopaminergic activity but the converse has also been suggested. The observation that SSRI antidepressants can occasionally cause dystonias may reflect the role of the serotonergic system in modulating dopaminergic transmission. Further, there is preclinical evidence that cholinergic agonists such as acetylcholine and carbachol can induce dystonias, and combined with the clinical efficacy of anticholinergics, it is suggested that increased striatal cholinergic activity may play a role in the development of dystonia. This notion is further supported by evidence that the acute administration of antipsychotics increases striatal acetylcholine release.

Differential diagnosis

The introduction of several atypical antipsychotics since the mid-1990s means that acute dystonias are encountered less frequently and many younger doctors and nurses may not have direct clinical experience of the syndrome. The bizarre movements associated with an acute dystonia may be misdiagnosed as somatoform problems, behaviour intended to obtain anticholinergic medication or seizures. Cunningham Owens (1999) has emphasized that the 'bizarre' appearance of many dystonias is in itself a pointer to the diagnosis. The true diagnosis is usually obvious once the patient is examined. The recent introduction, or abrupt discontinuation, of an antipsychotic drug is a strong indicator.

Management

The treatment of choice is an anticholinergic drug e.g. biperiden or procyclidine.

If symptoms are mild, medication may be given orally e.g. procyclidine 10 mg. If symptoms are severe, medication can be given intravenously (iv) e.g. procyclidine 10 mg iv over 1 minute. Intramuscular (im) medication acts more slowly but the im route may need to be used if the patients is agitated and there are problems in gaining safe iv access.

The patient should be observed for some time afterwards, as the symptoms may remit only to reappear as the effect of medication wears off. If the patient has been treated in the Accident and Emergency department and is to be discharged it may be advisable to give the patient oral procyclidine to take prn should there be any signs of a recurrence over the coming days (Barnes and McPhillips 1996).

To minimize the risk of recurrence, wherever possible, the dose of an antipsychotic drug should not be increased for several days after a dystonia has occurred.

Risk factors

Risk factors for dystonia include:

1 Use of high potency conventional antipsychotics

2 Male gender

3 Younger age

4 Drug naïve patient

5 Rapid escalation in drug dose

6 Recent abrupt discontinuation of antipsychotic medication.

Prevention

The incidence of dystonias is less with atypical antipsychotics than with conventional agents. The use of lower dosages and a more gradual titration following initiation of conventional drug will reduce the risk. We do not advocate the routine prescription of anticholinergics as a prophylaxis against dystonia in individuals prescribed oral antipsychotics unless dystonia has proved to be a problem in the past. However, when haloperidol is administered im for rapid tranquillization, consideration should be given to simultaneously administering im procyclidine. This is consistent with the recommendations on rapid tranquillization in the NICE (2002*b*) schizophrenia treatment guideline.

Akathisia

Clinical features

Akathisia has both subjective and objective components (Barnes and Braude 1985). The subjective component consists of inner restlessness, unease and dysphoria and can be extremely distressing for patients (Halstead *et al.* 1994). The objective component consists of motor restlessness which appears to be the patient's attempt, largely unsuccessful, to reduce the state of inner unease. Unlike other EPS, the movements seen with akathisia are semi-voluntary though patients feel that thay are 'forced' to move. Lying down sometimes eases the symptoms. During sleep akathisia can manifest with myoclonic jerks.

Both the subjective and objective components of akathisia may be localized to the lower limbs and patients may complain of abnormal sensations in their legs such as 'cramping' or 'stretching' feelings. Patients often move their legs incessantly and when trying to sit still they may stand up and then sit down repeatedly. When standing they may shift their weight from one foot to the other or walk on the spot (Braude *et al.* 1983). One of the authors recalls a male patient with schizophrenia, prescribed flupenthixol depot, who had akathisia and spent much of his day trying to sit in an armchair in his lounge. The fidgeting movements of his feet wore holes in two successive lounge carpets in front of his chair.

Possible associations between akathisia and both suicide (Hansen 2001; Atbasoglu *et al.* 2001) and violence to others have been suggested. Presumably such associations would be partly mediated by the distress, irritability and dysphoria of the condition. However, on the basis of the existing literature, these associations remain uncertain.

In populations prescribed conventional antipsychotics, the reported prevalence of akathisia has been around 20 to 25 per cent (Barnes 1992), although figures as high as 32 per cent (Kennedy *et al.* 1971) have been reported. Akathisia can emerge a few hours after a single dose of an antipsychotic and it may be more common after parenteral administration of antipsychotics as opposed to oral administration.

Although antipsychotics are the main cause of akathisia, the syndrome can occur with SSRIs (Lane 1998; Leo 1996), as already mentioned. Case reports have documented the syndrome appearing when SSRIs and antipsychotics are combined (Lane 1998). This may reflect a pharmacodynamic additive effect or a pharmacokinetic interaction. Some SSRIs inhibit the metabolism of certain antipsychotics leading to higher plasma levels. As akathisia is a dose-related phenomenon, this interaction may cause its appearance or worsening.

Pharmacological basis

The pathophysiology is unclear. The dopaminergic and adrenergic systems are presumed to be involved. This is based on the observation that most drugs that cause akathisia are D_2 receptor antagonists and that akathisia can be treated with central beta-adrenergic antagonists. An imbalance in cholinergic-dopaminergic transmission has also been suggested. An association between low serum iron and akathisia has been reported but attempts to replicate this have produced inconsistent and contradictory findings.

Differential diagnosis

An important differential diagnosis is psychomotor agitation. Differentiation can be extremely difficult not least because patients are often agitated as part of their their illness, when they commence antipsychotic medication. A vicious circle can develop whereby an antipsychotic drug causes akathisia, the features of which are then attributed to agitation as a symptom of their psychiatric illness, leading to the administration of higher doses of medication which in turn exacerbates the akathisia, and so on. Markers to assist differentiation include (i) akathisia usually commences within days of starting an antipsychotic or increasing its dose, (ii) people with akathisia will tend to locate the restlessness in the legs, and (iii) akathisia has an egodystonic or 'driven' quality (the patient feels compelled to move). Another aid to differentiation is to observe how symptoms alter with a change in dose of antipsychotic medication; a reduction in dose should lead to an improvement in akathisia, an increase in dose will rapidly worsen akathisia but may reduce agitation.

Ekboms syndrome, or restless legs syndrome, is another diagnosis to consider. However, other than by coincidence, the onset of this syndrome will not coincide with starting or increasing the dose of an antipsychotic. Further, Ekbom's syndrome tends to be experienced only at night, while akathisia is usually also present during the day (Blom and Ekbom 1961). Insomnia is a feature of both conditions.

Management

Treatment options include:

1 Reducing the dose of the antipsychotic.

2 Switch to an antipsychotic drug with a lower liability for akathisia.

3 Prescribing an anticholinergic drug (e.g procyclidine 5 mg tds), a benzodiazepine (e.g. diazepam 2 to 4 mg tds) or propranolol (initially 20 mg bd but the dose may need to be increased to 80 mg bd). The evidence base for these interventions is weak though it appears strongest for propranolol. Propranolol is contraindicated in those with asthma or peripheral vascular disease.

Risk factors

Risk factors for akathisia include:

1 Use of high potency conventional antipsychotics

2 Higher dosage

3 Drug naive patient

4 Rapid escalation in drug dose.

Prevention

The incidence of akathisia is less with atypical antipsychotics than with conventional agents. The use of lower dosages and gradual dose titration of conventional drugs will reduce the risk.

Parkinsonism

Clinical features

Parkinsonism comprises a triad of bradykinesia, rigidity, and tremor. Bradykinesia is probably the core feature, and manifests as difficulty initiating movements, slowness of movement, interruption of the normal flow of movements and a poverty of background motor activity. Rigidity can be of the lead pipe or cogwheel type. The tremor is worse at rest and comprises regular oscillatory movements with a frequency of 6 Hz. Tremor is usually present in the hands, but can also affect the head causing it to nod backwards and forwards or from side to side in a repetitive manner.

The signs of parkinsonism include a mask-like expression, lack of gesticulation, stooped posture, shuffling gait and a reduction in the normal arm swing that accompanies walking. In severe cases, the arms may be held motionless at the sides. Difficulty initiating movements can manifest in several ways, for example a patient may have difficulty getting out of a chair and require several attempts. When a patient is walking they may have difficulty stopping and this can lead to falls. Symptoms can be symmetrical or more marked on one side of the body. The voice can become deeper in tone, quieter and there may be difficulty in articulating words. When severe, these features make it difficult for the patient's speech to be understood. Other features include sialorrhoea and seborrhoea.

The onset of drug-induced parkinsonism tends to be gradual over several weeks. With conventional antipsychotics, 90 per cent of cases are manifest within 10 weeks of commencing treatment (Ayd 1961).

Pharmacological basis

The predominant abnormality is the impaired dopaminergic neurotransmission in the basal ganglia due to excessive striatal D_2 receptor blockade by the antipsychotic drug. However, it is unlikely that a single system and receptor can account for all the symptoms of parkinsonism and there is evidence implicating the cholinergic and GABA-ergic systems.

Differential diagnosis

Parkinsonism can have many causes; examples include Wilson's disease, Huntington's disease, idiopathic Parkinson's disease and carbon monoxide poisoning. Two common differential diagnoses for clinicians to consider are negative symptoms of schizophrenia and psychomotor retardation due to depression (Barnes and McPhillips 1995). Facial expression can be particularly helpful in differentiating parkinsonism from psychomotor retardation. In depression with psychomotor retardation, the expression is one of unhappiness, the mouth is down-turned, the brow may be furrowed and the patient may avoid eye contact, i.e. the face is expressive in that it shows unhappiness. In contrast, with parkinsonism there is a lack of expression, the face is mask-like, the lips may be slightly parted, the brow is smooth and the eyes often have a staring quality reflecting the reduced blink rate ('reptilian stare'). Impaired articulation can occur in parkinsonism but not in psychomotor retardation or a defect state.

Clinicians need to be alert to the possibility that the appearance of rigidity may represent the early stages of neuroleptic malignant syndrome rather than parkinsonism (see Chapter 2; Neuroleptic malignant syndrome). This is particularly important if stiffness appears within the first week of starting an antipsychotic. Consideration of the other features of the two syndromes will usually allow diagnosis but if there is any uncertainty it is essential the patient is carefully monitored.

Management

1   Reducing the dose of the causal drug.

2   Switch to an antipsychotic associated with a lower risk of parkinsonism. Symptoms generally resolve within a few days to a few weeks after stopping an oral drug, but resolution may take several months after a depot antipsychotic is stopped.

3   Prescribe an anticholinergic drug (e.g. procyclidine 5 mg tds initially, though higher doses may be needed). Anticholinergic use should be regularly reviewed as these drugs are associated with their own unwanted effects (Barnes and McPhillips 1996).

4   Occasionally symptoms are persistent after drug discontinuation. This may reflect the coincidental onset of idiopathic Parkinson's disease. In these cases a neurology referral is indicated.

Risk factors

Risk factors for parkinsonism include:

1   Use of high potency conventional antipsychotics

2   Higher dosage

3   Advancing age

4   Female gender.

Prevention

The risk of parkinsonism is reduced by avoiding high doses of high potency conventional antipsychotics or by selecting an atypical antipsychotic. It is not good practice to routinely prescribe prophylactic anticholinergic drugs (Barnes and McPhillips 1996).

Tardive dyskinesia

Clinical features

Tardive dyskinesia refers to a syndrome of various involuntary movements associated with the administration of antipsychotic drugs that appears late in the course of treatment. The condition most commonly affects the bucco-linguo-masticatory (BLM) muscles but virtually all parts of the body can be involved including the neck, trunk, limbs, pharyngeal muscles, intercostal muscles and diaphragm. All forms of abnormal movement, except tremor, can occur including myoclonic jerks, tics, chorea and dystonia. TD is most pronounced when patients are aroused. It eases during states of relaxation and disappears during sleep. TD can result in considerable social and physical disability.

The syndrome is very variable in its presentation. Abnormal 'worm-like' movements on the surface of the tongue are sometimes mentioned as an early sign of the condition, but consistent evidence for this is lacking. Complex and repetitive movements of the oro-facial muscles are the most common and characteristic feature of the condition. The tongue can show irregular darting protrusions ('fly catcher' sign), regular horizontal protrusions ('tromboning') and may sweep the buccal surfaces ('bon bon' sign). The lips can be puckered, pout or smack together. Abnormal movements of the jaw include grinding of the teeth, clenching of the teeth and forward and lateral protrusion of the jaw. Patients are usually unaware of these movements.

Abnormal movements of the facial muscles include blepharospasm, grimacing, frowning and 'up and down' movements of the eyebrows. The arms may show choreoathetoid movements. Involvement of the oro-pharyngeal muscles can result in dysphagia while involvement of the intercostal muscles and diaphragm can cause irregular breathing and grunting noises. This may lead to an increased mortality and morbidity due to respiratory tract infections and cardiovascular disorders (Youssef and Waddington 1987).

TD can involve dystonic elements. However, as well as occurring as part of a more generalized TD, tardive dystonia can occur as a distinct syndrome

(Barnes 1990). This most commonly effects the face or neck, and can be disabling (Wojcik *et al.* 1991). Spontaneous remission is rare.

With conventional antipsychotic treatment, the mean reported prevalence of tardive dyskinesia was around 15–20 per cent worldwide, although in older patients the figure could reach 60 per cent (Kane *et al.* 1992). The condition is not usually progressive, but rather waxes and wanes over time, with spontaneous remissions being relatively common, particularly in younger patients. Prospective studies of treatment with conventional antipsychotic drugs suggested that the cumulative incidence of TD was about 5 per cent per year over the first decade (Kane *et al.* 1992; Glazer *et al.* 1993). The incidence continues to rise, though less steeply, with continued antipsychotic drug treatment beyond 10 years.

It used to be thought that TD was irreversible but recent studies indicate that the prognosis is not so bleak. If the causal drug is stopped, most cases will gradually improve. However, in the first month or so symptoms may be exacerbated by stopping the drug or reduction in drug dosage. Conversely, an increase in drug dosage can lead to a temporary improvement in TD.

Pharmacological basis

The most widely accepted theory is that TD reflects super-sensitivity of the striatal post-synaptic D_2 receptors secondary to their blockade by antipsychotics (Carlson 1970). However, there is also evidence implicating the cholinergic and GABA-ergic systems.

Differential diagnosis

The diagnosis is usually obvious. Possible differential diagnoses include Huntington's disease and Wilson's disease.

Management

1 The most effective treatment is to stop the offending drug., but whether this is clinically indicated will depend on the nature of the psychiatric condition for which antipsychotic medication was prescribed. Thus, the clinician must judge how necessary it is to continue antipsychotic treatment. If such treatment is not essential it can be stopped altogether.

2 In many cases, particularly in patients with schizophrenia, antipsychotic medication will need to continue, but it may be possible to reduce the dose or to switch to an atypical agent with evidence for a lower liability for the condition (Llorca *et al.* 2002). If the patient is receiving a depot antipsychotic, it may be prudent to stop this and switch to oral medication. The latter allows the dose to be adjusted more finely and avoids the long lag times before

a change in depot injection dosage or frequency translates to a change in serum levels.

Many specific anti-dyskinetic treatments have been proposed, including tetrabenazine, vitamin E, benzodiazepines and sodium valproate (Gupta *et al.* 1999). Although these treatments may help some patients, the success rate appears low. A Cochrane review (McGrath *et al.* 2003) concluded that there was no strong evidence to support the use of any of a range of miscellaneous treatments (ceruletide, essential fatty acids, oestrogen, lithium and insulin) for TD, although the small sample sizes meant that results must be considered inconclusive.

Risk factors

Several risk factors have been identified for TD (Barnes 1990). These include:

1 Advancing age
2 Female gender
3 Dementia
4 Susceptibility to acute extrapyramidal side effects.

Use of anticholinergic drugs and affective illness have also been suggested as risk factors but their respective roles require confirmation. With regard to antipsychotic drug treatment variables, there is tentative evidence that intermittent treatment may be a risk factor, but factors such as duration of treatment or maximum dosage have not generally been found to be associated with an increased risk of developing TD. Those few studies where a relationship has been found between duration of drug treatment and the emergence of tardive dyskinesia have tended to be in samples of either younger patients early in treatment or elderly patients. However, the relative lack of evidence may partly reflect the limitations of cross-sectional surveys with retrospective assessment of the drug history. That duration of antipsychotic exposure and dosage may be important risk factors for TD is supported by the higher prevalence of the condition observed with increasing years of treatment with conventional antipsychotics and the findings of studies involving random assignment to different dosages of antipsychotic drug (Kane 1999).

Prevention

Avoid high doses of high potency conventional antipsychotics. Keep the duration of conventional antipsychotic treatment to the minimum. There is tentative evidence that long term use of some of the atypical antipsychotic may be associated with a lower incidence of tardive dyskinesia than those reported with the conventional drugs (Llorca *et al.* 2002). Avoid the unnecessary use of anticholinergic drugs.

Summary: Acute dystonia

Definition	An involuntary sustained contraction of a muscle to its maximum degree.
Incidence	Variable depending on drug, dose, rate of increase and subject characteristics.
	Up to 33% in some studies (Singh *et al.* 1990; Chakos *et al.* 1992).
Drugs causing syndrome	Highest incidence is with high potency conventional antipsychotics e.g. haloperidol. Rare with atypical antipsychotics. Occasionally occur with SSRIs. May occur on antipsychotic withdrawal.
Key symptoms/signs	Muscular contraction leading to postural distortion which often has a bizarre quality. Most common sites are neck followed by jaw/tongue though any site may be involved including trunk and limbs. Associated with subjective distress.
Pharmacological mechanism	Unknown; ?increased or decreased dopaminergic transmission
Investigations to confirm diagnosis	History and examination are key. Syndrome usually appears within 5 days of starting or increasing dose of antipsychotic. Resolution within minutes with anticholinergic treatment.
Management	Anticholinergic (oral, im or iv)
	Consider switching antipsychotic
	Avoid further increases in antipsychotic for next few days.
Further reading	Owens DGC (1990). Dystonia – a potential psychiatric pitfall. *Br J Psychiatry*, **156**, 620–34.
	Singh H, Levinson DF, Simpson GM, *et al.* (1990). Acute dystonia during fixed-dose neuroleptic treatment. *J of Clinical Psychopharmacology*, **10**, 389–96.
	Swett C (1975). Drug-induced dystonia. *Am J Psychiatry*, **132**, 532–4.

Summary: Akathisia

Definition	Increased restlessness, often located to lower limbs, associated with a subjective feeling of unease and often irritability, and distress and dysphoria in more severe cases.
Incidence	Variable depending on drug, dose and rate of dosage increase. Up to 32% in some studies (Kennedy *et al.* 1971).

Drugs causing syndrome	Highest incidence is with high potency conventional antipsychotics e.g. haloperidol. Rare with atypical antipsychotics. Occasionally occurs with SSRIs.
Key symptoms/signs	Objective restlessness, particularly of legs. The patient may shuffle his feet, walk on the spot, rock from foot to foot, walk around or, if sitting, stand up repeatedly. Subjective distress. Irritability.
Pharmacological mechanism	Unclear. May reflect combination of a depressed dopaminergic system and an overactive noradrenergic system.
Investigations to confirm diagnosis	History and examination are key. Usually appears soon after starting/increasing dose of antipsychotic. Worsens with further dose increase, lessens with dose decrease.
Management	Reduce antipsychotic dose
	Switch antipsychotic
	Prescribe either an anticholinergic, benzodiazepine or propranolol.
	Try to prevent the condition by gradual titration of dosage when starting or increasing amount of antipsychotic medication.
Further reading	Braude WM, Barnes TRE, and Gore SM (1983). Clinical characteristics of akathisia: a systematic investigation of acute psychiatric inpatient admissions. *British Journal of Psychiatry*, **143**, 139–50.
	Halstead SM, Barnes TRE, and Speller JC (1994). Akathisia: prevalence and associated dysphoria in an inpatient population with chronic schizophrenia. *British Journal of Psychiatry*, **164**, 177–83.
	Lane RM (1998). SSRI-induced extrapyramidal side-effects and akathisia: implications for treatment. *J Psychopharmacol*, **12**, 192–214.

Summary: Parkinsonism

Definition	Triad of bradykinesia, tremor and rigidity caused by psychotropic medication.
Incidence	Variable depending on drug and dose. Parkinsonian *symptoms*, as opposed to the full syndrome, are probably present in the majority of patients prescribed conventional antipsychotic drugs.
Drugs causing syndrome	Highest incidence is with high potency conventional antipsychotics e.g. haloperidol. Less common with atypical antipsychotics, though the problem is dose related to some extent with several of these agents. Occasionally occurs with SSRIs.

Key symptoms/signs	Mask-like expression, characteristic gait (slow, shuffling, small steps), lack of arm swing, resting tremor of hands, slowness of movements, absence of 'blink', sialorrhoroea, seborrhoea. Subjectively patients often complain of tiredness.
Pharmacological mechanism	D_2 blockade in striatum
Investigations to confirm diagnosis	History and examination are key. Usually appears within 3 months of starting/ increasing an antipsychotic. On examination: observe bradykinesia, resting tremor, and symptoms as listed previously. Test for leadpipe or cogwheel rigidity & reduced glabellar tap.
Management	Reduce antipsychotic dose
	Switch antipsychotic
	Prescribe an anticholinergic
Further reading	Ayd FJ (1961). A survey of drug-induced extrapyramidal reactions. *JAMA*, **175**, 1054–60.
	Barnes TRE and McPhillips MA (1995). How to distinguish between the neuroleptic-induced deficit syndrome, depression and disease-related negative symptoms in schizophrenia. *International Clinical Psychopharmacology*, **10**, (Suppl. 3), 115–21.
	Osser DN (1999). Neuroleptic induced parkinsonism. In AB Joseph and RR Young (ed.) *Movement Disorders in Neurology and Neuropsychiatry*, 2nd edn, pp. 61–8. Blackwell Science: Malden, MA.

Summary: Tardive dyskinesia

Definition	Various involuntary movements (including myoclonic jerks, tics, chorea and dystonia but not tremor) caused by a psychotropic drug and appearing late in the course of treatment.
Incidence	Cumulative incidence of about 5% per years in patients starting conventional antipsychotic treatment (Kane *et al.* 1992; Glazer *et al.* 1993).
Drugs causing syndrome	Conventional antipsychotics. Some evidence for lower incidence with some atypical antipsychotics.
Key symptoms/signs	Most commonly affects the bucco-linguo-masticatory muscles but abnormal involuntary movements (usually described as choreiform) of the trunk and limbs are seen. Patients are typically unaware of the movements.
Pharmacological mechanism	Super-sensitivity of the striatal post-synaptic D_2 receptors, secondary to their blockade by antipsychotics.

Investigations to confirm diagnosis	History and examination are key. Rare with less than 6 months antipsychotic treatment. If diagnosis is in doubt consider neurology referral.
Management	Reduce dose of causal drug
	Switch to an atypical (lowest risk is with clozapine)
	A wide range of drugs have been advocated but efficacy is uncertain. Options include vitamin E and low-dose tetrabenazine.
Further reading	Glazer WM, Morgenstern H, and Doucette JT (1993). Predicting the long-term risk of tardive dyskinesia in outpatients maintained on neuroleptic medications. *J Clinical Psychiatry*, **54**, 133–9.
	Llorca P-M, Chereau I, Bayle F-J, *et al*. (2002). Tardive dyskinesias and antipsychotics: a review. *European Psychiatry*, **17**, 129–38.
	McGrath JJ and Soares-Weiser KVS (2003). Miscellaneous treatments for neuroleptic-induced tardive dyskinesia (Cochrane Review). In: *The Cochrane Library*, Issue 1, 2003. Update software: Oxford.

References

Addonizio G, Roth SD, Stokes PE, *et al*. (1988). Increased extrapyramidal symptoms with addition of lithium to neuroleptics. *J Nerv Ment Dis*, **176**, 682–5.

Arvanitis LA, Miller BG, and the Seroquel Trial 13 Study Group (1997). Multiple fixed doses of Seroquel (quetiapine) in patients with acute exacerbation of schizophrenia: a comparison with haloperidol and placebo. *Biol Psychiatry*, **42**, 233–46.

Atbasoglu C, Schultz SK, and Andreasen NC (2001). The relationship of akathisia with suicidality and depersonalization among patients with schizophrenia. *J Neuropsychiatry Clin Sci*, **13**, 336–41.

Ayd FJ (1961). A survey of drug-induced extrapyramidal reactions. *JAMA*, **175**, 1054–60.

Barnes TRE (1990). Movement disorder associated with antipsychotic drugs: the tardive syndromes. *Int Rev Psychiatry*, **2**, 355–66.

Barnes TRE (1992). Neuromuscular effects of neuroleptics: akathisia. In *Adverse Effects of Psychotropic Drugs*, J Lieberman and JM Kane (ed.), pp. 201–17. Guilford Publications: New York.

Barnes TRE, Andrews D, and Awad G (2000). Poor compliance with treatment in people with schizophrenia: causes and management. In *Schizophrenia and Mood Disorders*, Peter F Buckley and John L Waddington (ed.), pp. 317–29. Butterworth-Heinemann: Oxford.

Barnes TRE and Braude WM (1985). Akathisia variants and tardive dyskinesia. *Arch Gen Psychiatry*, **42**, 874–8.

Barnes TRE and McPhillips MA (1995). How to distinguish between the neuroleptic-induced deficit syndrome, depression and disease-related negative symptoms in schizophrenia. *Int Clin Psychopharmacol*, **10** (Suppl. 3), 115–21.

Barnes TRE and McPhillips MA (1996). Antipsychotic-induced extrapyramidal symptoms: role of anticholinergic drugs in treatment. *CNS Drugs*, **6**, 315–30.

Beasley CM Jr, Tollefson G, Tran P, *et al.* (1996). Olanzapine versus placebo and haloperidol: acute phase results of the North American double-blind olanzapine trial. *Neuropsychopharmacology*, **14**, 111–23.

Blom S and Ekbom KA (1961). Comparison between akathisia developing on treatment with phenothiazine derivatives and the restless legs syndrome. *Acta Med Scand*, **170**, 689–94.

Boumans CE, de Mooij KJ, Koch PAM, *et al.* (1994). Is the social acceptability of psychiatric patients decreased by orofacial dyskinesia? *Schizophr Bull*, **20**, 339–44.

Braude WM, Barnes TRE, and Gore SM (1983). Clinical characteristics of akathisia: a systematic investigation of acute psychiatric inpatient admissions. *Br J Psychiatry*, **143**, 139–50.

Carlson A (1970). Biochemical implications of dopa-induced actions on the central nervous system with particular reference to abnormal movements. In *L-dopa and Parkinsonism*, A Barbeau and FH McDowell (ed.). Davis: Philadelphia.

Caroff SN, Mann SC, Campbell EC, *et al.* (2002). Movement disorders associated with atypical antipsychotic drugs. *J Clin Psychiatry*, **63** (Suppl. 4), 12–19.

Chakos MH, Mayerhoff DL, Loebel AD, *et al.* (1992). Incidence and correlates of acute extrapyramidal symptoms in first episode of schizophrenia. *Psychopharmacol Bull*, **28**, 81–6.

Claus A, Bollen J, De Cuyper H, *et al.* (1992). Risperodine versus haloperidol in the treatment of chronic schizophrenic inpatients: a multi-centre double-blind comparative study. *Acta Psychiatr Scand*, **85**, 295–305.

Coukell AJ, Spencer CM, and Benfield P (1996). Amisulpride: a re-view of its pharmacodynamic and pharmacokinetic properties and therapeutic efficacy in the management of schizophrenia. *CNS Drugs*, **6**, 237–56.

Cunningham Owens DG (1999). *A Guide to the Extrapyramidal Side-Effects of Antipsychotic Drugs*. Cambridge University Press: Cambridge.

Dolder CR and Jeste DV (2003). Incidence of tardive dyskinesia with typical versus atypical antipsychotics in very high risk patients. *Biol Psychiatry*, **53**, 1142–5.

Flaherty JA and Lahmeyer HW (1978). Laryngeal-pharyngeal dystonia as a possible cause of asphyxia with haloperidol treatment. *Am J Psychiatry*, **135**, 1414–15.

Geddes J, Freeemantle N, Harrison P, *et al.* (2000). Atypical antipsychotics in the treatment of schizophrenia: systematic overview and meta-regression analysis. *BMJ*, **321**, 1371–6.

Gerlach J and Peacock L (1995). Intolerance to neuroleptic drugs: the art of avoiding extrapyramidal syndromes. *Eur Psychiatry*, **10** (Suppl. 1), 27–33.

Gervin M, Browne S, Lane A, *et al.* (1998). Spontaneous abnormal involuntary movements in first-episode schizophrenia and schizophreniform disorder: baseline rate in a group of patients from an Irish catchment area. *Am J Psychiatry*, **155**, 1202–6.

Gill HS, De Vane CL, and Risch SC (1997). Extrapyramidal symptoms associated with cyclic antidepressant treatment: a review of the literature and consolidating hypotheses. *J Clin Psychopharmacol*, **17**, 377–89.

Glazer WM, Morgenstern H, and Doucette JT (1993). Predicting the long-term risk of tardive dyskinesia in outpatients maintained on neuroleptic medications. *J Clin Psychiatry*, **54**, 133–9.

Gupta S, Mosnik D, Black DW, *et al.* (1999). Tardive dyskinesia: review of treatments past, present and future. *Ann Clin Psychiatry*, **11**, 257–66.

Halliday J, Farrington S, MacDonald S, *et al.* (2002). Nithsdale schizophrenia surveys 23: movement disorders. *Br J Psychiatry*, **181**, 422–7.

Hansen L (2001). A critical review of akathisia and its possible association with suicidal behaviour. *Hum Psychopharmacol*, **16**, 495–505.

Halstead SM, Barnes TRE, and Speller JC (1994). Akathisia: prevalence and associated dysphoria in an inpatient population with chronic schizophrenia. *Br J Psychiatry*, **164**, 177–83.

Hummer M and Fleischhacker WW (1996). Compliance and outcome in patients treated with antipsychotics. *CNS Drugs*, **5** (Suppl. 1), 13–20.

Kane JM, Jeste DV, Barnes TRE, *et al.* (1992). *Tardive Dyskinesia: A Task Force Report of the American Psychiatric Association.* The American Psychiatric Association: Washington, DC.

Kane JM (1999). Tardive dyskinesia. In *Movement Disorders in Neurology and Neuropsychiatry*, 2nd edn, AB Joseph and RR Young (ed.), pp. 31–5. Blackwell Science: Malden, MA.

Kapur S, Zipursky R, Jones C, *et al.* (2000). Relationship between dopamine D(2) occupancy, clinical response, and side effects: a double-blind PET study of first-episode schizophrenia. *Am J Psychiatry*, **157**, 514–20.

Kennedy PF, Hershon HI, and McGuire RJ (1971). Extrapyramidal disorders after prolonged phenothiazine therapy, including a factor analytic study of clinical features. *Br J Psychiatry*, **118**, 509–18.

Kurz M, Hummer M, Oberbauer H, *et al.* (1995). Extrapyramidal side-effects of clozapine and haloperidol. *Psychopharmacology (Berl.)*, **118**, 52–6.

Lane RM (1998). SSRI-induced extrapyramidal side-effects and akathisia: implications for treatment. *J Psychopharmacol*, **12**, 192–214.

Leo RJ (1996). Movement disorders associated with the serotonin selective reuptake inhibitors. *J Clin Psychiatry*, **57**, 449–54.

Llorca P-M, Chereau I, Bayle F-J, *et al.* (2002). Tardive dyskinesias and antipsychotics: a review. *Eur Psychiatry*, **17**, 129–38.

Marder SR, McQuade RD, Stock E, *et al.* (2003). Aripiprazole in the treatment of schizophrenia: safety and tolerability in short-term, placebo-controlled trials. *Schizophr Res*, **61**, 123–36.

McGrath JJ and Soares-Weiser KVS (2003). Miscellaneous treatments for neuroleptic-induced tardive dyskinesia (Cochrane Review). In *The Cochrane Library*, Issue 1, 2003. Oxford: Update Software.

Modestin J, Stephan PL, Erni T, *et al.* (2000). Prevalence of extrapyramidal syndromes in psychiatric inpatients and the relationship of clozapine treatment to tardive dyskinesia. *Schizophr Res*, **42**, 223–30.

NICE (National Institute for Clinical Excellence) (2002*a*). Guidance on the use of newer (atypical) antipsychotic drugs for the treatment of schizophrenia. *Technology Appraisal*, No. 43, June 2002.

NICE (National Institute for Clinical Excellence) (2002*b*). Schizophrenia: core interventions in the treatment and management of schizophrenia in primary and secondary care. *Clinical Guide* 1, December 2002.

Newton-John H (1988). Acute upper airway obstruction due to supraglottic dystonia induced by a neuroleptic. *BMJ*, **297**, 964–5.

Osser DN (1999). Neuroleptic induced parkinsonism. In *Movement Disorders in Neurology and Neuropsychiatry*, 2nd edn, AB Joseph and RR Young (ed.), pp. 61–8. Blackwell Science: Malden, MA.

Owens DGC (1990). Dystonia – a potential psychiatric pitfall. *Br J Psychiatry*, **156**, 620–34.

Pato CN, Wolkowitz OM, Rapaport M, *et al.* (1989). Benzodiazepine augmentation of neuroleptic treatment in patients with schizophrenia. *Psychopharmacol Bull*, **25**, 263–6.

Peuskens J (1995). Risperidone in the treatment of patients with chronic schizophrenia: a multinational, multicentre double-blind, parallel-group study versus haloperidol. *Br J Psychiatry*, **166**, 712–26.

Puri BK, Barnes TR, Chapman MJ, *et al.* (1999). Spontaneous dyskinesia in first episode schizophrenia. *J Neurol Neurosurg Psychiatry*, **66**, 76–8.

Schillevoort I, van Puijenbroek EP, de Boer A, *et al.* (2002). Extrapyramidal syndromes associated with selective serotonin reuptake inhibitors: a case-control study using spontaneous reports. *Int Clin Psychopharmacol*, **17**, 75–9.

Singh H, Levinson DF, Simpson GM, *et al.* (1990). Acute dystonia during fixed-dose neuroleptic treatment. *J Clin Psychopharmacol*, **10**, 389–96.

Small JG, Hirsch SR, Arvanitis LA, *et al.* (1997). Quetiapine in patients with schizophrenia. *Arch Gen Psychiatry*, **54**, 549–57.

Steck H (1954). Le syndrome extrapyramidal et diencephalique au cours des traitements au Largactil et au Serpasil. *Ann Med Psychol*, **112**, 737–44.

Stones M, Kennedy DC, and Fulton JD (1990). Dystonic dysphagia associated with fluspirilene. *BMJ*, **301**, 668–9.

Swett C (1975). Drug-induced dystonia. *Am J Psychiatry*, **132**, 532–4.

Tarsy D, Baldessarini RJ, and Tarazi FI (2002). Effects of newer antipsychotics on extrapyramidal function. *CNS Drugs*, **16**, 23–45.

Tyrer P, Alexander MS, Regan A, *et al.* (1980). An extrapyramidal syndrome after lithium therapy. *Br J Psychiatry*, **136**, 191–4.

Umbricht D and Kane JM (1996*a*). Understanding the relationship between extrapyramidal side-effects and tardive dyskinesia. In *Serotonergic Mechanisms in Antipsychotic Treatment*, JM Kane, HJ Moller and F Awouters (ed.), pp. 221–51. Marcel Dekker: New York.

Umbricht D and Kane JM (1996*b*). Medical complications of new antipsychotic drugs. *Schizophr Bull*, **22**, 475–83.

Wojcik JD, Falk WE, Fink JS, *et al.* (1991). A review of 32 cases of tardive dystonia. *Am J Psychiatry*, **148**, 1055–9.

Wolkowitz OM and Pickar D (1991). Benzodiazepines in the treatment of schizophrenia: a review and reappraisal. *Am J Psychiatry*, **148**, 714–26.

Wright P, Birkett M, David SR, *et al.* (2001). Double-blind, placebo-controlled comparison of intramuscular olanzapine and intramuscular haloperidol in the treatment of acute agitation in schizophrenia. *Am J Psychiatry*, **158**, 1149–51.

Youssef HA and Waddington JL (1987). Morbidity and mortality in tardive dyskinesia: associations in chronic schizophrenia. *Acta Psychiatr Scand*, **75**, 74–7.

Chapter 2

Neuroleptic malignant syndrome

Dora Kohen

Neuroleptic malignant syndrome (NMS) is an increasingly rare but potentially fatal disorder. Since the original description of the syndrome in the 1960s (Delay *et al.* 1960; Delay and Deniker 1965) there have been numerous descriptive clinical and epidemiological publications and reviews enhancing the recognition, understanding and management of this condition. Most cases involve antipsychotic drugs and virtually all conventional and atypical agents have been implicated (Hasan and Buckley 1998; Caroff *et al.* 2000; Farver 2003). Occasional reports have involved other drugs including lithium (e.g. Gill *et al.* 2003) and antidepressants (Baca and Martinelli 1990; Heyland and Sauve 1991; Heinemann *et al.* 1997). The syndrome can also occur on sudden withdrawal of dopamine agonist treatment in Parkinson's disease (Fujitake *et al.* 1984; Friedman *et al.* 1985).

The reported incidence of NMS has varied widely in the past decades. This partly reflects methodological factors, including the diagnostic criteria adopted and whether these are restricted to the full syndrome or encompass partial cases. Although some retrospective studies have quoted quite high incidences, for example 2.4 per cent of patients treated with antipsychotics (Addonozio *et al.* 1986), the ranges in prospective studies are between 0.15 per cent (Keck *et al.* 1991) to 0.07 per cent (Gelenberg *et al.* 1988) with a figure of about 0.2 per cent being widely accepted (Caroff and Mann 1993). Men outnumber women twofold (Caroff 1980; Addonizio *et al.* 1987) and this has been attributed to the tendency to medicate men with higher doses than women. Although there are well documented cases of NMS occurring in elderly patients, over 80 per cent of cases are under 40 years of age (Caroff 1980), a finding that has been attributed to the use of higher doses of psychotropics in younger age groups.

Recently, increased awareness of NMS, better understanding of psychopharmacological issues, decreased use of antipsychotic polypharmacy and of high doses of antipsychotic drugs have all assisted in decreasing the incidence of NMS (Gelenberg *et al.* 1988; Keck *et al.* 1991). The increasing use of atypical antipsychotics may also be relevant. As well as a decrease in incidence there has been a decrease in the reported mortality rates. Studies of NMS before 1984 quote mortality rates of up to 30 per cent but in more recent studies death is a rare occurrence (Keck *et al.* 1991; Bristow and Kohen 1993; Kohen and Bristow 1996). The more benign course may be due to better recognition of the syndrome and more appropriate treatment and management methods.

Clinical features

Key symptoms

NMS comprises four key components (see Table 2.1):

- alteration of consciousness,
- autonomic disturbance,
- elevated temperature and
- severe muscular rigidity.

Alteration of consciousness can vary from mild confusion to coma. In the early stages of NMS mild confusion can be missed or incorrectly ascribed to the sedating effect of antipsychotic medication.

Autonomic instability may produce fluctuations in blood pressure, tachycardia, diaphoresis, hypersalivation and incontinence. Some of these symptoms may be attributed to side effects of the psychotropic medication.

Table 2.1 DSM-IV Research criteria for neuroleptic malignant syndrome (adapted from American Psychiatric Association 1994)

A The development of severe muscle rigidity and elevated temperature associated with neuroleptic medication

B Two or more of the following:
  1 Diaphoresis
  2 Dysphagia
  3 Tremor
  4 Incontinence
  5 Changes in level of consciousness ranging from confusion to coma
  6 Mutism
  7 Tachycardia
  8 Elevated or labile blood pressure
  9 Leucocytosis
  10 Laboratory evidence of muscle injury (e.g. elevated CPK)

C The symptoms in criteria A and B are not due to another substance (e.g. phencyclidine) or a neurological or other general medical condition (e.g. viral encephalitis)

D The symptoms in criteria A and B are not accounted for by a mental disorder (e.g. Mood disorder with catatonic features)

Hypertension should raise suspicion, especially in patients who have been on continuous psychotropic treatment that is expected to produce a drop in blood pressure. Urinary incontinence is uncommon in young psychotic patients and can be one of the first manifestations of NMS.

Fever is present in almost all cases but can range from mild pyrexia to a temperature over 42 °C (Kellam 1990). Hyperpyrexia, like severe rigidity, predisposes to higher mortality. In severe cases systemic complications ensue with renal failure, acidosis and coagulopathies.

Muscle rigidity can be very prominent and may not respond to anticholinergic treatment. It is usually of the lead pipe rather than the cogwheel type. Sometimes rigidity is localized to the tongue, facial and masticatory muscles and can manifest as dysarthria and dysphagia. In some reports limitations in speaking, eating and swallowing have been the initial signs of NMS before the full-blown picture became apparent and have been misinterpreted as lack of cooperation from the patient. Abnormal postures and movements, such as opisthotonus and myoclonus, can occur. Severe rigidity is associated with high mortality due to its association with myoglobinuria and renal failure.

Alteration of consciousness and many of the autonomic symptoms of NMS can fluctuate during the course of a day or even over several hours. This means that a patient with high blood pressure, tachycardia, diaphoresis or even mild confusion may give the semblance of normality when assessed at one time point leading to a delay in diagnosis. Some well-documented fatalities have occurred in the period of fluctuation when staff were trying to make sense of the changes and antipsychotics continued to be prescribed.

The spectrum concept of NMS regards NMS as shading imperceptibly into the well recognized extrapyramidal symptoms that occur with antipsychotic drugs. Adityanjee et al. (1988) have drawn attention to the controversies that surround this concept. They argue that the spectrum concept could be an artefact of arbitrary definition and that it may contribute to the mismanagement of extrapyramidal disorders with neuroleptics. They recommend that NMS is viewed as a definite clinical identity and a unitary concept and suggest strict criteria, including a fever in excess of 39 °C, clouding of consciousness, rigidity and autonomic dysfunction, as being necessary for diagnosis. However, they accept there are reports of NMS characterized by milder symptoms such as localized rigidity, lower temperature, mild autonomic symptoms, milder changes in the level of consciousness and lower creatinine phosphate kinase (CPK) levels (Caroff et al. 2000; Kohen 2000). The advantage of a strict definition is that it defines a severe syndrome where urgent treatment is needed. However it risks neglecting partial cases that may shed light on how the syndrome develops and how it can be aborted.

Most psychiatric patients are managed in the community and antipsychotic medication is often commenced or switched on an outpatient basis. This applies to patients with first-onset psychosis and those with established psychotic illnesses that follow a relapsing course. Consequently many patients will show initial symptoms of NMS in the community. To facilitate early diagnosis it is important that community staff, particularly community psychiatric nurses, are familiar with the disorder.

Laboratory investigations

Although laboratory changes can help to confirm the diagnosis, there are no findings that are pathognomonic to NMS. Laboratory tests are usually used to rule out other disorders that may have similar clinical pictures to NMS. They also help to identify concurrent medical conditions that require treatment alongside NMS.

Creatine phosphokinase (CPK) is often elevated in NMS with levels usually between 2000 and 15 000 IU/l. CPK is an enzyme widely distributed in skeletal muscle. It has several isoenzymes that are not significant in the diagnosis or follow-up of muscular hyperactivity and not specific to NMS. Most laboratories measure the pooled enzyme level of CPK. CPK is usually elevated following strenuous exercise, trauma, muscular injuries, intramuscular injection and other situations where the individual has been involved in high physical activity, such as restraint or exertion. Hence it is not a reliable diagnostic test but it can be considered a reasonable marker for clinical progression of the syndrome. Mild elevation of other enzymes such as lactate dehydrogenase, alkaline phosphatase and transaminases have been noted but are not of any clinical significance in NMS.

In severe cases of NMS, there can be widespread breakdown of skeletal muscle (rhabdomyolysis) leading to uraemia, myoglobinuria and acute renal failure. Leucocytosis occurs in most cases (Shalev and Munitz 1986). Other biochemical findings such as hypo- or hypernatraemia or metabolic acidosis and low serum iron levels have been noted (Rosebush and Stewart 1989; Rosebush and Mazurek 1991).

Studies on central nervous system imaging, electroencephalogram (EEG) and lumbar puncture have not yielded any significant results but only non-specific and non-conclusive changes. Post-mortem findings usually show renal failure and other serious systemic complications but no characteristic changes.

Clinical course

NMS usually occurs 4 to 11 days after commencing an antipsychotic or increasing its dosage. However there are cases which commence long after medication has been started and without any change to the dose. If the features of NMS are severe and dramatic they are easily recognisable, but in some patients the symptoms are mild and fluctuating and it is easy for diagnosis to be delayed.

When antipsychotic medication is withdrawn and supportive measures instituted, the majority of patients will recover in around two weeks. Only a small minority of patients today will need transfer to a medical ward. Regular two-hourly clinical and nursing observations give a good understanding of the course of the syndrome.

Follow up with CPK levels can be helpful in establishing the rate of amelioration and the time when the patient is ready to be further re-challenged with antipsychotic medication.

Pharmacological basis

The central dopamine hypoactivity hypothesis has been accepted as a valid explanation of NMS by many researchers (Henderson and Wooten 1981; Addonizio *et al.* 1987; Mann *et al.* 2000). According to this model decreased dopamine (DA) transmission in different brain circuits accounts for the features of the disorder. Antagonized dopamine receptors in the anterior hypothalamus impair thermoregulation while decreased dopamine transmission in the striatum mediates muscular rigidity. Muscle rigidity also increases heat production peripherally. Decreased dopaminergic input to the anterior cingulate-medial orbito-frontal circuit might lead to decreased arousal, mutism and akinesia which are key clinical features of NMS.

Supportive evidence for the dopamine hypoactivity theory comes from several sources. Virtually all known antipsychotics, including the atypicals, have been reported to cause NMS and all antipsychotics have the property of dopamine-2 (D_2) receptor blockade (Lazarus *et al.* 1989; Mann *et al.* 1991). Antipsychotics with greater potency as D_2 receptor blockers, in particular haloperidol, have been more frequently implicated in causing NMS. Other medications that reduce dopaminergic transmission have been linked to NMS. Examples include the withdrawal of dopamine agonists or levodopa treatment in patients with Parkinson's disease and treatment with non-neuroleptic dopamine blocking medication such as metoclopramide, all of which have been reported to cause NMS (Mann *et al.* 1991). NMS has been successfully treated with several dopamine agonists including bromocriptine (Caroff *et al.* 1998*a*). Finally, HVA levels are significantly lower in the acute phase of NMS indicating a reduced state of functioning of the dopaminergic system (Nisijima and Ishiguro 1995).

A comprehensive model needs to explain why NMS only develops only in certain individuals. Mann *et al.* (2000) had proposed that facilitating state- and trait-related factors act in conjunction with the 'causal drug' to trigger NMS. Facilitating state factors include interactions or relative imbalances between DA and other neurotransmitters (including serotonin, norepinephrine, GABA and acetylcholine), postsynaptic second messenger system abnormalities, underlying psychiatric illness, and miscellaneous factors such as dehydration, exhaustion, medical conditions and hot weather. Central pre-existing dopamine hypoactivity has been suggested as a trait vulnerability marker for NMS (Mann *et al.* 2000). It is postulated that baseline hypodopaminergia would render individuals susceptible to a marked suppression of dopaminergic activity on exposure to antipsychotic drug-induced DA receptor blockade.

Caroff *et al.* (1998*a*) hypothesize that catatonia, lethal catatonia, parkinsonism and NMS may represent a spectrum of overlapping clinical syndromes in which the exact presentation of each is determined by the degree or extent of inhibition of dopamine activity across dopaminergic pathways in the brain. Parkinsonism and simple catatonia may involve dopaminergic midbrain projections to the corpus striatum and nucleus accumbens while NMS and lethal catatonia may reflect more widespread interruption of dopamine neurotransmission in the ascending mesencephalic pathways, diencephalic tracts and hypothalamus (Mann *et al.* 1991).

Another theory that attempts to explain the pathophysiology of NMS centres on the role of sympathoadrenal hyperactivity (Gurrera and Romero 1992; Gurrera 1999; Gurrera 2000). According to this model, a predisposition to extreme sympathetic nervous system hyperactivity may act as a trait vulnerability for NMS. In the presence of state variables, such as neuroleptic-induced DA system hypoactivity or psychological distress, this leads to the clinical picture of NMS. This model needs to be tested in clinical studies to verify its validity.

Differential diagnosis

Lethal catatonia

Following the original description by Kahlbaum in 1874 catatonia was described by many authors in the pre-neuroleptic era (Mann *et al.* 1986). There is an overlap of symptoms between catatonia and NMS and some authors consider that the two entities are variants of the same syndrome (White and Robins 1991; White 1992). In particular, lethal catatonia, a condition described by many authors in the pre-neuroleptic era (e.g. Stauder 1934), can simulate the clinical picture of NMS. Patients develop motor excitement, muscular rigidity, confusion, fever, tachycardia, diaphoresis and labile blood pressure. It has high mortality rates (Mann *et al.* 1986). NMS is considered by some to be a neuroleptic-induced iatrogenic form of lethal catatonia with a similar pathophysiology (Fricchione 1985; Fricchione *et al.* 2000). Others regard this as simplistic and have emphasized apparent differences between the two syndromes, for example that lethal catatonia often begins with excitement progressing to exhaustion whereas NMS begins with muscular rigidity (Castillo *et al.* 1989).

Malignant hyperthermia

Malignant hyperthermia (MH) is a condition with a high mortality seen after the administration of halogenated inhalation anaesthetic agents or the depolarizing muscle relaxant succinylcholine. In MH body temperature rises over minutes following the administration of anaesthetic agents. In contrast in NMS fever rises over hours and sometimes over a period of 24–48 hours and there is no relationship to anaesthetic agents. MH has a strong genetic component related to chromosome 19 and about 80 per cent of family members are susceptible to MH. The pathogenesis is though to relate to a defect in the cell membrane of muscle that leads to increased intracellular calcium and severe muscle contractions. There are no reports of MH and NMS developing in the same patient.

Heat exhaustion

Heat exhaustion or heat stroke is a potentially lethal disorder that can occur in patients on neuroleptics in a hot environment. Sufferers of heat exhaustion may have hyperpyrexia, alteration of consciousness and agitation. However the muscles are usually flaccid and the skin red, hot and dry. In contrast, rigidity is one of the cardinal symptoms of NMS and the skin is often moist with sweat. Obtaining a history from the patient or the carers can be of assistance in the diagnosis.

Serotonin syndrome

Serotonin syndrome (SS) is a syndrome caused by serotonergic drugs, often in combination. Some symptoms of SS, including fever, tremor, changes in the mental state and fluctuating blood pressure, can mimic NMS. However several features aid differentiation. In particular, NMS is characterized by bradykinesia and rigidity whereas patients with SS are usually hyperkinetic and marked rigidity is unusual. Also patients with SS often show myoclonus but this is absent in NMS. Recent drug use is a helpful guide to differentiation; in NMS the causative agents are usually neuroleptics (though other drugs including antidepressants can be responsible), in serotonin syndrome serotonergic agents are implicated. For more information on serotonin syndrome see Chapter 3.

Miscellaneous conditions

Central nervous system infections, akinetic mutism, thyrotoxicosis, intermittent acute porphyria and tetanus can have phases that resemble NMS (Addonizio and Susman 1991). Anticholinergic delirium (atropinism) may also resemble NMS. High doses of anticholinergic drugs taken as an overdose or as part of prescribed treatment may cause confusion and pyrexia but a key distinguishing feature is that the skin and mucous membranes are dry whereas diaphoresis is common in NMS. Improvement with physostigmine distinguishes atropinism from NMS (see Chapter 16 for a more detailed description of anticholinergic delirium).

Management

General measures and treatment

On suspicion of NMS neuroleptic medication should be discontinued immediately. If the patient is on any other psychotropic medication such as antidepressants or lithium, or even anticholinergic treatment, this should be stopped as well. Tricyclic antidepressants affect the autonomic nervous system and SSRI's can reduce dopaminergic transmission and may contribute to the clinical picture of NMS.

At the same time two-hourly nursing observations of pulse, blood pressure and temperature should be commenced. CPK levels need to be established promptly. Supportive measures such as rehydration, cooling the patient and antibiotic treatment for concurrent infection are important. Levels of CPK should be checked repeatedly on a daily basis, generally for the first week, to note the direction of the trend. After the first week every two days will be sufficient to note the changes until the levels fall within normal limits.

The patient should be referred to a physician for advice on any concurrent medical condition and any deterioration that may occur 48–72 hours following the diagnosis of NMS. Psychiatric units may not be able to offer all the medical treatment the patient needs and in severe cases transfer to a medical ward or even an intensive care unit may be necessary. In such cases the psychiatric team should support the medical team who may find it difficult to cope with the demands of an agitated and psychotic patient.

Benzodiazepines can be effective as both muscle relaxants and as sedatives for the agitated patient (Fink 1996) but they may not prevent NMS from developing (Shalev and Munitz 1986; Keck *et al.* 1989). Bromocriptine and amandatine are dopamine agonists and will counteract the action of antipsychotic drugs at dopamine receptors. In NMS bromocriptine has been shown to shorten time to clinical response compared to supportive treatment

(Rosenberg and Green 1989; Shalev *et al.* 1989). Dantrolene is a muscle relaxant. Its mechanism of action is to inhibit calcium release from the sarcoplasmic reticulum thereby decreasing the availability of calcium for muscle contraction. It has been used in NMS to treat rigidity, induce muscle relaxation and minimize heat production in skeletal muscle. Rosenberg and Green (1989) found that dantrolene reduced mortality in NMS when compared to supportive care alone. Shalev *et al.* (1989) found significantly reduced mortality in reported NMS cases treated with bromocriptine, amantadine or dantrolene compared to cases reported before these agents were used in NMS.

Electroconvulsive therapy (ECT) is effective in treating catatonic states. Its use in NMS is controversial though some case reports have reported it being effective (Mann *et al.* 1990).

In view of the heterogeneity of reported cases and the lack of prospective, controlled trials it is difficult to recommend one mode of treatment over the other. Supportive care, benzodiazepines, dantrolene, bromocriptine and possibly ECT play a role. It is important that treatment should be individualized for each patient and based on the duration and severity of clinical symptoms.

Recurrence

In NMS recurrence is common. Estimate studies of recurrence vary from 1 per cent (Pope *et al.* 1991) to 43 per cent (Susman and Addonizio 1988). Premature reintroduction of neuroleptics in cases where the original episode of NMS has not completely resolved poses the greatest risk of recurrence. Rapid and dramatic dosage increment lead to more episodes of NMS (Shalev and Munitz 1986).

Rechallenge

Most NMS patients encountered in psychiatric practice have a diagnosis of severe mental illness and an episode of acute exacerbation at the time they develop NMS. One of the most important issues in the treatment of NMS is the reintroduction of psychotropics following an episode of NMS. Withdrawal of antipsychotics during the crisis of NMS may cause a worsening of psychotic symptoms. The length of the antipsychotic free phase has been debated widely. Early, rapid or dramatic dosing increments of medication may lead to recurrence while a longer drug-free period may increase the suffering and bring difficulties into the management of a patient that may pose dangers to himself or the others.

Studies looking at the outcome of rechallenge show that at least 50 per cent of the cases may be rechallenged successfully while a further 20 per cent have a successful reintroduction of the medication when the first rechallenge led to a

Table 2.2 Key principles in antipsychotic rechallenge

- ◆ Allow signs and symptoms of NMS to totally resolve before commencing antipsychotic medication
- ◆ Consider using an antipsychotic with a different pharmocodynamic profile
- ◆ Avoid depots
- ◆ Avoid high potency conventional antipsychotics
- ◆ Start with a low dose
- ◆ Titrate slowly
- ◆ Be vigilant for reappearance of NMS:
    - – regular monitoring of temp, pulse and blood pressure
    - – consider monitoring creatinine kinase

---

recurrence of NMS. In 15 per cent there seems to be longer susceptibility to NMS in the form of rising in the CPK levels and return of some of the NMS symptoms (Bristow and Kohen 2002). In the same cohort of patients, the last 15 per cent are the group who were not rechallenged with antipsychotics, possibly because they originally presented with transient and reversible psychotic symptoms and so did not require further antipsychotic treatment.

In the same study, the comparison of successful versus failed rechallenges showed that a switch from traditional to atypical antipsychotics, lower CPK levels at the time of rechallenge, and shorter periods of hospitalization were associated with lower risks of NMS at the time of rechallenge. Other significant factors associated with lower risk of recurrence of NMS at rechallenge were no previous history of NMS, no previous history of catatonia, and less severe symptoms during the original episode of NMS. Table 2.2 summarizes some key principals in the management of an antipsychotic rechallenge.

Risk factors and prevention

Diagnosis as a risk factor

NMS occurs in neuroleptic treated patient from all psychiatric diagnostic groups. Most cases have a diagnosis of schizophrenia or bipolar affective disorder but NMS has occurred in patients with other affective disorders and organic brain disease (Caroff 1980; Rosebush and Stewart 1989). All disorders that may effect cortico-hypothalamic circuits, such as major depression and mania, and have an association with elevated sympathetic nervous system activity increase the risk of NMS (Gurrera 2000). Patients with learning disabilities and infections of the central nervous system may be predisposed to NMS (Caroff *et al.* 1998*b*). Parkinson's disease, Lewy body dementia and other basal ganglia disorders may also increase the risk of NMS with antipsychotic treatment or withdrawal of dopamine agonists (Davis *et al.* 2000).

Beside the actual diagnosis, various factors in the physical state and mental state of the patient are significantly linked to the risk of developing NMS (Keck *et al.* 1989; Kohen and Bristow 1996). Catatonic symptoms were shown to increase the risk of NMS in a case control study (Berardi *et al.* 1998). Dehydration, agitation, confusion, disorganized behaviour and overactivity also increase the risk (Berardi *et al.* 1998) as does a previous history of a NMS episode (Keck *et al.* 1989; Berardi *et al.* 1998).

Pharmacological risk factors

Virtually all traditional antipsychotics have been associated with NMS. The risk is highest with high potency agents, especially haloperidol. A rapid increase in antipsychotic dose is a well recognized risk factor for NMS. Despite their reduced affinity for D_2 receptors, all the atypical antipsychotics have been associated with NMS (Hasan and Buckley 1998; Caroff *et al.* 2000; Farver 2003). Even in monotherapy, clozapine, olanzapine, risperidone and quetiapine all have been reported as causing NMS.

Other psychotropic drugs including lithium (e.g. Gill *et al.* 2003), tricyclic antidepressants (e.g. Baca and Martinelli 1990), mono-amine oxidase inhibitors (e.g. Heyland and Sauve 1991), selective serotonin reuptake inhibitors (Heinemann *et al.* 1997) and venlafaxine (Nimmagadda *et al.* 2000) have occasionally been reported as causing NMS. However the concomitant use of antipsychotics in some of these reports makes it difficult to attribute causality to any single agent. Patients with Parkinson's disease after withdrawal of dopamine agonists (Fujitake *et al.* 1984, 1985) and patients with Huntington's disease after starting tetrabenazine can develop NMS (Burke *et al.* 1981). The syndrome has also been reported with metoclopramide, an antiemetic that is a D2 antagonist (Donnet *et al.* 1991).

Biochemical and other risk factors

There are several non-specific risk factors that have been associated with the emergence of NMS. Dehydration is a risk factor for the development of NMS in patients on antipsychotic treatment and rehydration on its own can improve the clinical picture of NMS. Low serum iron in patients with NMS has been noted in many cases but its relevance is unclear (Rosebush and Mazurek 1991). Unlike malignant hyperthermia, NMS carries no known familial risk and there are no reports of cases occurring in the same family. However despite this genetic factors are likely to be relevant to the pathogenesis.

Prevention

Preventive measures to lower the incidence of NMS include good practice, such as avoiding unnecessarily high doses of psychotropic medication and increasing doses gradually. This is particularly important when high potency D_2 receptor blocking agents are used. Better understanding of augmentation strategies and adherence to guidelines on the rapid tranquillization should also help minimize incidence. It is now recognized that high doses of antipsychotics should not be used for sedating purposes but benzodiazepines should be used when necessary.

Early recognition of prodromal symptoms of NMS is essential in preventing the syndrome becoming severe. A clear understanding of differential diagnosis will help the clinician to recognize NMS and instigate prompt management. Appropriate education for inpatient and community psychiatric staff could help to further reduce associated morbidity. Further prevention strategies will depend on future research findings and clarification of the patho-physiology of NMS.

Summary: Neuroleptic malignant syndrome

Definition	A rare but potentially fatal disorder characterized by changes in consciousness, rigidity, autonomic disturbance and fever. Associated with high doses and/or fast incremental increases in antipsychotic medication.
Incidence	Ranges from 0.15% to 0.07% but is decreasing in frequency and severity.
Drugs causing syndrome	Strong association with haloperidol but virtually all conventional antipsychotics and atypical antipsychotics (including clozapine) have been implicated in causing NMS. Other drugs associated with NMS include lithium, tricyclic antidepressants, MAOIs, SSRIs, metoclopramide and sudden stoppage of dopaminergic drugs in Parkinson's disease.
Key symptoms/signs	Changes in consciousness range from mild confusion to coma.
	Rigidity: can be localized but in later stages usually severe and generalized.
	Autonomic disturbance: pallor, tachycardia, labile blood pressure, sweating, urinary incontinence
	Pyrexia: can exceed 42 °C in extreme cases.
	Partial forms of NMS can occur.
Pharmacological mechanism	Dopamine receptor blockade and central dopamine hypoactivity.
Investigations to confirm diagnosis	History is important as NMS usually occurs within a few days of commencing the causal agent. Examination will reveal the key signs. Creatine phosphokinase levels usually elevated.

Management	Discontinue all psychotropic medication on suspicion of NMS. Rehydrate the patient and seek advice from physicians for the treatable causes of high temperature i.e. systemic infections. Benzodiazepines, bromocriptine, dantrolene and possibly electroconvulsive therapy may be helpful in individual patients.
Further reading	Bristow M and Kohen D (2002). Predicting the effects of re-challenge with antipsychotics following NMS: A review of cases from Neuroleptic Malignant Syndrome database. *Brain Pharmacology*, **1**, 181–7.
	Caroff SN (1980). The neuroleptic malignant syndrome. *Journal of Clinical Psychiatry*, **41**, 79–83.
	White DA (1992). Catatonia and the neuroleptic malignant syndrome – a single entity? *British Journal of Psychiatry*, **161**, 558–60.

References

Addonozio G, Susman VL, and Roth SD (1986). Symptoms of neuroleptic malignant syndrome in 82 consecutive inpatients. *Am J Psychiatry*, **143**, 1587–90.

Addonizio G, Susman VL, and Roth SD (1987). Neuroleptic malignant syndrome; review and analysis of 115 cases. *Biol Psychiatry*, **22**, 1004–20.

Addonizio G and Susman VL (1991). *Neuroleptic Malignant Syndrome; A Clinical Guide.* Mosby-Year Book: St Louis, MO.

Adityanjee, Singh S, Sing G, *et al.* (1988). Spectrum concept of neuroleptic malignant syndrome. *Br J Psychiatry*, **153**, 107–11.

American Psychiatric Association (1994). *Diagnostic and Statistical Manual of Mental Disorders*, 4th edn (DSM-1V). American Psychiatric Press: Washington, DC.

Baca L and Martinelli L (1990). Neuroleptic malignant syndrome: a unique association with a tricyclic antidepressant. *Neurology*, **40**, 1797–8.

Berardi D, Amore M, Keck PE, *et al.* (1998). Clinical and pharmacological risk factors for neuroleptic malignant syndrome; a case control study. *Biol Psychiatry*, **44**, 748–54.

Bristow MF and Kohen D (1993). How 'malignant' is neuroleptic malignant syndrome? *BMJ*, **307**, 1223–4.

Bristow M and Kohen D (2002). Predicting the effects of re-challenge with antipsychotics following NMS. A review of cases from Neuroleptic Malignant Syndrome database. *Brain Pharmacol*, **1**, 181–7.

Burke RE, Fahn S, Mayeux R, *et al.* (1981). Neuroleptic malignant syndrome caused by domapine depleting drugs in a patient with Huntingdon's chorea. *Neurology (NY)*, **31**, 1022–6.

Caroff SN (1980). The neuroleptic malignant syndrome. *J Clin Psychiatry*, **41**, 79–83.

Caroff SN and Mann SC (1993). Neuroleptic malignant syndrome. *Med Clin North Am*, **77**, 185–202.

Caroff SN Mann SC, and Keck PE (1998a). Specific treatment of the neuroleptic malignant syndrome. *Biol Psychiatry*, **44**, 378–81.

Caroff SN, Mann SC, McCarthy M, *et al.* (1998*b*). Acute infectious encephalitis complicated by neuroleptic malignant syndrome. *J Clin Psychopharmacol*, **18**, 349–51.

Caroff SN, Mann SC, and Campbell EC (2000). Atypical antipsychotics and neuroleptic malignant syndrome. *Psychiatric Ann*, **30**, 314–21.

Castillo E, Rubin RT, and Holsboer-Trachsler E (1989). Clinical differentiation between lethal catatonia and neuroleptic malignant syndrome. *Am J Psychiatry*, **146**, 324–8.

Davis JM, Caroff SN, and Mann SC (2000). Treatment of neuroleptic malignant syndrome. *Psychiatric Ann*, **30**, 325–31.

Delay J, Pichot P, Lemperiere T, *et al.* (1960). Un neuroleptique majeur non phenothiazine et non reserpinique, l'haloperidol, dans le traitement des psychoses. *Ann Med Psychol* (Paris), **118**, 145–52.

Delay J and Deniker P (1965). Sur quelques erreurs de prescription des medicaments psychiatriques. *Soc Med Hop Paris*, **116**, 487–93.

Donnet A, Harle JR, Dumont JC, *et al.* (1991). Neuroleptic malignant syndrome induced by metoclopramide. *Biomed Pharmacother*, **45**, 461–2.

Farver DK (2003). Neuroleptic malignant syndrome induced by atypical antipsychotics. *Expert Opin Drug Saf*, **2**, 21–35.

Fink M (1996). Neuroleptic malignant syndrome and catatonia: One entity or two? *Biol Psychiatry*, **39**, 1–4.

Fricchione G (1985). Neuroleptic catatonia and its relationship to psychogenic catatonia. *Br J Psychiatry*, **20**, 304–13.

Fricchione G, Mann SC, and Caroff SN (2000). Catatonia, lethal catatonia, and neuroleptic malignant syndrome. *Psychiatric Ann*, **30**, 347–55.

Friedman JH, Feinberg SS, and Feldman RG (1985). A neuroleptic malignant-like syndrome due to levodopa therapy withdrawal. *JAMA*, **254**, 2792–5.

Fujitake J, Kuno S, and Nishitani H (1984). Neuroleptic malignant syndrome-like state in eight patients with parkinsomnism. *Rinsho Shinkeig'aku (Clin Neurol)*, **24**, 371–8.

Gelenberg AJ, Bellinghausen B, Wocjik JD, *et al.* (1988). A prospective survey of neuroleptic malignant syndrome in a short term psychiatric hospital. *Am J Psychiatry*, **145**, 517–18.

Gill J, Singh H, and Nugent K (2003). Acute lithium intoxication and neuroleptic malignant syndrome. *Pharmacotherapy*, **23**, 811–15.

Gurrera RJ (1999). Sympathoadrenal hyperactivity and the etiology of neuroleptic malignant syndrome. *Am J Psychiatry*, **156**, 169–80.

Gurrera RJ (2000). The role of calcium and peripheral catecholamines in the pathophysiology of neuroleptic malignant syndrome. *Psychiatric Ann*, **30**, 356–62.

Gurrera RJ and Romero JA (1992). Sympatho-adrenomedullary activity in neuroleptic malignant syndrome. *Biol Psychiatry*, **32**, 334–43.

Hasan S and Buckley P (1998). Novel antipsychotics and the neuroleptic malignant syndrome; a review and critique. *Am J Psychiatry*, **155**, 1113–16.

Henderson VW and Wooten GF (1981). Neuroleptic malignant syndrome: a pathogenetic role for the dopamine receptor blockade? *Neurology*, **13**, 132–7.

Heinemann F, Assion HJ, Hermes G, *et al.* (1997). Paroxetine-induced neuroleptic malignant syndrome (Article in German). *Nervenarzt*, **68**, 664–6.

Heyland D and Sauve M (1991). Neuroleptic malignant syndrome without the use of neuroleptics. *CMAJ*, **145**, 817–19.

Keck PE, Pope HG, Cohen BM, *et al.* (1989). Risk factors for neuroleptic malignant syndrome; a case control study. *Arch Gen Psychiatry*, **46**, 914–18.

Keck PE, Pope HG, and McElroy SL (1991). Declining frequency of neuroleptic malignant syndrome in a hospital population. *Am J Psychiatry*, **148**, 880–2.

Kellam AMP (1990). The (frequently) neuroleptic (potentially) malignant syndrome. *Br J Psychiatry*, **157**, 169–73.

Kohen D and Bristow M (1996). Neuroleptic malignant syndrome. *Adv Psychiatr Treat*, **2**, 151–7.

Kohen D and Bristow M (1999). Atypical antipsychotics and neuroleptic malignant syndrome. *Br J Psychiatry*, **175**, 392–3.

Kohen D (2000). Novel antipsychotics and NMS: The United Kingdom NMS database. *APA Proceedings*, **84**, 150.

Lazarus A, Mann SC, and Caroff SN (1989). *The Neuroleptic Malignant Syndrome and Related Conditions*. American Psychiatric Association: Washington, DC.

Mann SC, Caroff SN, Bleier HR, *et al.* (1986). Lethal catatonia. *Am J Psychiatry*, **143**, 1374–81.

Mann SC, Caroff SN, Bleier HR, *et al.* (1990). Electroconvulsive therapy of the lethal catatonia syndrome; case report and review. *Convuls Ther*, **6**, 239–47.

Mann SC, Caroff SN, and Lazarus A (1991). Pathogenesis of neuroleptic malignant syndrome. *Psychiatric Ann*, **21**, 175–80.

Mann SC, Caroff SN, Fricchione G, *et al.* (2000). Central dopamine hypoactivity and the pathogenesis of neuroleptic malignant syndrome. *Psychiatric Ann*, **30**, 363–74.

Nimmagadda SR, Ryan DH, and Atkin SL (2000). Neuroleptic malignant syndrome after venlafaxine. *Lancet*, **355**, 289–90.

Nisijima K and Ishiguro T (1995). Cerebrospinal fluid levels of monoamine metabolites and gamma-aminobutiryric acid in neuroleptic malignant syndrome. *J Psychiatr Res*, **29**, 233–44.

Pope HG Jr, Aizley HG, Keck PE Jr, *et al.* (1991). Neuroleptic malignant syndrome: long-term follow-up of 20 cases. *J Clin Psychiatry*, **52**, 208–12.

Rosebush P and Stewart T (1989). A prospective analysis of 24 episodes of neuroleptic malignant syndrome. *Am J Psychiatry*, **146**, 717–25.

Rosebush P and Mazurek I (1991). Serum iron and neuroleptic malignant syndrome. *Lancet*, **338**, 149–51.

Rosenberg MR and Green M (1989). Neuroleptic malignant syndrome review of response to therapy. *Arch Intern Med*, **149**, 1927–31.

Shalev A and Munitz H (1986). The neuroleptic malignant syndrome; agent and host interaction. *Acta Psychiatr Scand*, **73**, 337–47.

Shalev A, Hermesh H, and Munitz H (1989). Mortality from neuroleptic malignant syndrome. *J Clin Psychiatry*, **50**, 18–25.

Stauder KH (1934). Die Toldliche katatinie. *Arch Psychiatr Nervenkranke*, **102**, 614–34.

Susman VL and Addonizio G (1988). Recurrence of neuroleptic malignant syndrome. *J Nerv Ment Dis*, **176**, 234–41.

White DA and Robins AH (1991). Catatonia: harbinger of the neuroleptic malignant syndrome. *Br J Psychiatry*, **158**, 419–21.

White DA (1992). Catatonia and the neuroleptic malignant syndrome – a single entity? *Br J Psychiatry*, **161**, 558–60.

Chapter 3

Serotonin syndrome

Ken Gillman and Ian M Whyte

Introduction

There have been many deaths caused by serotonin (5-hydroxytryptamine, 5-HT) toxicity (serotonin syndrome) approximately 50 of which have been described in the literature. This book will arrive in time to mark the fiftieth anniversary of the first of these reported fatalities (Mitchell 1955). Serotonin toxicity reactions continue to result from therapeutic drug combinations that predictably cause this interaction. These instances demonstrate both the difficulty and the importance of communicating complex knowledge to health professionals and also of implementing procedures to prevent predictable adverse interactions and reactions. Serotonin toxicity is one of the rare situations in medicine where the administration of a single therapeutic dose of a drug can lead to death.

The adverse effects of excess serotonin occur on a spectrum that ranges from mild dose-related effects that occur during routine therapy and require no specific treatment (or occasionally dose reduction) to severe, potentially life-threatening serotonin toxicity that requires early recognition and urgent intervention with specific treatment. The term 'serotonin syndrome' is loosely used to refer to significant serotonin toxicity. The authors prefer the term serotonin toxicity but it seems likely that both 'serotonin syndrome' and 'serotonin toxicity' will continue to be used interchangeably. The key issue is not the term that is used but an appreciation that toxicity occurs on a spectrum.

Some observations about the history of serotonin toxicity will provide perspective and help to clarify the current state of the literature and research. A useful body of animal work demonstrating the occurrence of serotonin toxicity had been performed before 1970 including the recognition that chlorpromazine (a $5\text{-HT}_2\text{A}$ antagonist) could suppress serotonin toxicity as early as 1958 (Bogdanski *et al.* 1958). Oates, a neurologist, described the human clinical picture in 1960 and proposed the mechanism as excess 5-HT (Oates *et al.* 1960). Early usage of therapeutic combinations of monoamine oxidase inhibitors (MAOIs) and tricyclic antidepressants (TCAs) led to reports of toxic reactions. Similar reactions occurred when MAOIs were combined with the analgesic pethidine. Both reactions are now known to be examples of serotonin toxicity (Gillman 1998). Debate ensued concerning the safety of 'combined antidepressant treatment'.

Imipramine, the TCA involved in the early reports, possesses weak serotonin reuptake inhibitor (SRI) capacity which is usually insufficient to precipitate serotonin toxicity, even if combined with MAOIs. Following the introduction of clomipramine, more severe reactions were reported in combination with MAOIs, reflecting the fact that clomipramine is a more potent blocker of serotonin reuptake than imipramine. This variation, and the unpredictability of reactions with imipramine, caused confusion in the literature, especially because the mechanism of the reaction was not widely understood by clinicians until the 1980s (despite extensive evidence from animal work). This legacy of confusion still permeates psychiatric opinion and practice and incorrect information remains in both current textbooks and journal reviews about MAOI interactions with analgesics and serotonin reuptake inhibitors (SRIs). Aspects of this are analysed in Gillman (1998).

Clinical features

The spectrum of serotonin toxicity

Serotonin toxicity is an iatrogenic reaction mediated by drug induced excess of intra-synaptic 5-hydroxytryptamine (5-HT). The degree of elevation of 5-HT determines the severity of the reaction, which occurs on a spectrum progressing from mild side-effects through to toxicity. The predictability of serotonin toxicity differentiates it from its idiosyncratic drug reactions such as NMS or malignant hyperthermia (Bodner *et al.* 1995; Lane *et al.* 1997; Gillman 1998; Radomski *et al.* 2000; Whyte *et al.* 2002).

The spectrum concept makes some simple and important predictions about the frequency and severity of toxicity. It indicates there will be a dose–effect relationship and toxicity will be progressively more common with larger doses and overdoses of a single drug, than with therapeutic doses. As with all dose–effect relationships there appears to be a maximum (plateau) effect for each individual mechanism of serotonin elevation. Predictably, combinations of drugs having different mechanisms of action (which raise serotonin levels higher) will cause more frequent and more severe toxicity. Conversely the toxicity of drugs with different mechanisms of action may tell us something about their role in affecting 5-HT.

A dose–effect relationship has been demonstrated in animal work (see Gillman 1998). Increased death rates were observed in animals with more

Table 3.1 Severity of serotonergic effects with individual drugs and combinations

Drug and dose	Serotonin side effects (mild/moderate)	Serotonin toxicity (severe with risk of fatality)
SRI therapeutic dose	Mild**	None*
SRI overdose	Moderate in 16.3%*	None*
Nefazodone and mirtazapine (therapeutic dose and overdose)	None**	None*
Moclobemide therapeutic dose	Rare**	None*
Moclobemide overdose	Rare (moderate in 3%)*	None*
MAOI + TCA (excluding imipramine and clomipramine)	Few**	None*
MAOI + SRI therapeutic dose	Commonly severe **	Frequent*, fatalities occur**
MAOI (moclobemide) + SRI in overdose	Very common (moderate or greater in 55%)*	Frequent (severe in 29%)*

* HATS data (Whyte and Dawson 2002; Isbister *et al.* 2003).

** Estimates from other published data (see www.psychotropical.com/SerotoninToxicity.doc for full details).

potent SRIs given in combination with an MAOI. There is also evidence that in humans the extent and severity of serotonin toxicity is dose-related and occurs with increasing frequency with larger doses of selective serotonin reuptake inhibitors (SSRIs) and with even greater frequency in overdoses. Experience also indicates that fatalities occur almost exclusively with combinations of MAOIs and SRIs. Experience of overdoses with different serotonergic drugs also fits this pattern (Table 3.1).

In humans prescribed MAOIs, the addition of drugs with potent serotonergic effects, usually SRIs, is likely to cause severe serotonin toxicity and risk of death (Oefele *et al.* 1986). Conversely, drugs that can be combined with a MAOI without frequent serotonin toxicity have weak serotonergic effects; neither do they cause serotonin toxicity if ingested by themselves in overdose. Hence combining amitriptyline (a weak serotonin reuptake inhibitor) with a MAOI does not cause serotonin toxicity; neither does amitriptyline in overdose present with serotonin toxicity (Gillman 2003*a*). Conversely clomipramine, a clinically effective serotonin reuptake inhibitor, does cause serotonin side effects by itself, serotonin toxicity in overdose and fatalities if combined with MAOIs. Trazodone and nefazodone, as well as mianserin and mirtazapine (all very low potency SRIs thought to have other weak serotonergic effects) have no serotonin side-effects, do not cause serotonin toxicity in overdose, and can be combined safely with an MAOI. These basic observations serve to illustrate why case reports positing the involvement of trazodone, nefazodone and mirtazapine (and also olanzapine) are likely to represent artefactual and erroneous observations and misleading reasoning (Whyte *et al.* 2001; Gillman 2003*b*).

It is important to note that there is now sufficient high quality prospectively collected data from human studies of serotonin toxicity to support the spectrum concept (Table 3.1) (Whyte 2002; Whyte *et al.* 2002; Whyte and Dawson 2002; Isbister *et al.* 2003; Whyte *et al.* 2003). This provides a framework for a significantly increased degree of predictability about drug interactions and gives clearer guidance to clinicians concerning which drug combinations may have a favourable risk benefit ratio in particular clinical circumstances.

The clinical picture

Serotonin toxicity may be characterized as a triad of neuroexcitatory features which occur on a spectrum ranging from mild to life threatening features (Sternbach 1991; Bodner, Lynch *et al.* 1995; Gillman 1998; Radomski, Dursun *et al.* 2000; Whyte and Dawson 2002; Dunkley *et al.* 2003). The triad comprises:

- **Altered mental status;** agitation, excitement and confusion
- **Neuromuscular hyperactivity;** tremor, clonus, myoclonus, hyperreflexia, and (in the advanced stage) pyramidal rigidity
- **Autonomic hyperactivity;** diaphoresis, fever, mydriasis, tachycardia and tachypnoea.

The onset of frank toxicity is usually rapid because it results from drug combinations and starts when the second drug is introduced. The symptoms are often alarming and usually occur within hours of one of the first few doses of the second serotonergic drug in the patient's regime. Typically the serotonin toxic patient is initially alert, even hypervigilant, with tremor and hyperreflexia. Ankle clonus may be demonstrable and also myoclonus, which may be generalized. Neuromuscular signs are initially greater in the lower limbs then become more generalized as the toxicity increases when the autonomic features also become more evident with fever, sweating and tachycardia. The autonomic features of tachypnoea, tachycardia and hypertension may fluctuate and are not usually a management problem. Other symptoms may include shaking, shivering often including chattering of the teeth and trismus. Pyramidal rigidity is a late development and when it affects truncal muscles this impairs respiration. Rigidity and a fever of $> 38\,^{\circ}\text{C}$ heralds life-threatening toxicity.

The clinical picture is strongly influenced by the potency of the combination causing the symptoms and the stage at which the patient is observed.

Table 3.2 Serotonin related signs stratified by severity

Severity of reaction	Examples of causal drugs	Signs		
		Mental state	Neuromuscular	Autonomic
Mild	SSRI + Li or buspirone	No abnormality	Shivering, occasional myoclonus, tremor, hyperreflexia	Fever (37.5 °C to 38.5 °C)
Moderate	Overdose of SSRI	Confusion/ agitation	Regular myoclonus, inducible ankle clonus,hyperreflexia	Fever (38.5 °C to 39.5 °C)
Severe	MAOI or RIMA + SRI	Marked confusion	Generalised myoclonus, sustained ankle clonus, hypertonia/rigidity, marked hyperreflexia	Fever (>39.5 °C)

The mild cases seen in outpatient settings represent a different problem to the obtunded, rigid, feverish patient in the emergency department. This highlights the importance of the spectrum concept, the stage of presentation, and the mechanism of action of different drugs that may be implicated.

As noted above, the quality of the clinical signs and symptoms data from which deductions are made is most important. Whyte and colleagues at the Hunter Area Toxicology Service (HATS) have systematically recorded prospective data in detail concerning all cases of drug overdose and toxicity over a number of years and published various findings in relation to drug toxicity and serotonin toxicity. An important advantage of this approach is that it ensures an improved quality of clinical examination and recording of data by a team of doctors experienced in this field and avoids the selective bias inherent in analysing case reports and other similar data sources (Whyte 2002; Whyte *et al.* 2002; Whyte and Dawson 2002). The HATS database is now sufficiently large to allow useful analysis in relation to a number of different drugs and the frequency with which they are associated with different clinical features. This has produced a clear picture of features that are associated with serotonin toxicity specifically, as opposed to features that are characteristic of other types of drug toxicity. The HATS data indicate the features that distinguish serotonergic drug overdose from overdose with other drugs are clonus (inducible, spontaneous or ocular), hyperreflexia, agitation, diaphoresis and tremor, and in severe toxicity temperature > 38 °C and hypertonia/pyramidal rigidity (pyramidal rigidity is clasp-knife progressing to fixed rigidity).

Pharmacological basis

Mechanisms

By definition the pharmacology involves central nervous system (functional) serotonin excess. There is no natural mechanism by which this occurs; it is always the result of the ingestion of drugs. The most powerful mechanisms appear to be blocking serotonin reuptake (e.g. SSRIs), preventing serotonin metabolism by inhibiting monoamine oxidase (e.g. MAOIs) and promoting presynaptic release (e.g. L-5-hydroxytryptophan). Drugs having direct effects at postsynaptic serotonin receptors may have relevant but more specific effects, e.g. tryptans.

The interconnections of neural pathways suggests that serotonin will modulate other pathways and also be modulated by them. Norepinephrine, dopamine (DA) and gamma-aminobutyric acid (GABA) pathways may play some part in modulating symptoms, and alterations in these pathways may play a role in the expression of symptoms and therefore be relevant in relation to treatment (Nisijima *et al.* 2003).

There are a number of mechanisms that may currently be expected to be relevant to the expression of serotonergic effects. 5-HT levels are crucial, and second directly acting agonists such as tryptans may be of relevance. Third, the sensitivity of postsynaptic receptors can vary and denervation supersensitivity induced by potent 5-HT$_2$A antagonists may be clinically relevant. Lastly, modulation of 5-HT by other pathways may influence the expression of serotonergic symptoms; but we do not yet know sufficient about norepinephrine, dopamine and GABA to conclude whether they have a significant influence on the development of toxicity.

Blockade of postsynaptic serotonin receptors produces denervation supersensitivity as occurs with DA receptors following chronic administration of neuroleptics (Green 1977). A variety of drugs used clinically, including antidepressants (clomipramine, doxepin, nefazodone, mirtazapine), and various neuroleptics are potent blockers of 5-HT$_2$A receptors (Gillman 1999). Cessation of any of these drugs may lead to rebound increased activity when either normal, or elevated, levels of serotonin act on both unmasked and supersensitized receptors. Several case reports suggest this mechanism may be relevant (Gillman 1998; Zerjav-Lacombe *et al.* 2001). The use of olanzapine with SSRIs may be expected to demonstrate this, if the olanzapine is ceased first, thereby exposing supersensitive 5-HT$_2$A receptors to enhanced levels of serotonin.

Both human and animal evidence indicates that *severe* serotonin toxicity, as manifest by fever and neuroexcitatory symptoms, is optimally suppressed by blockade of 5-HT$_2$A receptors (but not by blockade of 1A receptors).

Our knowledge of the 5-HT receptor subtypes and their anatomical location and function remains imperfect and future developments will increase the depth of our understanding. A range of structurally different drugs that are currently thought to be 5-HT$_2$A antagonists, both specific and non-specific, suppress serotonin toxicity more effectively than other drugs: these include chlorpromazine, cyproheptadine, risperidone, ketanserin and methysergide. Most of these drugs are one hundred times more potent as 5-HT$_2$A, than as 5-HT$_1$A, antagonists.

Implicated drugs

Table 3.3 shows the common and important drugs that might be involved in serotonin toxicity, as well as those that have already been implicated in toxicity or fatalities. Chlorpheniramine and brompheniramine are widely available 'over the counter' antihistamines and are structurally related to the TCAs and like clomipramine are SRIs. Chlorpheniramine is available in an intravenous form and has been implicated in serotonin toxicity via this route. Dexamphetamine can be a problem, particularly in combination with an SRI. Pethidine, dextromethorphan and tramadol are the main analgesics possessing significant serotonin reuptake inhibitor capacity and have been associated with severe toxicity and fatalities.

Table 3.3 Serotonergic drugs

Selective serotonin reuptake inhibitors
Citalopram, fluoxetine, fluvoxamine, paroxetine, sertraline

Non-selective serotonin reuptake inhibitors
Brompheniramine, chlorpheniramine, clomipramine, dextromethorphan, dextropropoxyphene, duloxetine, imipramine, minalcipran, pentazocine, pethidine, St John's Wort (*Hypericum perforatum*), sibutramine, tramadol, venlafaxine

Serotonin precursors
5-hydroxytryptophan, L-tryptophan

Serotonin agonists
Buspirone, dihydroergotamine, LSD, tryptans

Serotonin releasers
Amphetamine and derivatives (MDMA MDEA MDA), fenfluramine, methylphenidate

Monoamine oxidase inhibitors
Clorgyline, furazolidone, iproniazid, isocarboxazide, isoniazid, linezolid, moclobemide, nialamide, pargyline, phenelzine, procarbazine, selegiline, toloxatone, tranylcypromine

Other drugs
Bromocriptine, S-adenosylmethionine, ginseng (panax ginseng)

NB: Some drugs may have uncertain and/or multiple mechanisms of action.

All amphetamine derivatives and cocaine have the potential to cause serotonin toxicity, although deaths involving single drugs seem rare. Ecstasy (3,4-methylenedioxymethamphetamine, MDMA) is the most serotonergic and may pose the greatest risk; there have been fatalities (Brown *et al.* 1987; Mueller *et al.* 1998). Other reports implicate MDMA in combination with antidepressants, including four recent deaths with moclobemide (Vuori *et al.* 2003); as is predicted from the risk analysis herein.

Differential diagnosis

A key differential diagnosis is neuroleptic malignant syndrome (NMS) (see Chapter 2). NMS is a hypo-dopaminergic state, where progressive bradykinesia results in a state of immobilization, akinesia and 'stupor' accompanied by 'lead pipe' or 'cogwheel' rigidity, fever, and autonomic instability. It may also occur following cessation of dopaminergic drugs and in this situation the receptor adaptation of subsensitivity may play a role in symptoms just as supersensitivity may in serotonin toxicity.

Features differentiating serotonin toxicity and NMS include the following:

- **Causal agents:** SS is caused by serotonergic drugs. NMS usually occurs in association with neuroleptics; it can also occur with other drugs and following cessation of dopaminergic agents.

- **Speed of onset and progression:** SS, rapid onset and progression. NMS, slow onset and progression.

- **Motor signs:** SS, hyperkinesia and hyperreflexia/clonus, pyramidal rigidity. NMS, bradykinesia and extrapyramidal rigidity.

- **Aetiology:** SS, a predictable manifestation of toxicity. NMS, an idiosyncratic reaction to therapeutic dosages.

The differentiation of serotonin toxicity and NMS is further discussed in an analysis of controversial published cases in Gillman (1998) and also by Whyte and colleagues in various subsequent publications.

Another important differential diagnosis is anticholinergic delirium (see Chapter 16). Both anticholinergic delirium and SS can manifest with impairment of consciousness, tachycardia and pyrexia. The key distinguishing signs of SS are diaphoresis, clonus and hyperreflexia. In contrast in anticholinergic toxicity the skin and also the mucous membranes are dry, and increased tone and hyperreflexia are not present. The characteristric signs of diaphoresis, clonus, and hyperreflexia also make it difficult to confuse serotonin syndrome with drug withdrawal, e.g. alcohol or benzodiazepines.

Exclusion criteria for the diagnosis of serotonin toxicity have been suggested, including recent administration of a neuroleptic and substance withdrawal.

There is not a satisfactory logical explanation of why those, or any other features, should assume a hierarchical precedence over signs of serotonin toxicity.

Management

The spectrum concept and a knowledge of the drugs involved guides assessment of the likely severity of reactions and therefore the setting in which assessment and treatment is appropriate (Tables 3.1 and 3.2). Two pieces of information best predict the course of action:

1 a knowledge of the quantity and type of drugs ingested and

2 the current symptoms and their rate of change over time.

When both an MAOI and an SRI have been co-ingested (even in low doses) rapid deterioration is well documented, indicating a conservative approach to treatment is unjustified.

If serotonin side effects are mild, or moderate, then they may be managed by adjustment of the dose of medication or by switching medication. However, in certain instances it may be appropriate to consider cyproheptadine, a 5-HT$_2$A antagonist. An overdose of an SSRI alone produces moderately severe serotonin toxicity in 10–20 per cent of cases (sufficient to warrant active medical treatment), but serious sequelae and fatalities appear to be extremely unlikely and none have yet been reliably documented. Analysis of the HATS data shows that it is those cases where a MAOI or reversible inhibitor of monoamine oxidase-A (RIMA) has been taken in conjunction with a SRI that are likely to experience severe serotonin toxicity (more than 50 per cent of such cases) (Isbister *et al.* 2003). It is these combinations that are most likely to require active medical intervention including intensive care admission, cooling, 5-HT$_2$A antagonists, such as cyproheptadine or chlorpromazine, as well as intubation and neuromuscular paralysis. Details of these treatments are available in toxicology texts.

A brief overview indicates that cyproheptadine is effective for the milder cases who are able to take oral medication. Current experience suggests that 12 mg orally or by nasogastric tube, followed by 4–8 mg every four to six hours, is an appropriate dose range. For severe toxicity chlorpromazine has been used in many cases with apparent good effect. Current experience indicates fluid resuscitation is required prior to administration of chlorpromazine and that the dose is probably in the range of 12.5–25 mg IV initially, followed by 25 mg orally or iv every six hours. Severe late stage serotonin toxicity progresses to rigidity of the lower limbs and then truncal muscles, which can produce impairment of breathing and a rise in PaCO$_2$ requiring intubation and neuromuscular paralysis.

The obtunded, rigid, hyperpyrexic emergency that requires immediate intensive medical resuscitation represents a different diagnostic problem, which is beyond the scope of this review.

Risk factors

The most important risk factor is the degree to which the drugs involved can enhance serotonin transmission; this depends on the pharmacology of the individual drugs, the doses involved and the potential for pharmacological interactions that can enhance serotonin transmission. Data from HATS (Table 3.1) now provides us with a relative estimate of the incidence of serotonin toxicity with different drugs taken alone in overdose. Moclobemide alone has a low propensity to cause serotonin toxicity (Isbister *et al.* 2003). As suggested by Finberg, this may because it is both reversible and competitive so the higher it raises 5-HT the more 5-HT competes with it for MAO binding. The spectrum concept guides an interpretation of the risk with doses and combinations.

Case reports suggest that patients with organic brain disease may be especially susceptible and this is consonant with the sensitivity of those with Lewy Body dementia to neuroleptics and anti-muscarinics. It would also be expected that poor metabolizers for various cytochrome P450 enzymes that are responsible for metabolizing relevant drugs would be more susceptible as a result of higher drug levels. However, there is no direct evidence for this as yet since blood levels are rarely performed, either routinely or in cases of overdose.

There have been about 50 deaths from serotonin toxicity reported in the medical literature (not counting MDMA – 'ecstasy' – deaths). So far the only fatalities reported have been with MAOIs (including RIMAs like moclobemide and tolaxatone) when combined with any drug that acts as a serotonin reuptake inhibitor (SRI), note this does include (Table 3.3) some analgesics that are also SRIs (e.g. tramadol) and antihistamines (e.g. chlorpheniramine).

The risk of severe reactions occurring with moclobemide, when combined with SRIs, is significant even at 'therapeutic' doses. The low toxicity of moclobemide alone may create a false sense of security concerning its interactions with other serotonergic drugs, particularly SRIs. Even a small overdose of moclobemide, if combined with a serotonin reuptake inhibitor, may produce a severe or fatal reaction. The short half-life of moclobemide lessens the risk when the transition is from it to another serotonergic drug and a washout period of 24–48 hours is likely to be quite sufficient. However more caution is required when changing to moclobemide from SRIs which have longer half-lives, especially fluoxetine, which also markedly elevates moclobemide levels (Gillman 2003*c*).

Prevention

Prevention follows logically from the concepts discussed above. Continuing education of health and medical personnel will help to ensure that potentially risky combinations are avoided. At the primary care level it is worthwhile practitioners being aware of, and taking steps to avoid, the possession of MAOIs/RIMAs and SRIs of any type in the same household and making sure that supplies are returned to the pharmacist prior to swapping to a different treatment.

At the specialist level it is an increasing challenge for psychopharmacologists to keep up with the intricate developments in the field. Numerous case reports of drug toxicity illustrate the pitfalls of combining different psychotropic medications, even in the most expert hands. Fostering a full appreciation of the complexities of pharmacokinetic and pharmacodynamic interaction amongst all specialists remains important.

At the intensive care admission level disseminating the latest knowledge about treatment of serotonin toxicity is relevant and the network of toxicologists that exists in most countries is the appropriate avenue for this. The spectrum concept contributes to this by helping to identify the high-risk cases (MAOI plus SRI) that are likely to require aggressive intervention with chlorpromazine or cyproheptadine. Chlorpromazine may be life-saving in severe cases of toxicity, its value has been under-recognized and it has been under-utilized over the last 50 years; this contention is supported from systematic treatment data emerging from the HATS database.

Summary

Definition	Serotonin toxicity is an iatrogenic reaction mediated by drug-induced excess of intra-synaptic serotonin (5-HT). The term serotonin syndrome is usually used to refer to clinically significant toxicity.
Incidence	Dependent on the type and dose of the drugs ingested and the threshold used to define toxicity (e.g. occurs in approx. 15% of SSRI overdoses).
Drugs causing syndrome	Usually occurs with combinations of serotonergic drugs (see Table 3.3) but can occur with single drugs in overdose. Most severe cases have involved combinations of MAOIs (any type) with drugs having the property of serotonin reuptake inhibition; this includes some narcotic analgesics and antihistamines.
Key symptoms	Altered mental status; agitation, anxiety, hypomania and confusion Neuromuscular hyperactivity; tremor, clonus, myoclonus, hyperreflexia and (in the advanced stage) rigidity.

	Autonomic hyperactivity; diaphoresis, fever, tachycardia and tachypnoea.
Pharmacological mechanism	Drug-induced serotonin excess and post-synaptic receptor supersensitivity.
Investigations to confirm diagnosis	History and examination especially neurological examination for clonus, hyperreflexia and rigidity.
Management	Cease causal agents. Cyproheptadine; chlorpromazine; if severe refer to ICU.
Further reading	Bodner RA, Lynch T, Lewis L, *et al.* (1995) Serotonin syndrome. *Neurology* **45**, 219–23.
	Dunkley E, Isbister G, Sibbritt D, *et al.* (2003) Hunter serotonin toxicity criteria: a simple and accurate diagnostic decision rule for serotonin toxicity. *Quarterly Journal of Medicine* **96**, 635–42.
	Gillman PK (1998) Serotonin syndrome: history and risk. *Fundamental and Clinical Pharmacology* **12**, 482–91.

References

Bodner RA, Lynch T, Lewis L, *et al.* (1995). Serotonin syndrome. *Neurology*, **45**, 219–23.

Bogdanski DF, Weissbach H, and Udenfriend S (1958). Pharmacological studies with the serotonin precursor 5-hydroxytryptophan. *J Pharmacol Exp Ther*, **122**, 182–94.

Brown C and Osterloh J (1987). Multiple severe complications from recreational ingestion of MDMA ('Ecstasy'). *JAMA*, **258**, 780–1.

Dunkley E, Isbister G, Sibbritt D, *et al.* (2003). Hunter serotonin toxicity criteria: a simple and accurate diagnostic decision rule for serotonin toxicity. *Q J Med*, **96**, 635–42.

Gillman PK (1998). Serotonin syndrome: history and risk. *Fund Clin Pharmacol*, **12**, 482–91.

Gillman PK (1999). The serotonin syndrome and its treatment. *J Psychopharmacol*, **13**, 100–9.

Gillman PK (2003*a*). Amitriptyline: dual-action antidepressant? *J Clin Psychiatry*, **64**, 391.

Gillman PK (2003*b*). Mirtazapine: unable to induce serotonin toxicity? *Clin Neuropharmacol*, **26**, 288–9.

Gillman PK (2003*c*). Serotonin toxicity (serotonin syndrome): a current analysis. Psychopharmacology Update Notes online available at: www.psychotropical.com/ SerotoninToxicity.doc.

Green AR (1977). Repeated chlorpromazine administration increases a behavioural response of rats to 5-hydroxytryptamine receptor stimulation. *Br J Pharmacol*, **59**, 367–71.

Isbister G, Hackett L, Dawson A, *et al.* (2003). Moclobemide poisoning: toxicokinetics and occurrence of serotonin toxicity. *Br J Clin Pharmacol*, **56**, 441–50.

Lane R and Baldwin D (1997). Selective serotonin reuptake inhibitor-induced serotonin syndrome: review. *J Clin Psychopharmacol*, **17**, 208–21.

Mitchell RS (1955). Fatal toxic encephalitis occurring during iproniazid therapy in pulmonary tuberculosis. *Ann Intern Med*, **42**, 417–24.

Mueller PD and Korey WS (1998). Death by 'ecstasy': the serotonin syndrome? *Ann Emerg Med*, **32**, 377–80.

Nisijima K, Shioda K, Yoshino T, et al. (2003). Diazepam and chlormethiazole attenuate the development of hyperthermia in an animal model of the serotonin syndrome. *Neurochem Int*, **43**, 155–64.

Oates JA and Sjoerdsma A (1960). Neurologic effects of tryptophan in patients receiving a monoamine oxidase inhibitor. *Neurology*, **10**, 1076–8.

Oefele KV, Grohmann R, and Ruther E (1986). Adverse drug reactions in combined tricyclic and MAOI therapy. *Pharmacopsychiatry*, **19**, 243–4.

Radomski JW, Dursun SM, Reveley MA, et al. (2000). An exploratory approach to the serotonin syndrome: an update of clinical phenomenology and revised diagnostic criteria. *Med Hypotheses*, **55**, 218–24.

Sternbach H (1991). The serotonin syndrome. *Am J Psychiatry*, **148**, 705–13.

Vuori E, Henry JA, Ojanpera I, et al. (2003). Death following ingestion of MDMA (ecstasy) and moclobemide. *Addiction*, **98**, 365–8.

Whyte IM (2002). Introduction: research in clinical toxicology – the value of high quality data. *J Toxicol Clin Toxicol*, **40**, 211–12.

Whyte IM, Buckley NA, and Dawson AH (2002). Data collection in clinical toxicology: are there too many variables? *J Toxicol Clin Toxicol*, **40**, 223–30.

Whyte IM and Dawson AH (2002). Redefining the serotonin syndrome. *J Toxicol Clin Toxicol*, **40**, 668–9.

Whyte IM, Dawson AH, and Buckley NA (2003). Relative toxicity of venlafaxine and selective serotonin reuptake inhibitors in overdose compared to tricyclic antidepressants. *Q J Med*, **96**, 369–74.

Whyte IM and Isbister GK (2001). Misdiagnosis of myoclonus in antidepressant induced serotonin excess. *Vet Hum Toxicol*, **43**, 375–6.

Zerjav-Lacombe S and Dewan V (2001). Possible serotonin syndrome associated with clomipramine after withdrawal of clozapine. *Ann Pharmacother*, **35**, 180–2.

Chapter 4

Torsade de pointes and sudden death

Nicol Ferrier

Introduction

Antipsychotic drugs have transformed the management of patients with psychosis. A link between these drugs, ventricular tachycardia and sudden death was made soon after their use in clinical care became widespread (Reinert and Hermann 1960; Kelly *et al.* 1963; Desautels *et al.* 1964). In the intervening four decades no consensus has been achieved on the frequency of these events, or even whether a true causal association exists. For example the Working Group of the Royal College of Psychiatrists' Psychopharmacology SubGroup (1997) said 'there is uncertainty regarding the mechanisms underlying sudden death . . . and a lack of any systematic data relevant to an individual patient's risk, or the relative risk with various antipsychotics'. There is therefore a dilemma of balancing the unknown risk of a rare but lethal adverse reaction against the undoubted and life-saving benefits of long-term treatment.

A possible mechanism for the association with sudden death was recognized at an early stage, since ECG abnormalities indicating abnormal repolarization were present in significant proportions of patients on neuroleptics (Ban and St Jean 1965). These ECG effects were found to result from quinidine-like effects of the antipsychotic drug on the ventricular myocardium, specifically potassium channel blockade and delayed ventricular repolarization (Hollander and Cain 1971). The conventional measure of ventricular repolarization is the QT interval, i.e. the time from the onset of ventricular depolarization to completion of repolarization. Prolongation of the QT interval indicates that the individual may be at increased risk of cardiac arrhythmias, including a potentially fatal arrhythmia termed 'torsade de pointes'.

This chapter explores the relationship between antipsychotics and torsade de pointe and sudden death. QTc prolongation is considered in detail as it is a marker of arrhythmic risk. Arrhythmias and sudden death are not adverse events unique to antipsychotics but are recognized with an ever increasing number of drugs.

Clinical features

Torsade de pointes

Torsade de pointes (TDP) is a polymorphic ventricular tachycardia character-ized by QRS complexes of changing amplitude. It may be asymptomatic or cause dizziness, palpitations or syncope. In rare cases it may progress to ven-tricular fibrillation which presents clinically as a cardiac arrest and, unless resuscitation is successful, sudden death.

Sudden unexplained death

Sudden unexplained death has been defined as

> Death within the hour of symptoms (excluding suicide, homicide and accident), which is both unexpected in relation to the degree of disability before death and unexplained because clinical investigation and autopsy failed to identify any plausible cause.
>
> (Jusic and Lader 1994)

Various conditions can cause sudden death but are usually identifiable at post-mortem. For example both myocardial infarction and rupture of a cerbral aneurysm can lead to sudden death. However the former may be associated with total occlusion of a coronary artery, while the latter will be associated with intracranial haemorrhage. These causes of sudden death are therefore *explained* on autopsy. In contrast drug-related arrhythmic deaths are not asso-ciated with anatomical changes, the deaths are *unexplained* and in each indi-vidual case, diagnosis is usually by exclusion and the existence of circumstantial evidence.

QTc prolongation

The QT interval is subject to a number of influences including gender, age, time of day and heart rate. The latter effect has led to the adoption of the QTc interval which is the QT interval with a correction for heart rate. The most commonly employed correction is Bazett's formula (QTcB) but this method has limitations, particularly when studying drugs that may effect heart rate. The Fridericia formula (QTcF) appears to correct more accurately when the heart rate is increased. There are also problems in the interpretation of QT and there is only weak consensus on the cut-off points for abnormality (Moss 1993).

QT interval prolongation may be congenital or acquired. Congenital long QT syndromes result from mutations of genes that code for specific compon-ents of cardiac ion channels. In healthy unmedicated subjects, the evidence linking QT prolongation with increased cardiovascular risk is conflicting. Schoeten *et al.* (1991) showed an increase relative risk of all causes of mortality over 15 years with QTc prolongation of 440 ms (relative risk 1.7 in men and 1.6 in women). Cardiovascular mortality largely accounted for this increase in risk. Algara *et al.* (1991) found that QT prolongation was an independent risk factor for sudden death in patients without intraventricular conduction defects. Conversely, Goldberg *et al.* (1991) showed no statistically significant increase in overall relative risk of death (relative risk 1.02, 95 per cent CI 0.70–1.49) or sudden death (relative risk 1.31, 95 per cent CI 0.60–2.86) in patients with QTc interval > 440 ms in data derived from the Framingham Heart Study. In a study involving almost 2000 patients with congenital long QT syndrome and their relatives, 52 per cent of affected probands, 22 per cent of affected relatives and 0 per cent of unaffected relatives had a QTc interval of more than 500 ms. The risk of a cardiac event increased by an average of 5.2 per cent (95 per cent confidence intervals 1.7, 8.8 per cent) for every 10 ms increase in QTc (Moss *et al.* 1991). In patients with both cardiovascular and liver disease there is good evidence that QT prolongation is associated with increased risk of arrhythmia or death (Yap and Camm 2000).

The relationship between the degree of drug-induced QT interval prolongation and the extent of the increase in risk of arrhythmia has not been subject to formal epidemiological study. However risk appears to increase with more extreme QT interval prolongation, though the relationship is non-linear. Torsade appears unusual if the QT interval is less than 500 ms and in one study the mean QT interval prior to the onset of torsade was 580 ms (Stratmann and Kennedy 1987). However QTc prolongation is only a surrogate marker or signal of arrhythmic risk. Drugs which produce the same degree of QT prolongation may provide different risks of arrhythmia. For example, the class III antiarrhythmic drug amiodarone is less commonly associated with torsade than other drugs, even though it causes QT prolongation which is just as marked (Hii *et al.* 1992).

The Committee for Proprietary Medicinal Products (1997) provided guidance on 'signal' values for drug-induced QT prolongation after Bazett's correction. Individual changes less than 30 msec relative to drug-free baseline measurements are regarded as unlikely to raise significant concerns about the proarrhythmic potential of a drug. In contrast, an individual change in the QTc greater than 60 msec relative to drug-free baseline measurements or an absolute QTc value, or at lower heart rates an uncorrected QT value, greater than 500 msec are identified as raising 'clear concerns' regarding the risk of drug-induced arrhythmias. Of these two signals, the absolute QTc value is regarded as having greater prognostic significance. QTc dispersion greater than 100 per cent across a 12-lead ECG is also regarded as raising concern about the potential for arrhythmias.

Pharmacological basis of torsade de pointes

The most important mechanism underlying the arrhythmic action of antipsychotic drugs is blockade of the delayed rectifier potassium channel I_{Kr} in the myocardium. This prevents the outward movement of potassium that is responsible for ventricular depolarization. As far as antipsychotics are concerned, this is an entirely separate mechanism from their primary pharmacological action and therefore a risk of arrhythmia is entailed which is not associated with any clinical advantage. Prolonged ventricular repolarization predisposes to arrythmias as the myocardium is more susceptible to the occurrence of early after depolariations.

The cloning of the human 'ether-a-go-go' (HERG) gene which encodes for this channel has resulted in studies confirming the specific I_{kr} blocking potency of haloperidol, droperidol, pimozide and sertindole. Antipsychotics bind to the I_{kr} channel with varying affinities which may prove to be associated with their potential for arrhythmogenesis. Animal studies of I_{kr} blockade with thioridazine have shown a concentration dependent effect. Hence the prospect now exists for newly developed antipsychotics to be screened by manufacturers for their relative potential to block I_{kr}, and to be excluded if affinity is high. However, the extent to which pre-clinical models are predictive of arrhythmias during the clinical use of the drug remains to be established.

Those drugs which produce heterogeneous prolongation of QT interval across the myocardium (increased QT dispersion) may carry a higher risk, compared to those which produce a homogeneous QT prolongation (Hii et al. 1992). Some drugs have ancillary properties that may either increase or decrease the risk of arrhythmia. For example drugs that are associated with tachycardia may be less likely to produce torsade, since torsade occurs most often when the heart rate is slow. There is also evidence that torsade de pointes most often occurs disproportionately early during therapy which has implications for monitoring, since it would be logical to focus this at the time of highest risk.

Differential toxicity of antipsychotic drugs

Evidence suggests that the pro-arrhythmic actions of antipsychotic drugs vary, with some agents being particularly potent at causing arrhythmias and sudden death. The data comprises case reports and open studies, ECG studies and epidemiological studies of sudden deaths. Each will be considered in turn.

Case reports and open studies

Initial data consisted of case reports or open studies. Interpretation of case reports of arrythnia and sudden death in patients receiving antipsychotic drugs is further complicated because psychiatric patients are known to be at a high risk of cardiovascular death (Baxter 1996; Hensen *et al.* 1997; Ruschena *et al.* 1998; Sims and Prior 1980) as they have a high prevalence of risk factors for cardiovascular disease. It should also be noted that there are also other possible mechanisms for sudden death in psychiatric patients related to their medication. These include convulsions, choking due to food bolus obstruction, as a result of anticholinergic-induced dry mouth and hypotension because of drug-induced alpha receptor antagonism.

A disproportionate number of case reports of arrhythmia or sudden death involved thioridazine and doses of 100 mg daily or more caused QT interval abnormalities in over half of recipients (Buckley *et al.* 1995). A study in Finland of 49 cases of sudden death affecting patients taking psychiatric drugs found that 46 were exposed to a phenothiazine and in 28 cases this was thioridazine. This figure was out of proportion to the local use of the drug (Mehtonen *et al.* 1991).

Reports of 13 sudden deaths in recipients of pimozide prompted the United Kingdom Committee on Safety of Medicines (CSM) to issue specific recommendations on the use of this drug, including gradual dose escalation and recording an ECG before and periodically during treatment in those receiving high doses. Affected patients were often receiving high doses of pimozide or concurrent treatment with other neuroleptic drugs. In view of the long and variable plasma half-life of the drug, rapid dose escalation may have caused drug accumulation and toxicity.

More recently the atypical antipsychotic drug sertindole was linked with QT interval prolongation with 36 suspected fatal adverse drug reactions and 13 episodes of serious but non-fatal arrhythmia reported (CSM 1999). The drug was withdrawn by the manufacturers in 1998. However, restrictions in the European Union were lifted in June 2002 following the receipt of further epidemiological and *in vitro* data.

Despite the frequency of reported associations between antipsychotics and sudden cardiac death, until recently there were few, if any, compelling, controlled data supporting an association (Psychopharmacology Working Party, Royal College of Psychiatrists 1997). However, data are now emerging which better support the association between antipsychotics and cardiac mortality. This data comprises (1) ECG studies demonstrating differential effects between antipsychotic with regard to QTc prolongation and (2) recently systematically-collected epidemiological evidence has examined the risk of sudden deaths between different drugs.

ECG studies

Warner *et al.* (1996) performed ECGs in 111 patients receiving neuroleptic therapy, as well as 42 untreated controls. QTc prolongation (defined as >420 ms) was more common in the treated patients, and particularly in those taking high doses (more than 2000 mg chlorpromazine (CPZ) equivalents).

To investigate the possible differential cardiotoxic effects of antipsychotic drugs, ECGs were collected from 495 psychiatric patients in various inpatient and community settings in the north-east of England (Reilly *et al.* 2000). Details of their clinical histories and drug treatment were taken, together with a 12-lead ECG. Normal limits for ECG variables were defined from a reference group of healthy individuals. Logistic regression was used to investigate factors predictive of QTc prolongation. These were found to be age over 65 years, use of tricyclic antidepressants and use of either thioridazine or droperidol. For antipsychotic drugs as a whole, the risk of QT prolongation was significantly greater if high or very high doses were used, compared to low doses. This relationship persisted even if thioridazine and droperidol recipients were excluded from the analysis. This study showed a significant increase in risk for QTc prolongation if the dose prescribed was greater than 1000 mg CPZ equivalents providing independent retrospective support for the level at which the Royal College of Psychiatrists guidelines suggested should invoke caution and careful monitoring of therapy. For thioridazine, QT prolongation was more common in recipients of more than 600 mg daily. Significant relationships between QT interval prolongation and other individual antipsychotic drugs were not found, although there was a low level of exposure for some neuroleptics in this population.

Other non-phenothiazine antipsychotics may also cause cardiac abnormalities and QTc prolongation. Haloperidol exhibits no clear effect on QTc at low (around 5 mg/day) or at moderate (5–20 mg) daily doses but has been associated with cases of QTc prolongation and torsade de pointes at higher clinical doses (above 20 mg a day) and in overdose. High dose intravenous haloperidol seems particularly likely to prolong QTc. Lower intravenous doses (5–25 mg) have also been associated with QTcB prolongation to values exceeding 500 ms and intramuscular therapy has been shown to prolong QTcB by a mean of 15 ms. These prolongations may be underestimates since, as haloperidol increases heart rate, QTcF maybe a more appropriate correction. Sudden death has also been reported in patients taking haloperidol. These risks are higher in patients who are medically ill (Lawrence and

Nasraway 1997; O'Brien *et al.* 1999). Intravenous droperidol, a chemically similar butyrophenone, has also been shown to exhibit dose-dependent pro-longation of QTc ranging from 37 ms or 8 per cent over baseline (0.1 mg/kg) to 59 ms or 14.9 per cent over baseline (0.25 mg/kg) (Lischke *et al.* 1994). These observations support the findings with oral droperidol in patients (Reilly *et al.* 2000).

These data suggesting differential effects of antipsychotic drugs on the QT interval are supported by a randomized open parallel comparison of the effects of six antipsychotic drugs on the QT interval at steady state in 185 patients with stable psychotic disorders. Drugs were introduced after tapering of previous medication and a 5 day placebo run-in. The largest mean increases in QTc interval were seen with thioridazine 150 mg twice daily (35.6 ms), while changes with ziprasidone 80 mg twice daily (20.3 ms), queti-apine (14.5 ms), risperidone (11.6 ms) olanzapine (6.8 ms) and haloperidol 15 mg daily (4.7 ms) were less marked (Glassman and Bigger 2001).

Epidemiological studies of sudden deaths

Ray and colleagues (2001) investigated the rates of sudden cardiac death in Tennessee Medicaid enrolees aged 15–84 years without life-threatening non-cardiac illness between 1988 and 1993. The cohort comprized 481,744 per-sons, 1.3 million person years of follow-up (including 53,614 of current antipsychotic drug use) and a total of 1,487 sudden cardiac deaths. In the unexposed group there were 11.3 deaths per 10^4 person years of follow-up. This figure increased to 14.4 and 26.9 per 10^4 person years for current users of low and high doses of antipsychotics respectively. Multivariate-adjusted risk of death was increased 2.4 times in recipients of antipsychotic drugs. Risk was highest with thiothixene (RR 4.23, 95 per cent CI 2.00–8.91), chlorpromazine (3.64, 1.36–9.74), thioridazine (3.19, 1.32–7.68) and haloperidol (1.90, 1.10–3.30).

A case control epidemiological study was performed in the north-east of England to investigate the link between sudden death and drug therapy (Reilly *et al.* 2002). A retrospective notes review was conducted of all inpatient deaths occurring in 5 psychiatric hospitals over the 12 years between 1984 and 1995. Sudden deaths were defined as deaths occurring within 1 hour of the patient being observed in their usual state of health or found dead more than 1 hour after having been seen, but having been seen in their usual state of health within the last 24 hours. Patients with a proven a non-cardiac cause or acute myocardial infarction were excluded. Of 1202 deaths reviewed, 77 (6.4 per cent) met these criteria for sudden death. Most of these patients were elderly (median age 69 years) and most had been in hospital for more than a year (median duration of admission 633 days). Using conditional logistic regression, factors associated with sudden death included the presence of an organic psychiatric disorder, the presence of hypertension or previous myocardial infarction and treatment with thioridazine. No relationship between sudden death and thioridazine dose was observed in this comparatively small study.

Although this study is comparatively small and retrospective, it raised serious concerns about the safety of thioridazine, particularly when viewed in the presence of the other epidemiological evidence. Thioridazine is a potent blocker of the delayed rectifier potassium channel (Drolet *et al.* 1999) and has been shown to be more toxic than other antipsychotic drugs when taken in overdose (Buckley *et al.* 1995). These data have resulted in regulatory changes which have restricted indications for thioridazine in both the United Kingdom and USA. The manufacturers of droperidol have suspended marketing of this product.

The epidemiological studies described above were all conducted before the widespread introduction of atypical antipsychotic drugs, and provide no evidence about their relative safety. Summaries of the available open human volunteer and patient studies on atypical neuroleptics are given in Taylor's (2003) review. There appears to be only small effects at low doses but at higher doses there are modest effects on Qtc for the majority of atypicals. This effect is better established for clozapine. The risk of sudden death with these drugs is unknown but probably low, and a further case control study is currently underway in the UK which may provide more systematic information (Appleby *et al.* 2000).

Putting the risk in perspective

In order to estimate the risk of sudden death attributable to a drug using an odds ratio obtained from a case-control study, an estimate of the absolute risk of sudden death in an unmedicated population is needed. Three recent epidemiological studies have estimated the underlying crude risk of sudden death per 10,000 patient years in people without apparent cardiovascular disease as 5.5–11.3 (Ray *et al.* 2001). The Medicaid data (Ray *et al.* 2001) provide an estimate of the overall additional risk of sudden death attributable to high doses of antipsychotic drugs as 15.6 deaths per 10^4 patient years of treatment. A higher risk would be expected for more toxic drugs. However, attributable risks would be substantially higher in patients with increased underlying level of risk due to age or heart disease or other risk factors identified in these studies. These include increased body mass index, smoking, diabetes, parental history of sudden death and increases in heart rate, blood pressure or cholesterol (Jouven *et al.* 1999). Such patients were often prescribed thioridazine until recent changes were made to its licensing.

Differential diagnosis

TDP may manifest with dizziness, palpitations, and syncope. In patients prescribed antipsychotics, the sudden appearance of these symptoms should
prompt physical examination and an ECG. Examination will help exclude
other causes of these symptoms while an ECG may show the characteristic
trace of TDP. If symptoms are episodic it may be necessary to request a
24 hour ECG.

Clinicians sometimes encounter a sudden unexplained death in patients
prescribed an antipsychotic and are faced with the uncertainty of whether the
drug was a causal factor. It is usually impossible to make a dogmatic statement
in such cases. Arrhythmic deaths occur in unmedicated patients and the death
may be coinicidental. If the patient was on a high dose of an antipsychotic or
was prescribed other drugs that could increase the arrhythmic risk, this is
indirect evidence that the drug may have been a factor. Similarly death shortly
after an increase in antipsychotic dose is suggestive. Conversely the presence of
other risk factors, such as substance misuse or pre-existing heart disease,
increases the likelihood that the drug was not involved or at least was not the
sole factor in causing death. It needs to be stressed that in many cases death
will result from a combination of pro-arrhythmic factors of which the drug is
just one.

Management

If excessive QTc prolongation is identified on an ECG then the responsible
drug should be stopped and a cardiac opinion should be sought. If TDP is
identified on the ECG then an immediate cardiac opinion is necessary on
whether specific treatment needs to commence. Given the sudden and potentially life-threatening nature of ventricular arrhythmias, prevention is more
relevant to psychiatrists than the management of arrhythmias, which is the
expertize of physicians. All mental health professionals should receive regular
training in cardiopulmonary resuscitation.

Risk factors

A range of clinical and pharmacological risk factors can act to increase the risk
of drug-induced arrhythmia (see Table 4.1).

Clinical risk factors

Patients who have pre-existing abnormal ventricular repolarization are at
higher risk of drug-induced cardiac arrhythmias. Indicators of abnormal
repolarization include abnormalities of the T wave or large U waves, as well as

Table 4.1 Risk factors for TDP

Clinical risk factors
Pre-existing repolarisation abnormality
Previous episode of TDP
Left ventricular hypertrophy
Cardiac failure
Electrolyte imbalance
Female gender
Liver disease
Restraint?
Psychological distress?
Drug and alcohol misuse?

Pharmacological risk factors
Overdose
Prescribed high dose of antipsychotic
Slow metaboliser status
Pharmacokinetic interactions
Pharmacodynamic interactions
Diuretics

QT prolongation. Patients who have had previous episodes of torsade are at particular risk, even if this was provoked by a different drug. Patients with pre-existing cardiac disease such as left ventricular dysfunction or hypertrophy are also at increased risk. It is not clear if age is an independent risk factor but it may be so in the case of antipsychotics. Torsade de pointes is most likely to occur when the heart rate is slow and in the presence of extrasystoles. Thus conditions associated with these factors, such as heart block, increase the risk of torsade. The arrhythmia is more likely to occur in the presence of electrolyte abnormalities, e.g. hypokalaemia, hypocalcaemia or hypomagnasemia. Treatment with diuretics appears to increase risk, perhaps by producing such electrolyte abnormalities.

Patients with alcohol dependence may be at increased risk because this may be associated with liver disease which increases the risk of sudden death (Day *et al.* 1993). The impact of recreational substances on cardiac repolarization and sudden cardiac death is unclear. QT interval prolongation has been reported with ecstasy (Drake and Broadhurst 1996) and cocaine (Perera *et al.* 1997) and sympathomimetic agents may increase the risk of ventricular arrhythmias independent of any effects on repolarization. However, there are few published data in this area and further research is needed.

Several of the case reports of sudden death involve agitated patients undergoing restraint (Jusic and Lader 1994; Lareya 1995). Concerns have been raised that patients may be at increased risk of arrhythmia during such physiological activation as a result of increased sympathomimetic activity. To date, epidemiological studies suggest that, if this mechanism exists, it is uncommon (Reilly *et al.* 2002).

Women have a longer QT interval on average than men (Merri *et al.* 1989; Rautaharju 1992) and epidemiological studies have consistently shown that a disproportionate number of episodes of drug-induced torsade de pointes occur in women (Makkar *et al.* 1993). There is evidence that sex steroids have effects on the numbers and function of potassium channels in cardiac membranes (Drici *et al.* 1996).

A group combining several risk factors are patients with anorexia nervosa. These patients are at increased risk not only because they are usually female and often have electrolyte abnormalities but also because doses of antipsychotic drugs employed are often high relative to body weight.

Pharmacological risk factors

There is ample evidence that QT prolongation and resulting arrhythmias are concentration-related effects. Recent epidemiological studies in psychiatric patients have confirmed this association (Warner *et al.* 1996; Reilly *et al.* 2000; Ray *et al.* 2001). Any factor that increases drug concentration at the site of action will increase risk. Arrhythmia is more common in patients who have taken overdoses or who are prescribed high therapeutic doses of certain drugs (Thomas *et al.* 1994). The latter situation should be avoided unless there is ample clinical justification. Impaired hepatic and renal function may enhance plasma and tissue drug concentrations and substantial QT interval prolongation may occur with resulting risk of arrhythmia.

There are genetic polymorphisms for some hepatic p450 oxidative enzymes and for N-acetyl transferase, the enzymes responsible for the metabolism of drugs that cause QT prolongation and torsade de pointes. As a result, some patients who do not express individual isoforms may experience enhanced (parent drug causes QT prolongation) or attenuated (metabolite causes QT prolongation) ECG effects. There is, as yet, no direct clinical evidence that reduced expression of hepatic enzymes predisposes the individual to arrhythmia. However, this is an important area for further research since it offers the possibility of identifying patients at increased risk before drug exposure. Several antipsychotic and antidepressant drugs are hydroxylated via CYP2D6 (debrisoquine hydroxylase). Thioridazine is an important example. Slow hydroxylators of debrisoquine achieve higher plasma concentrations of the parent drug and its ring sulphoxide metabolite than rapid hydroxylators (von Bahr *et al.* 1991) and thioridazine-induced QT prolongation has been linked to plasma concentration (Hartigan Go *et al.* 1996).

There is an increased risk of provoking arrhythmia in some subjects if the metabolism of the drug is highly variable between individuals. Individuals with comparatively slow metabolism or excretion are at risk of unusually high plasma and tissue drug concentrations and marked QT prolongation in spite of the use of modest drug doses. If the elimination half-life is long there is a risk of accumulation in susceptible groups, particularly the elderly.

Pharmacokinetic drug interactions resulting in increased plasma or tissue concentrations of a QT interval-prolonging drug are a particularly important source of torsade. The most common interaction is via inhibition of the hepatic cytochrome p450 isoform CYP3A4. This isoform is important because it is very abundant in human liver and is primarily responsible for the metabolism of many QT-prolonging drugs.

The most important pharmacodynamic interaction is from the combined use of two drugs that prolong ventricular repolarization, since these may have an additive affect on QT interval. It is important to note that some hepatic enzyme inhibitors (e.g. erythromycin, ketoconazole) also delay cardiac repolarization and this effect increases the severity of the interaction.

In the context of antipsychotic drug therapy, there is increasing evidence of significant interaction with selective serotonin reuptake inhibitors and tricyclic antidepressants. Interaction with the latter is of particular importance since these drugs also produce QT prolongation independently. There is also emerging evidence of a link between dothiepin use and ischaemic heart disease (Hippisley-Cox *et al.* 2001) which, if confirmed, would further augment the risk of sudden death.

A non-sedating antihistamine, astemizole, and the prokinetic drug cisapride have also been withdrawn due to their association with QT prolongation, and ventricular arrhythmias and interactions with CYP3A4 inhibitors were implicated with both these drugs. A similar interaction precipitating torsade de pointes has been described between pimozide and clarithromycin (Flockhart *et al.* 2000). A more detailed account of important interactions between psychotropics with potential for alterations of the QTc can be found in Taylor's review (2003).

Prevention

Although the risk of sudden death with antipsychotic drugs is small, it is important that all reasonable steps are taken to minimize the risk of this devastating adverse drug reaction. Preventative measures stem from a knowledge of the differential arrhythmic risk of antipsychotic drugs and risk factors for arrhythmia – both topics have already been covered in depth.

In the first instance, it is important that attention is paid to the general health of patients with psychosis, since reduction in the prevalence of heart disease will reduce the intrinsic risk of sudden death, as well as the risk of drug-induced arrhythmia. Modifiable risk factors for ischaemic heart disease should be identified and managed appropriately, including smoking, hypertension, hyperlipidaemia, sedentary lifestyle and obesity. It is important to recognize that obesity, hyperlipidaemia and glucose intolerance may be exacerbated by antipsychotic drug therapy (Koro *et al.* 2002) and in some cases this may be a more important risk for the patient than that of prolonged QTc. It is, however, prudent to ensure that the neuroleptics drugs given to such patients should not further increase the risk of adverse cardiovascular events.

The choice of antipsychotic therapy is important in determining risk. The use of drugs with more pronounced effects on cardiac repolarization can only be justified if the drug has specific advantages for the patient in comparison to antipsychotic drugs with less marked electrophysiological risks. High doses and drug combinations should only be used when there is a clinical justification, particularly if the combination may result in inhibition of clearance or additive ECG effects.

To further reduce the risk of arrhythmia, all patients should be assessed for cardiovascular disease prior to the institution of antipsychotic drug therapy. This should, whenever possible, include an ECG, which should be examined for evidence of ischaemic heart disease, left ventricular hypertrophy and repolarization abnormalities. The presence of such factors may affect the choice of antipsychotic drug chosen or increase the frequency of monitoring required, as well as prompt a more detailed cardiac assessment. An ECG prior to antipsychotic therapy is particularly important if higher risk antipsychotic drug treatment is contemplated (e.g. thioridazine, sertindole, and pimozide), if high dose or parenteral antipsychotic drug therapy is to be used or in people with a history of cardiovascular disease. It is also prudent to check the blood biochemistry, particularly plasma potassium, before embarking on such therapy, especially in patients at higher risk of electrolyte abnormalities, due, for example, to anorexia nervosa, diuretic use, or dehydration.

As discussed above there is little direct evidence that there is a disproportionate increase in sudden death in situations of acute disturbed behaviour or restraint. Nonetheless there are numerous case reports of such events and it is conceivable that increased arousal and possibly noradrenaline levels may be involved in sensitizing the myocardium to arrhythmias. Under the circumstances of rapid tranquillization (RT) where assessment of cardiovascular disease and status is difficult and ECGs impossible it is prudent to avoid high doses of antipsychotics, particularly parentally. There is evidence for the usefulness of droperidol in rapid tranquillization but it is no longer available in the UK. There is evidence that haloperidol may increase the risk for QTc prolongation (see above). Under these circumstances emphasis should be put on the first line use of short acting benzodiazepines (McAllister-Williams and Ferrier 2002).

Periodic monitoring of the ECG and electrolytes during therapy is advocated when high risk antipsychotic drug therapy is to be used. The most recent Maudsley guidelines (Taylor *et al.* 2003) recommend ECG monitoring following the administration of parenteral antipsychotic therapy, especially when higher doses are used. The summaries of product characteristics of several higher risk drugs recommend periodic ECG monitoring during therapy, which should also be considered in patients at increased risk because of underlying heart disease. However, if ECGs are to be done, it is not clear how often this should occur and whether this would have any impact on cardiac mortality. A case can be made for these to be performed every few days following initiation of therapy or dose escalation until steady state concentrations are thought to have been reached. Thereafter ECG and electrolyte assessment could be recommended every few months, at times of acute illness, when potentially interacting drugs are introduced or if the patient experiences symptoms that could be due to arrhythmia, e.g. syncope or fits. Although such monitoring may help prevent some episodes of drug-induced torsade, the numbers prevented will be very small in comparison to the huge numbers of ECG and blood tests required and the cost-effectiveness of this approach is very uncertain. Further research is needed before such an approach is widely adopted.

A major source of drug-induced arrhythmia is from drug interactions and strategies are needed to minimize the risk of this. One suggestion has been that the patient carry a warning card that lists the risk factors, precautions and contraindications for co-prescriptions (Yap and Camm 2000). Certainly, those involved in prescribing drugs to people receiving these agents need to be aware of the potential for drug interactions and those agents most commonly implicated.

Summary

Definition	A polymorphic ventricular arrhythmia characterized by QRS complexes twisting round the isoelectric line.
Incidence	Unknown with psychotropics. 1 in 100,000 prescriptions with cisapride (ADR data). Up to 8% of post-MI patients treated with class III antiarrhythmics (various clinical trials).
Key drugs causing syndrome	Thiordiazine and other phenothiazines

	Other antipsychotics e.g. pimozide
	Tricyclic antidepressants
Key symptoms	Syncope, palpitations, sudden death (may be asymptomatic).
Pharmacological mechanism	Blockade of cardiac I_{kr} channels.
Investigations to confirm diagnosis	ECG
Management	Consult cardiologist, stop causal agent, correct any electrolyte imbalance, magnesium infusion.
Further reading	Reilly JG, Ayis SA, Ferrier IN, *et al.* (2000) QT interval abnormalities and psychotropic drug therapy in psychiatric patients. *Lancet*, **355**, 1048–52.
	Taylor DM (2003) Antipsychotics and QT prolongation. *Acta Psychiatrica Scandinavica*, **107**, 85–95.
	Yap YG and Camm J (2000) Risk of torsades with non-cardiac drugs. *British Medical Journal*, **320**, 1158–9.

References

Algra A, Tijsien J, Roelandt J, *et al.* (1991). QTc prolongation measured by standard 12-lead electrocardiography is an independent risk factor for sudden death due to cardiac arrest. *Circulation*, **83**, 1888–94.

Appleby L, Thomas S, Ferrier IN, *et al.* (2000). Sudden unexplained death in psychiatric in-patients. *Br J Psychiatry*, **176**, 405–6.

Ban TA and St-Jean A (1965). Electrocardiographic changes induced by phenothiazine drugs. *Am Heart J*, **70**, 575–6.

Baxter DN (1996). The mortality experience of individuals in the Salford psychiatric case register. I. All cause mortality. *Br J Psychiatry*, **168**, 772–9.

Buckley NA, Whyte IM, and Dawson AH (1995). Cardiotoxicity more common in thioridazine overdose than other neuroleptics. *Clin Toxicol*, **33**, 199–204.

Committee for Proprietary Medicinal Products of the European Agency for Evaluation of Medicinal Products (1997). Points to consider: the assessment of the potential for QT interval prolongation by non-cardiovascular medicinal products (12.17.1997). Committee for Proprietary Medicinal Products of EAEMP: London. www.emea.eu.int/pdfs/ human/swp/098696cn.pdf.

Committee on Safety of Medicines (1999). Suspension of the availability of sertindole. *Curr Prob Pharmacovigilance*, **25**, 1.

Day CP, James OFW, Butler TJ, *et al.* (1993). QT prolongation and sudden death in patients with alcoholic liver disease. *Lancet*, **341**, 1423–8.

Desautels S, Filteau C, and St Jean A (1964). Ventricular tachycardia associated with administration of thioridazine hydrochloride (Mellaril). *Can Med Assoc J*, **90**, 1030–1.

Drake WM and Broadhurst PA (1996). QT-interval prolongation with ecstasy. *SAMJ*, **86**, 180–1.

Drici MD, Burklow TR, Haridasse V, *et al.* (1996). Sex hormones prolong the QT interval and downregulate potassium channel expression in the rabbit heart. *Circulation*, **94**, 1471–4.

Drolet B, Vincent F, Rail J, *et al.* (1999). Thioridazine lengthens repolarization of cardiac ventricular myocytes by blocking the delayed rectifier potassium current. *J Pharmacol Exp Therap*, **288**, 1261–8.

Flockhart DA, Drici MD, Kerbusch T, *et al.* (2000). Studies on the mechanism of a fatal clarithromycin-pimozide interaction in a patient with Tourette syndrome. *J Clin Psychopharmacol*, **20**, 317–24.

Glassman AH and Bigger JT (2001). Antipsychotic drugs: prolonged QTc interval torsade de pointes, and sudden death. *Am J Psychiatry*, **158**, 1774–82.

Goldberg RJ, Bengtson J, Chen Z, *et al.* (1991). Duration of the QT interval and total cardiovascular mortality in healthy persons (The Framingham Study Experience). *Am J Cardiol*, **67**, 55–8.

Hartigan-Go K, Bateman DN, Nyberg G, *et al.* (1996). Concentration-related pharmacodynamic effects of thioridazine and its metabolites in humans. *Clin Pharmacol Ther*, **60**, 543–53.

Hensen V, Arnesen E, and Jacobsen BK (1997). Total mortality in people admitted to a psychiatric hospital. *Br J Psychiatry*, **170**, 186–90.

Hii JTY, Wyse DG, Gillis AM, *et al.* (1992). Precordial QT interval dispersion as a marker of torsade de pointes. Disparate effects of class 1a antiarrhythmic drugs and amiodarone. *Circulation*, **86**, 1376–82.

Hippisley-Cox J, Pringle M, Hammersley V, *et al.* (2001). Antidepressants as a risk factor for ischaemic heart disease: case-control study in primary care. *BMJ*, **323**, 666–9.

Hollander PB and Cain RM (1971). Effects of thioridazine on transmembrane potential and contractile characteristics of guinea pig hearts. *Eur J Pharmacol*, **16**, 129–35.

Jouven X, Desnoos NM, Guerot C, *et al.* (1999). Predicting sudden death in the population: the Paris prospective Study. I. *Circulation*, **99**, 1978–83.

Jusic N and Lader M (1994). Post-mortem antipsychotic drug concentrations and unexplained deaths. *Br J Psychiatry*, **165**, 787–91.

Kelly HQ, Fay JE, Laverty FG (1963). Thioridazine hydrochloride (Mellaril): its effect on the electrocardiogram and a report on two fatalities with electrographic abnormalities. *Can Med Assoc J*, **89**, 546–54.

Koro CE, Fedder DO, L'Italien GJ, *et al.* (2002). Assessment of independent effect of olanzapine and risperidone on risk of diabetes among patients with schizophrenia: population-based nested case-control study. *BMJ*, **325**, 243–5.

Lareya J (1995). Sudden death, neuroleptics and psychotic agitation. *Prog Neuropsychopharmacol Biol Psychiatry*, **19**, 229–41.

Lawrence KR and Nasraway SA (1997). Conduction disturbances associated with administration of butyrophenone anti-psychotics in the critically ill: a review of the literature. *Pharmacotherapy*, **17**, 531–7.

Lischke V, Behne M, Doelken P, *et al.* (1994). Droperidol causes a dose-dependent prolongation of the QT interval. *Anesth Analg*, **79**, 983–6.

McAllister-Williams RH, and Ferrier IN (2002). Rapid tranquillisation: time for a reappraisal of options for parenteral therapy. *Br J Psychiatry*, **180**, 485–9.

Makkar RR, Fromm BS, Steinman RT, *et al.* (1993). Female gender as a risk factor for torsade de pointes associated with cardiovascular drugs. *J Am Med Assoc*, **270**, 2590–7.

Mehtonen OP, Aranko K, Malkonen L, *et al.* (1991). Survey of sudden death associated with the use of antipsychotic or antidepressant drugs: 49 cases in Finland. *Acta Psychiatr Scand*, **84**, 58–64.

Merri M, Benhorin J, Alberti M, *et al.* (1989). Electrocardiographic quantitation of ventricular repolarization. *Circulation*, **80**, 1301–8.

Moss AJ, Schwartz PJ, Crampton RS, *et al.* (1991). The long QT syndrome. Prospective longitudinal study of 328 families. *Circulation*, **84**, 1136–44.

Moss AJ (1993). Measurement of the QT interval and the risk associated with QTc interval prolongation: a review. *Am J Cardiol*, **72**, 23–5.

O'Brien JM, Rockwood RP, and Suh KI (1999). Haloperidol-induced torsade de pointes. *Ann Pharmacother*, **33**, 1046–50.

Perera R, Kraebber A, and Schwartz M (1997). Prolonged QT interval and cocaine use. *J Electrocardiol*, **30**, 337–9.

Rautaharju P, Zhou SH, Wong S, *et al.* (1992). Sex differences in the evolution of the electrocardiographic QT interval with age. *Can J Cardiol*, **8**, 690–5.

Ray WA, Meredith S, Thapa PB, *et al.* (2001). Antipsychotics and the risk of sudden cardiac death. *Arch Gen Psychiatry*, **58**, 1161–7.

Reilly JG, Ayis SA, Ferrier IN, *et al.* (2000). QT interval abnormalities and psychotropic drug therapy in psychiatric patients. *Lancet*, **355**, 1048–52.

Reilly JG, Ayis SA, Ferrier IN, *et al.* (2002). Thioridazine and sudden unexplained death in psychiatric inpatients. *Br J Psychiatry*, **180**, 515–22.

Reinert RE and Hermann CG (1960). Unexplained deaths during chlorpromazine therapy. *J Nerv Ment Dis*, **131**, 435–42.

Ruschena D, Mullen PE, Burgess P, *et al.* (1998). Sudden death in psychiatric patients. *Br J Psychiatry*, **172**, 331–6.

Schoeten EG, Dekker JM, Meppelink P, *et al.* (1991). QT interval prolongation predicts cardiovascular mortality in an apparently healthy population. *Circulation*, **84**, 1516–23.

Sims ACP and Prior MP (1980). Arteriosclerosis-related deaths in severe neurosis. *Compr Psychiatry*, **23**, 181–5.

Stratmann HG and Kennedy HL (1987). Torsades de pointes associated with drugs and toxins: recognition and management. *Am Heart J*, **113**, 1470–82.

Taylor D, Paton C, and Kerwin R *The Maudsley 2003 Prescribing Guidelines*. Martin Dunitz Ltd: London.

Taylor DM (2003). Antipsychotics and QT prolongation. *Acta Psychiatr Scand*, **107**, 85–95.

Thomas SHL (1994). Drugs, QT interval abnormalities and ventricular arrhythmias. *Adverse Drug React T*, **13**, 77–102.

von Bahr C, Movin G, Nordin C, *et al.* (1991). Plasma levels of thioridazine and metabolites are influenced by the debrisoquin hydroxylation phenotype. *Clin Pharmacol Ther*, **49**, 234–40.

Waddington JL, Youssef HA, and Kinsella A (1998). Mortality in schizophrenia. *Br J Psychiatry*, **173**, 325–9.

Warner JP, Barnes TRE, and Henry JA (1996). Electrocardiographic changes in patients receiving neuroleptic medication. *Acta Psychiatr Scand*, **93**, 311–13.

Working Group of the Royal College of Psychiatrists' Psychopharmacology Sub-Group (1997). *The Association between Antipsychotic Drugs and Sudden Death* (Council Report CR 57). Royal College of Psychiatrists: London.

Yap YG and Camm J (2000). Risk of torsades with non-cardiac drugs. *BMJ*, **320**, 1158–9.

Chapter 5

Hyperprolactinaemia

Angelika Wieck and Peter M Haddad

The ability of antipsychotic drugs to elevate serum prolactin with resulting symptoms has been recognized since the 1970s (Beumont *et al.* 1974). However until recently the area received little attention. The introduction of the atypical antipsychotics, some of which are prolactin sparing, has acted as an impetus to research in this area. Recent cross-sectional studies indicate that the majority of women and more than one-third of men treated with prolactin-raising antipsychotics have hyperprolactinaemia (Smith *et al.* 2002*a*; Kinon and Gilmore 2001). Other psychotropic drugs, including tricyclic antidepressants, monoamine oxidase inhibitors, selective serotonin reuptake inhibitors and lithium can also stimulate prolactin secretion but this is much less common and severe (Checkley 1991). For clarity most of this chapter will refer to antipsychotics, but the clinical features of drug-induced hyperprolactinaemia and its differential diagnoses are the same irrespective of the drug that is responsible.

Hyperprolactinaemia can be symptomatic or asymptomatic, although this distinction is not often made in clinical trials. Some symptoms result from a direct effect of prolactin on target tissues (e.g. galactorrhoea) and others from disruption of the normal function of the hypothalamic–pituitary axis (e.g. menstrual cycle irregularities). Some symptoms (e.g. sexual dysfunction) can result from either a direct effect of raised prolactin and/or gonadal dysfunction. These symptoms can cause significant distress to patients and may lead to poor adherence with medication that can lead to exacerbations or recurrences of the underlying psychiatric illness. There is increasing evidence that chronic hyperprolactinaemia may also lead to initially 'silent' health problems. The evidence is strongest for bone loss but there may also be a small increase in the risk of female breast cancer.

Prolactin physiology

Serum levels and physiological functions

Prolactin is a polypeptide hormone that is secreted by the lactotroph cells of the anterior pituitary gland. It is released in a pulsatile manner with an interval of about 95 minutes between peak amplitudes. During sleep amplitudes increase and are highest in the second half of sleep. Levels fall gradually after awakening and reach a nadir at about noon that is approximately 40 per cent of the 24 hour mean (Veldhuis and Johnson 1988). The best estimation of average prolactin levels can therefore be obtained by taking blood samples about 2 to 4 hours after waking. During the daytime up to threefold transient increases of prolactin levels can be seen in response to stress, food intake, breast stimulation and sexual activity (Molitch 1995). If a prolactin assay reveals mild elevation, we recommend conducting a second estimation to clarify whether these factors are responsible. The effect of venepuncture on prolactin levels is small and can only be avoided by obtaining cannulated blood samples. In our opinion this is not necessary for clinical purposes but needs to be considered for research studies.

Prolactin hormone levels are usually measured by using standards that have been calibrated against international reference preparations. Units of measurement are mU/L, nmol/l or ng/ml whereby 1 ng/ml is approximately equivalent to 30 mU/L or 43 nmol/l. The upper limit of normal is usually around 500 mU/L or 15–25 ng/ml.

The main physiological function of prolactin is to cause breast enlargement during pregnancy and milk production during lactation. The reduction in libido and fertility that are associated with nursing may have evolutionary advantages. Prolactin is known to have an important function in promoting maternal behaviour in animals, but whether it has such a role in humans is not known.

Neuro-endocrine control

Dopamine is the predominant prolactin inhibiting factor in humans. It is produced by the tuberoinfundibular neurons in the hypothalamus and transported in the hypophyseal circulation to the anterior pituitary gland. By binding to the dopamine-2 (D_2) receptors on the membrane of lactotroph cells it inhibits prolactin gene transcription, synthesis and release in a complex fashion, involving several signal transduction systems (Gudelsky 1981). In this system dopamine is acting as a hormone and not as a neurotransmitter.

Serotonin (5-HT) is a stimulatory neurotransmitter in the regulation of prolactin secretion and mediates nocturnal surges and suckling-induced rises (Tuomisto and Mannisto 1985). The serotonergic neurons involved originate from the dorsal raphe nucleus and exert their effects via 5-HT1a and 5-HT2 receptor mechanisms in the medial basal hypothalamus, probably by stimulating releasing factors.

Gonadotrophin-associated protein, acetylcholine and gamma-aminobutyric acid (GABA) have been identified as prolactin inhibiting factors but their relevance in humans is uncertain. Substances that are known to increase prolactin secretion are thyrotropin releasing hormone and oestrogen, the latter being responsible for the higher levels in women at mid-cycle, the second half of the menstrual cycle and during pregnancy.

Prevalence of hyperprolactinaemia

Drug-free patients with depression and schizophrenia have normal prolactin levels and so hyperprolactinaemia cannot be a consequence of psychiatric illness (Meltzer *et al.* 1974; Linkwork *et al.* 1989). Longitudinal studies of patients either starting or switching antipsychotic drugs clearly show that hyperprolactinaemia is a consequence of antipsychotic treatment (e.g. Kim *et al.* 2002).

The prevalence of hyperprolactinaemia has recently been investigated in two large cross-sectional studies. Kinon and Gilmore (2001) assessed 402 patients treated with conventional antipsychotics or risperidone for at least 3 months. The prevalence of hyperprolactinaemia in men (>18.77 ng/ml) was 42.4 per cent and in women (>24.20 ng/ml) was 59.2 per cent. Smith *et al.* (2002*a*) assessed 101 patients prescribed conventional antipsychotics. The prevalence of hyperprolactinaemia (>480 IU/l) in men was 34 per cent and in women it was 75 per cent. The proportion of hyperprolactinaemic patients in each study who had symptoms as a result of their prolactin elevation is unclear. However in the Smith *et al.* (2002*b*) study hyperprolactinaemia was related to sexual dysfunction in both sexes, indicating that it was clinically significant.

The degree of prolactin elevation associated with antipsychotic drugs depends on various factors including the patient's gender, the drug being considered and its dose. Women are more susceptible than men when treated with comparable doses of antipsychotics (Kuruvilla *et al.* 1992). Higher drug doses are more likely to cause hyperprolactinaemia (Meltzer *et al.* 1983) but significant elevation can still occur with relatively low doses e.g. 200 mg chlorpromazine (Meltzer and Fang 1976).

Among the atypical antipsychotics risperidone (Peuskens 1995) and amisulpride (Grunder *et al.* 1995) cause a marked and sustained increase in serum prolactin levels in a sizeable proportion of patients. In contrast clozapine (Meltzer *et al.* 1979) and quetiapine (Small *et al.* 1997) do not elevate plasma prolactin levels across their full dose range. Aripiprazole causes a fall in prolactin levels consistent with it being a D_2 partial agonist (Goodnick and Jerry 2002). Olanzapine is generally regarded as prolactin sparing, although at higher doses hyperprolactinaemia can occur (Crawford *et al.* 1997). Although the division of atypicals into 'prolactin sparing' and 'prolactin raising' is useful, such a categorical division is a simplification. In reality the likelihood of each atypical causing prolactin elevation in any individual patient varies on a dimension. This is analogous to the likelihood of these drugs causing other side-effects such as extrapyramidal symptoms or weight gain.

Although a partial tolerance may develop, prolactin levels are usually still significantly elevated after several years of chronic treatment (Rivera *et al.* 1976; Zelaschi *et al.* 1996). When oral antipsychotics are discontinued baseline prolactin levels may take up to 3 weeks to return to the normal range depending on the half life of the drug and its metabolites as well as storage in fatty tissues. In the case of oil-based depots it may take as long as six months after stoppage of the depot for serum prolactin levels to normalize (Wistedt *et al.* 1981).

Clinical features

Hyperprolactinaemia can cause a wide range of symptoms (Table 5.1) and there is great individual variation as to the threshold at which they arise. Symptoms often appear within a few weeks of commencing an antipsychotic or increasing its dose but can also commence after long-term treatment with a stable dose.

Gynaecomastia

Gynaecomastia is a relatively uncommon manifestation of raised prolactin. It can occur in either sex and be unilateral or bilateral. Women may also develop breast tenderness and engorgement in association with galactorrhoea.

Table 5.1 Clinical manifestations of hyperprolactinaemia

- Galactorrhoea
- Gynecomastia
- Infertility
- Menstrual irregularities
  - oligomenorrhoea
  - amenorrhoea
- Sexual dysfunction
  - decreased libido
  - impaired arousal
  - impaired orgasm
- Decreased bone mineral density
- Increased risk breast cancer in women
- Acne and hirsutism in women

Galactorrhoea

Most women who have given birth can express small amounts of serous fluid from one or both breasts despite normal prolactin levels. Significant milk production is usually associated with prolactin levels that are above the normal reference range. Estimates of the prevalence of galactorrhoea in women treated with conventional antipsychotics vary widely from 10 per cent to over 50 per cent (Windgassen *et al.* 1996). A well-conducted prospective study of 150 female inpatients of premenopausal age found that 21 (14 per cent) developed galactorrhoea within 75 days of commencing typical antipsychotic treatment (Windgassen *et al.* 1996). Another 7 of the 150 women developed galactorrhoea during antipsychotic treatment in the month before entering the study resulting in a prevalence rate of 19 per cent (28/150). Twenty-four of the 28 women with galactorrhoea had a serum prolactin estimation. The median value was 37.5 ng/ml (range 10.0–246.0 ng/ml) and 20 of the 24 women had values above the upper limit of the reference range (16 ng/ml). Drug-induced galactorrhoea is rare in men (Kaneda *et al.* 2000).

Sexual dysfunction

There is indirect evidence that prolactin is involved in the regulation of sexual behaviour. First, men and women with hyperprolactinaemia unrelated to medication have been reported to have dysfunction in all phases of sexual activity, although it is not clear whether this is related to prolactin, hypogonadism or both (Lundberg and Hulter 1991). Second, prolactin receptors are distributed within CNS structures which are involved in the regulation of sexual behaviour and have also been identified in female and male reproductive organs (Krueger *et al.* 2002). Third, orgasm triggers a transient surge of prolactin secretion in men and women and this has been suggested to contribute to central or peripheral mechanisms of sexual refractoriness (Krueger *et al.* 2002).

Given this background it is not surprising that drug-induced hyperprolactinaemia can cause sexual dysfunction. However hyperprolactinaemia is only one of several mechanisms by which psychotropic drugs can influence sexual behaviour, with other central and peripheral drug effects also being relevant (see Chapter 7).

In a well-designed study Smith *et al.* (2002*a*) assessed 101 patients prescribed conventional antipsychotics. In the 67 men there was no correlation between prolactin levels and any measure of sexual response. However, when analysis was confined to the 34 per cent of men with hyperprolactinaemia, prolactin levels were negatively correlated with erectile dysfunction ($r = -0.562$,

$P = 0.023$) and quality of orgasm ($r = -0.56$, $P = 0.023$) and overrode the effects of age, depression and autonomic side effects. Thus prolactin appeared to be the main cause of sexual dysfunction in hyperprolactinaemic men. In the women prolactin correlated with physical arousal problems such as poor vaginal response ($r = 0.52$, $P = 0.02$), an association that was strengthened after controlling for the effect of dose of medication and depression.

A few cross-sectional studies have compared the effects of prolactin-raising with prolactin-sparing atypical antipsychotics on sexual function. The results have either shown no difference (Hummer *et al.* 1999) or have been in favour of the prolactin sparing agents (Aizenberg *et al.* 2001; Wirshing *et al.* 1992). Several case reports (Haddad *et al.* 2001; Dickson and Glazer 1999) and a small study (Kim *et al.* 2002) have noted improvements in sexual functioning when patients with antipsychotic induced hyperprolactinaemia are switched to prolactin-sparing agents and their prolactin level normalizes.

Menstrual abnormalities

Oligomenorrhoea and amenorrhoea are common symptoms of hyperprolactinaemia in female pre-menopausal patients. In cross-sectional studies of women with severe psychiatric illnesses, on chronic treatment with various conventional antipsychotics, the point prevalence of menstrual abnormalities varies between 26 per cent (Polishuk and Kulcsar 1956) and 78 per cent (Smith *et al.* 2002*b*). However, these figures need to be interpreted with caution due to the studies having small samples and in some cases the researchers not providing a clear definition of what constitutes oligomenorrhoea or amenorrhoea.

Recent studies suggest that some schizophrenic women may have an illness-related dysfunction in the hypothalamic–pituitary axis which predisposes them to menstrual irregularities (Wieck and Haddad 2003). Nevertheless prospective studies leave no doubt that antipsychotics frequently cause menstrual irregularities in female patients (Nonacs 2000) and that these resolve on switching to prolactin-sparing antipsychotics (Kim *et al.* 2002).

Other symptoms

Acne and hirsutism can occur in women and reflect relative androgen excess compared to low oestrogen levels. Several studies have reported an association of hyperprolactinaemia with hostility, anxiety and depression although the severity of these symptoms appears to be mild (Sobrinho 1993; Reavley *et al.* 1997). Binding sites for prolactin are widely distributed in the body and several hundred different actions have been described in animals (Bole-Feysot *et al.* 1998). Consequently it is possible that hyperprolactinaemia may have physical consequences that are not yet recognized.

Initially silent consequences

Reduced bone mineral density

In women it is well established that oestrogens have an important role in maintaining bone tissue and that hypo-oestrogenic states unrelated to drug treatment can lead to bone loss. The most obvious example is the acceleration in age-related bone loss that follows the menopause and the observation that this can be halted by oestogen replacement therapy (Kiel *et al.* 1987). The role of testosterone in maintaining skeletal integrity in men has attracted less research. Nevertheless there is evidence that testosterone deficiency can cause decreased bone mineral density (BMD). Men with congenital hypogonadism have significant bone loss and an increased risk of fractures (Finkelstein *et al.* 1983). Furthermore, both men (Greenspan *et al.* 1986) and women (Koppelman *et al.* 1984) with prolactin-secreting tumours and secondary hypogonadism show significant loss of both vertebral and radial bone density which correlates with the duration of the disease. Prospective follow-up studies of both men (Greenspan *et al.* 1989) and women (Schlechte *et al.* 1987; Klibanski and Greenspan 1986) with prolactinomas have shown that reversal of hypogonadism, independent of the prolactin concentration, is associated with an improvement in bone mass.

Given this background it is reasonable to postulate that antipsychotic-induced hyperproactinaemia, sufficient to cause hypogonadism, could cause reduced BMD. However, as yet only a few published studies have investigated this possibility and most have methodological shortcomings including small sample sizes, selecting patients with various diagnoses, therapy with drug combinations and failing to control for confounding variables such as alcohol intake, smoking, diet and exercise levels.

Halbreich *et al.* (1995) studied 68 men and women treated with various psychotropics including antipsychotics. In the 33 female patients BMD values were significantly lower in the lumbar spine ($P = 0.001$), but not in the femoral neck. The role of ovarian function in this result was difficult to interpret because some subjects were of postmenopausal age. There was no relationship between bone density and prolactin levels. In 10 pre-menopausal women with long-standing antipsychotic-induced hyperprolactinaemia and hypo-oestrogenism Ataya *et al.* (1988) found a reduction of BMD by about 12 per cent at three sites of the proximal femur. Femoral BMD was positively correlated with a vaginal maturation index, a measure of biological oestradiol activity, but not prolactin levels. In nine women with a shorter history of antipsychotic-induced hypo-oestrogenism (mean of 30 months) Akande *et al.* (2002) reported that BMD in the radial trabecular bone was reduced by 0.8 standard deviations compared to age and sex matched controls ($P > 0.002$) though BMD was not significantly different at other sites. There was no significant relationship of any bone measurement with age, body mass index, exercise levels, and alcohol and nicotine intake. Trabecular bone is particularly sensitive to oestrogen deficiency.

In the 35 men studied by Halbreich *et al.* (1995) significant reductions in BMD were found in the lumbar spine and the femoral neck. Indeed, age-related bone losses were greater in the men than in the women at all skeletal sites. In men there was a significant correlation between BMD and both free and total testosterone in the lumbar region ($P = 0.009$) and between BMD and free testosterone at the femoral neck ($P = 0.012$). BMD was also negatively correlated with prolactin levels in the lumbar spine ($P = 0.031$). In a small study of 16 male and female schizophrenic patients Abraham *et al.* (2002) found a significant negative correlation between prolactin levels in three sites of the proximal femur but not in the spine.

Despite their methodological shortcomings, these studies taken together, and in light of existing knowledge about endocrine involvement in skeletal integrity, strongly suggests that antipsychotic-induced hyperprolactinaemia is associated with reduced BMD. Furthermore the most likely mechanism is via reduced oestrogen levels in women and reduced testosterone levels in men. Other mechanisms may also be relevant, for example raised prolactin may have a direct effect on BMD in both sexes.

Breast cancer

In animals increased prolactin levels can cause malignant transformation of breast tissue (Welsch and Nagaasawa 1977) and promote tumour growth in induced mammary malignancies (Pearson *et al.* 1969). Several studies have assessed the rate of breast cancer in female psychiatric patients receiving treatment with antipsychotic drugs but have produced conflicting results (e.g. Kanhouwa *et al.* 1984; Gulbinat *et al.* 1992; Halbreich *et al.* 1996). However the most recent study, and probably the strongest methodologically, found that antipsychotic dopamine antagonists conferred a small but significant risk or breast cancer (Wang *et al.* 2002). This study had a retrospective cohort design and compared women exposed to prolactin-raising antipsychotics with age-matched women who were not. There were over 50 000 women in each group and the total follow-up period was more than 200 000 person years. Use of antipsychotics was associated with a 16 per cent increase in breast cancer with a dose-response relationship between larger cumulative dosages and greater risk. The increased risk was also seen in women who used dopamine antagonists as anti-emetics. Interestingly, the risk was only increased in women over 40 years of age, indicating that perhaps in younger women the antipsychotic-induced oestrogen-deficiency may have counteracted the effect of prolactin. However, the magnitude of the increased risk is small and the authors emphasize that the study requires replication.

Pharmacological basis

All antipsychotic drugs have the capacity to block D_2 receptors and in the mesolimbic and mesocortical areas this appears integral to antipsychotic efficacy. Blockade of D_2 receptors on lactotroph cells causes hyperprolactinaemia as it removes the main inhibitory influence on prolactin secretion. Positron emission tomographic (PET) studies cannot directly measure occupancy of pituitary D_2 receptors and consequently striatal D_2 receptor occupancy is usually used as a substitute. In patients treated with conventional antipsychotics, approximately 50 per cent striatal D_2 receptor occupancy is associated with hyperprolactinaemia (Nordstrom and Farde 1998; Baron *et al.* 1989). This is similar to the degree of occupancy associated with clinical efficacy and this explains the high rate of hyperprolactinaemia seen in naturalistic studies of patients treated with conventional antipsychotics (e.g. Smith *et al.* 2002*a*).

Several mechanisms may explain the differential effect of antipsychotics on serum prolactin including affinity for D_2 receptors, their dissociation coefficient from the D_2 receptor and their ability to penetrate the blood–brain barrier. Data from PET studies shows that atypical drugs associated with raised prolactin (e.g. risperidone) are associated with higher D_2 binding occupancies in the striatum than those that are prolactin-sparing (e.g. clozapine) (Kapur *et al.* 1999). A drug with a fast dissociation from the D_2 receptor may achieve a reduction in dopaminergic activity sufficient for an antipsychotic effect whilst at the same time allowing enough dopaminergic activity to inhibit prolactin secretion (Kapur and Seeman 2001). The pituitary gland is located outside the blood–brain barrier and one would expect that drugs with poor brain penetrability and higher serum concentrations, such as sulpiride, would have a greater effect on pituitary prolactin secretion.

The ability of certain antidepressants to cause hyperprolactinaemia is believed to reflect their enhancement of serotonergic function and the fact that serotonin stimulates prolactin release.

Differential diagnosis

If a patient is prescribed a drug known to cause hyperprolactinaemia and subsequently develops symptoms suggestive of this problem, then a serum prolactin level should be obtained. Mild to moderate elevations should be checked with a second sample. It is important for the clinician to consider other possible causes of raised prolactin (see Table 5.2). A history, physical

Table 5.2 Causes of hyperprolactinaemia

Cause	Examples
Drugs	**Psychiatric drugs** Antidepressants (particularly serotonergic agents) Conventional antipsychotics Some atypical antipsychotics (especially risperidone, amisulpride) **Antihypertensive drugs** Alpha-methyldopa Reserpine Verapamil **Anti-dopaminergic anti-emetics** Metoclopramide **H2 blockers** Cimetidine Ranitidine **Hormones** Oestrogens (e.g. oral contraceptives) Thyrotrophin-releasing hormone **Miscellaneous** Amphetamine Opiates
Physiological	Lactation Pregnancy Sleep Stress Sexual activity
Pituitary disease	Empty sella syndrome Prolactin secreting pituitary tumours (micro and macro-prolactinomonas) Pituitary stalk lesions (preventing dopamine reaching the pituitary)
Hypothalamic disease	Hypothalamic tumours Hypothalamic sarcoidosis Postencephalitis
Endocrine disease	Acromegaly Cushing's disease Polycystic ovary syndrome Primary hypothyroidism
Miscellaneous	Breast stimulation Chest wall lesions e.g. trauma, neoplasms Chronic renal failure Cirrhosis, severe liver disease Ectopic production of prolactin e.g. small cell bronchial carcinoma Idiopathic

examination, pregnancy test, thyroid function test, urea and creatinine level will help exclude these causes.

The following features suggest that an antipsychotic is the cause of hyperprolactinaemia:

- Use of an antipsychotic that is well documented to cause hyperprolactinaemia (i.e. any conventional agent, amisulpride, risperidone or zotepine).
- Onset of hyperprolactinaemic symptoms shortly after starting the antipsychotic drug or increasing its dose.
- Absence of signs and symptoms suggestive of a sellar space occupying lesion.
- A prolactin level <2500 mU/l (in the absence of pregnancy, levels >4500 mU/l suggest a prolactin secreting adenoma).
- Other laboratory tests are normal.

However these indicators can only serve as a guide. For example, although symptoms often begin shortly after either starting or increasing the dose of an antipsychotic drug, symptoms can commence after a long period of treatment with a stable dose (Haddad *et al.* 2001). In addition, prolactinomas can present with serum prolactin values within the range usually associated with antipsychotic-induced hyperprolactinaemia. The best confirmation that an antipsychotic is the cause of hyperprolactinaemia is when the drug is stopped or switched and this is followed by normalization of prolactin levels and resolution of symptoms. If there is concern that hyperprolactinaemia may have an organic cause then the patient should be referred to an endocrinologist. Assessment will usually include magnetic resonance imaging of the pituitary fossa to exclude a tumour.

Management

Is intervention warranted?

Not all patients with antipsychotic-induced hyperprolactinaemia will require intervention to reverse the hyperprolactinaemia. Whether or nor intervention is required will depend on an assessment, on an individual patient basis, of the risks and benefits of continuing the current antipsychotic. Whenever possible the patient should be fully involved in the assessment and discussion about management options. However, as with many other clinical issues, the degree to which this is done must be tailored to the individual patient taking account of their mental state, educational level, and how much information and involvement they want.

Factors to be considered in the risk: benefit assessment include the following:

- How distressing the patient finds the hyperprolactinaemic symptoms.
- In females, the duration of secondary amenorrhoea.

+ How long treatment with the antipsychotic drug is expected to continue.
+ The degree of benefit that the patient has gained from the antipsychotic drug.
+ The risk of an exacerbation of symptoms or recurrence should the antipsychotic be substantially reduced in dose or switched.

In accordance with the guidelines from the Royal College of Physicians (1999) in England we recommend that any woman with hyperprolactinaemia-related amenorrhoea of 12 months duration or more should have BMD measurements. An estimation of BMD based on one site can be misleading and so BMD measurements should be taken at several sites e.g. lumbar spine, proximal femur and forearm. The results should be incorporated into the assessment of risks and benefits of continuing the current antipsychotic. We would recommend that patients with either osteopenia or osteoporosis on one or more sites be referred for specialist advice on further management.

Assessing the risk of osteoporosis developing in men is hindered by the lack of an objective clinical indicator of gonadal function in the way that menstrual function acts in women. At present there is insufficient evidence to conclusively state that antipsychotic-induced hypogonadism in men leads to decreased BMD. If further data confirmed the association then there would be a case for routinely monitoring serum prolactin and testosterone in men prescribed antipsychotics.

Women treated with antipsychotic medication may be less likely to undergo breast cancer surveillance. Because the risk for breast cancer is possibly increased such women should be encouraged at least to participate in national breast screening programmes.

Treatment options

Several strategies are available to treat drug-induced hyperprolactinaemia. The simplest is to reduce the dose of the suspected offending drug. However the effect of dose reduction on prolactin levels is unpredictable and it may precipitate an exacerbation or recurrence of the underlying psychiatric illness. Another option is to switch medication. In the case of antipsychotics, switching the patient to a prolactin-sparing antipsychotic (i.e. aripiprazole, olanzapine, quetiapine or clozapine) usually proves effective though there is also a risk of relapse (Kim *et al.* 2002; Haddad *et al.* 2001). In the case of antidepressants one can consider switching from a serotonergic antidepressant to a noradrenegic agent (e.g. reboxetine).

There are sometimes good reasons to continue treatment with an antipsychotic drug that is causing hyperprolactinaemia. For example a patient may have had a good response to the drug but failed to respond to several previous antipsychotics. In this situation neither the patient nor the clinician may wish to take the risk of switching medication and causing a relapse. Another scenario relates to a patient whose illness is well controlled with a long acting intramuscular depot but who previously showed repeated poor adherence with oral medication. The treating team may conclude that a depot is the only way of ensuring adequate adherence with medication and that the risks of relapse are too high to justify stopping the depot (at present prolactin-sparing atypical drugs are not available as depot injections). This is particularly likely to be the view if the patient's illness has involved aggression or self-harm i.e. there are major issues of risk. In such cases one can consider prescribing a D_2 receptor agonist, such as bromocriptine or cabergoline, which will inhibit prolactin secretion. This approach has been investigated in several small studies of patients with antipsychotic-induced hyperprolactinaemia (Beumont et al. 1975; Siever 1981; Matsuoka et al. 1986; Smith 1992). These indicate that amenorrhoea responds better than galactorrhoea and that the risk of precipitating a psychotic relapse is fairly small in stable patients. Other side-effects depend on the drug employed e.g. bromocriptine can cause postural hypotension, gastrointestinal symptoms and vasospasm of the fingers and toes, especially in those with Raynaud's syndrome.

If there are good clinical reasons for a premenopausal female patient to remain on a prolactin-raising antipsychotic but this is causing amenorrhoea (i.e. a clinical marker of oestrogen deficiency) then one can consider prescribing a combined oral contraceptive. This will prevent symptoms associated with oestrogen deficiency, including possible loss of BMD, though symptoms directly due to hyperprolactinaemia (e.g. galactorhoea, gynaecomastia) will be unaffected. The main drawbacks of this approach are the health risks associated with oral contraceptive use, namely an increased risk of thromboembolism and breast cancer. In addition about 5–10 per cent of the general population has an asymptomatic microprolactinoma (Molitch 1995). The effect of hormone replacement in women who have both a prolactinoma and antipsychotic-induced hyperprolactinaemia is unknown. For this reason it has been recommended that prolactin levels are monitored every 2–3 months for the first six months of hormone replacement therapy followed by annual measurements (Molitch 2000).

Risk factors and prevention

Any patient prescribed a prolactin-raising antipsychotic is at risk of developing hyperprolactinaemia – however certain patient groups appear to have a higher risk. It has consistently been shown that women have significantly greater prolactin elevations than men during chronic treatment with the same antipsychotic dose (Kuruvilla *et al.* 1992). Women in the postnatal period also appear to be at higher risk (Goode *et al.* 1980).

A recent study suggested that children and adolescents might be more sensitive to the prolactin-raising effect of both haloperidol and olanzapine, though small patient numbers limited the study (Wudarsky *et al.* 1999). In contrast quetiapine did not cause any elevation of prolactin when used in adolecent patients, though this study was also limited by small numbers (Shaw *et al.* 2001).

Health professionals often fail to detect antipsychotic-induced hyperprolactinaemic symptoms (Hellewell 1998). There may be a variety of reasons for this, including the nature of the symptoms and the attitudes of both patients and health professionals. It is important that, when patients are prescribed drugs known to be associated with a high rate of hyperprolactinaemia, clinicians routinely ask patients about side-effects that may indicate this problem.

To help clarify the temporal link between an antipsychotic drug and future symptoms we would recommend that, whenever possible, a history of sexual functioning is taken before antipsychotic medication is initiated. With female patients one should also take a history of recent menstrual cycling (duration, amount, and intervals of menstruation) and note any recent lactation. When prolactin-elevating drugs are used it is helpful to obtain a pre-treatment prolactin level which one can compare with subsequent levels should the patient develop symptoms suggestive of hyperprolactinaemia. This can be helpful in deciding the likely aetiology of the symptoms if the levels taken at that time are only modestly elevated.

Summary: Hyperprolactinaemia

Definition	Serum prolactin above the upper limit of the normal range (ULN). ULN varies between laboratories but is approximately 500 mU/l . Hyperprolactinaemia may or may not cause symptoms.
Incidence	Depends on drug, dose, gender of subjects and whether asymptomatic or symptomatic hyperprolactinaemia is considered. In a recent cross-sectional study of patients prescribed conventional antipsychotics the point prevalence of prolactin >ULN was 75% in women and 34% in men (Smith *et al.* 2002a).
Drugs causing syndrome	Conventional antipsychotics
	Certain atypical antipsychotics (risperidone, amisulpride and occasionally olanzapine, particularly at high dosages)

	Occasional reports with SSRIs, MAOIs and TCAs
	Various non-psychiatric drugs: see Table 5.2.
Key symptoms	Menstrual irregularities (oligoamenorrhoea or amenorrhoea), sexual dysfunction, infertility, galactorrhoea, breast enlargement, possible reduced BMD. Increased risk of breast cancer queried in women.
Pharmacological mechanism	Antipsychotics: Blockade of D_2 receptors on pituitary lactotroph cells
	Antidepressants: Enhanced serotonergic tranmsision.
Investigations to confirm diagnosis	Serum prolactin level (repeat if marginal elevation) Exclude other causes of raised prolactin: see Table 5.2.
Management	Options include;
	◆ Reduce dose of causal agent
	◆ Switch to prolactin sparing antipsychotic (if caused by antipsychotic)
	◆ Switch to a noradrenergic antidepressant (if caused by antidepressant)
	◆ Dopamine agonist (enhances dopaminergic drive and so inhibits prolactin production)
	◆ Combined oral contraceptive (prevents symptoms of hypo-oestrogenism in female patients).
Further reading	Smith SM, O'Keane V, and Murray, R (2002a). Sexual dysfunction in patients taking conventional antipsychotic medication. *Br J Psychiatry*, **181**, 49–55.
	Smith S, Wheeler MJ, Murray R, *et al.* (2002b). The effects of antipsychotic-induced hyperprolactinaemia on the hypothalamic-pituitary-gonadal axis. *J Clin Psychopharmacol*, **22**, 109–14.
	Wieck A and Haddad PM (2003) Antipsychotic-induced hyperprolactinaemia in women: pathophysiology, severity and consequences. Selective literature review. *Br J Psychiatry*, **182**, 199–204.

References

Aizenberg D, Modai I, Landa A, *et al.* (2001). Comparison of sexual dysfunction in male schizophrenic patients maintained on treatment with classical antipsychotics versus clozapine. *J Clin Psychiatry*, **62**, 541–4.

Akande B, Wieck A, and Haddad PM (2002). Bone mineral density in premenopausal women with antipsychotic-induced hyperprolactinaemia. *Eur Neuropsychopharmacol*, **12**, (Suppl. 3), S311–12.

Ataya K, Mercado A, Kartaginer J, *et al.* (1988). Bone density and reproductive hormones in patients with neuroleptic-induced hyperprolactinemia. *Fertil Steril*, **50**, 876–81.

Baron JC, Martinot JL, Cambon H, *et al.* (1989). Striatal dopamine receptor occupancy during and following withdrawal from neuroleptic treatment: correlative evaluation by positron emission tomography and plasma prolactin levels. *Psychopharmacology*, **99**, 463–72.

Beumont P, Bruwer J, Pimstone B, *et al.* (1975). Brom-ergocryptine in the treatment of phenothiazine-induced galactorrhea. *Br J Psychiatry*, **126**, 285–8.

Beumont PJV, Gelder MG, Friesen HG, *et al.* (1974). The effects of phenothiazines on endocrine function: I. Patients with inappropriate lactation and amenorrhoea. *Br J Psychiatry*, **124**, 413–19.

Bole-Feysot C, Goffin V, Edery M, *et al.* (1998). Prolactin (PRL) and its receptor: actions, signal transduction pathways and phenotypes observed in PRL receptor knockout mice. *Endocr Rev*, **9**, 225–68.

Checkley S (1991). Neuroendocrine effects of psychotropic drugs. *Ballieres Clin Endocrinol Metab*, **5**, 15–33.

Crawford AM, Beasley CM Jr, and Tollefson GD (1997). The acute and long-term effect of olanzapine compared with placebo and haloperidol on serum prolactin concentrations. *Schizophr Res*, **26**, 41–54.

Dickson RA and Glazer WM (1999). Hyperprolactinaemia and male sexual dysfunction. *J Clin Psychiatry*, **60**, 125.

Finkelstein JS, Klibanski A, Neer RM, *et al.* (1983). Osteoporosis in men with idiopathic hypogonadotropic hypogonadism. *Ann J Med*, **75**, 977–83.

Goode DJ, Meltzer HY, and Fang VS (1980). Increased serum prolactin levels during phenothiazine and butyrophenone treatment of six postpartum women. *Psycho-neuroendocrinology*, **5**, 345–51.

Goodnick PJ and Jerry JM (2002). Aripiprazole; profile on efficacy and safety. *Expert Opin Pharmacother*, **3**, 1773–81.

Greenspan SL, Neer RM, Ridgway EL, *et al.* (1986). Osteoporosis in men with hyperprolactinemic hypogonadism. *Ann Intern Med*, **104**, 777–82.

Greenspan SL, Oppenheim DS, and Klibanski A (1989). Importance of gonadal steroids to bone mass in men with hyperprolactinemic hypogonadism. *Ann Intern Med*, **110**, 526–31.

Grunder G, Wetzel H, Schlosser R, *et al.* (1999). Neuroendocrine response to antipsychotics: effects of drug type and gender. *Biol Psychiatry*, **45**, 89–97.

Gudelsky GA (1981). Tuberoinfundibular dopamine neurons and the regulation of prolactin secretion. *Psychoneuroendocrinology*, **6**, 3–16.

Gulbinat W, Dupont A, Jablensky A, *et al.* (1992). Cancer incidence of schizophrenic patients: results of record-linkage studies in three countries. *Br J Psychiatry*, **161** (Suppl. 18), 75–85.

Haddad PM, Hellewell JSE, and Wieck A (2001). Antipsychotic-induced hyperprolacti-naemia: a series of illustrative case reports. *J Psychopharmacol*, **15**, 293–5.

Halbreich U, Rojansky N, Palter S, *et al.* (1995). Decreased bone mineral density in medicated psychiatric patients. *Psychosomat Med*, **57**, 485–91.

Halbreich U, Shen J, and Panaro V (1996). Are chronic psychiatric patients at increased risk for developing breast cancer? *Am J Psychiatry*, **153**, 559–60.

Hellewell JSE (1998). Antipsychotic tolerability: the attitudes and perceptions of medical professionals, patients and caregivers towards side-effects of antipsychotic therapy. *Eur Neuropsychopharmacol*, **8**, S248.

Hummer M, Kemmler G, Kurz M, *et al.* (1999). Sexual disturbance during clozapine and haloperidol treatment for schizophrenia. *Am J Psychiatry*, **156**, 631–3.

Kaneda Y, Fujii A, Yamaoka T, *et al.* (2000). Neither Gynaecomastia not galactorrhea is a common side effects of neuroleptics in male patients. *Neuroendocrinol Lett*, **21**, 447–51.

Kanhouwa S, Gowdy JM, and Solomon JD (1984). Phenothiazines and breast cancer. *J Nat Med Assoc*, **76**, 785–8.

Kapur S and Seeman P (2001). Does fast dissociation from the dopamine d(2) receptor explain the action of atypical antipsychotics?: a new hypothesis. *Am J Psychiatry*, **158**, 360–9.

Kapur S, Zipursky RB, and Remington G (1999). Clinical and theoretical implications of 5-HT2 and D2 receptor occupancy of clozapine, risperidone, and olanzapine in schizophrenia. *Am J Psychiatry*, **156**, 286–93.

Kiel DP, Felson DT, Andersen JJ, *et al.* (1987). Hip fractures and the use of estrogen in postmenopausal women: The Framingham Study. *New Engl J Med*, **317**, 1169–74.

Kim KS, Pae CU, Chae JH, *et al.* (2002). Effects of olanzapine on prolactin levels of female patients with schizophrenia treated with risperidone. *J Clin Psychiatry*, **63**, 408–13.

Kinon B and Gilmore J (2001). Prevalence of hyperprolactinemia in a large cohort of schizophrenic patients treated with conventional antipsychotic drugs or risperidone. *Arch Wom Ment Health*, **3** (Suppl. 2), S185.

Klibanski A and Greenspan SL (1986). Increase in bone mass after treatment of hyperprolactinemic amenorrhea. *New Engl J Medicine*, **315**, 542–6.

Koppelman MCS, Kurtz DW, Morrish KA, *et al.* (1984). Vertebral bone mineral density content in hyperprolactinemic women. *J Clin Endocrinol Metab*, **59**, 1050–3.

Krueger TCH, Haake P, Hartmann U, *et al.* (2002). Orgasm-induced prolactin secretion: feedback control of sexual drive? *Neurosci Biobehav Rev*, **26**, 31–44.

Kuruvilla A, Peedicayil J, Srikrishna G, *et al.*(1992). A study of serum prolactin levels in schizophrenia: comparison of males and females. *Clin Exp Pharmacol Physiol*, **19**, 603–6.

Linkwork P, Van Acuter E, L'Hermite-Baleriaux M, *et al.* (1989). The 24-hour profile of plasma prolactin in men with major endogenous depressive illness. *Arch Gen Psychiatry*, **46**, 813–19.

Lundberg PO and Hulter B (1991). Sexual dysfunction in patients with hypothalamo-pituitary disorders. *Exp Clin Endocrinol*, **98**, 81–8.

Matsuoka I, Nakai T, Miyaki M, *et al.* (1986). Effects of bromocriptine on neuroleptic-induced amenorrhea, galactorrhea and impotence. *JPN J Psychiatry Neurol*, **40**, 639–46.

Meltzer HY and Fang VS (1976). The effect of neuroleptics on serum prolactin in schizophrenic patients. *Arch Gen Psychiatry*, **33**, 279–86.

Meltzer HY, Goode DJ, Schyve PM, *et al.* (1979). Effect of clozapine on human serum prolactin levels. *Am J Psychiatry*, **136**, 1550–5.

Meltzer HY, Kane JM, and Kolakowska T (1983). Plasma levels of neuroleptics, prolactin levels, and clinical response. In *Neuroleptics: Neurochemical, Behavioural and Clinical Perspectives*, JT Coyle and SJ Enna (ed.), pp. 255–79. Raven Press: New York.

Meltzer HY, Sachar EJ, and Frantz AG (1974). Serum prolactin levels in unmedicated schizophrenic patients. *Arch Gen Psychiatry*, **31**, 564–9.

Molitch ME (1995). Prolactin. In *The Pituitary*, S Melmed (ed.), pp. 136–86. Blackwell Science: Oxford.

Molitch ME (2000). Antipsychotic drug-induced hyperprolactinemia: clinical implications. *Endocr Prac*, **6**, 479–81.

Nonacs RM (2000). *Antipsychotic Treatment and Menstrual Irregularity*, 153rd Annual Meeting of the American Psychiatric Association, New Research Abstracts, 245.

Nordstrom AL and Farde L (1998). Plasma prolactin and central D_2 receptor occupancy in antipsychotic drug-treated patients. *J Clin Psychopharmacol*, **18**, 305–10.

Pearson OH, Llerena O, and Llerena L (1969). Prolactin-dependent rat mammary cancer: a model for man? *Trans Assoc Am Physicians*, **82**, 225–38.

Peuskens J (1995). Risperidone in the treatment of patients with chronic schizophrenia: a multi-national, multi-centre, double-blind, parallel-group study versus haloperidol. *Br J Psychiatry*, **166**, 712–26.

Polishuk JL and Kulcsar S (1956). Effects of chlorpromazine on pituitary function. *J Clin Endocrinol*, **16**, 292–3.

Reavley A, Fisher AD, Owen D, *et al.* (1997). Psychological distress in patients with hyperprolactinaemia. *Clin Endocrinol*, **47**, 343–8.

Rivera JL, Lal S, Ettigi P, *et al.* (1976). Effect of acute and chronic neuroleptic therapy on serum prolactin levels in men and women of different age groups. *Clin Endocrinol*, **5**, 273–82.

Royal College of Physicians (1999). *Osteoporosis: Clinical Guidelines for Prevention and Treatment*. Royal College of Physicians: London.

Schlechte J, El-Khoury G, Kathol M, *et al.* (1987). Forearm and vertebral bone mineral density in treated and untreated hyperprolactinemic amenorrhea. *J Clin Endocrinol Metab*, **64**, 1021–6.

Shaw JA, Lewis JE, Pascal S, *et al.* (2001). A study of quetiapine: efficacy and tolerability in psychotic adolescents. *J Child Adolesc Psychopharmacol*, **11**, 415–24.

Siever L (1981). The effect of amantadine on prolactin levels and galactorrhea in neuroleptic-treated patients. *J Clin Psychopharmacol*, **1**, 2–7.

Small JG, Hirsch SR, Arvanitis LA, *et al.* (1997). Quetiapine in patients with schizophrenia: a high- and low-dose double-blind comparison with placebo. *Arch Gen Psychiatry*, **54**, 549–57.

Smith S (1992). Neuroleptic-associated hyperprolactinaemia. Can it be treated with bromocriptine? *J Reproductive Med*, **37**, 737–40.

Smith SM, O'Keane V, and Murray R (2002a). Sexual dysfunction in patients taking conventional antipsychotic medication. *Br J Psychiatry*, **181**, 49–55.

Smith S, Wheeler MJ, Murray R, *et al.* (2002b). The effects of antipsychotic-induced hyperprolactinaemia on the hypothalamic-pituitary-gonadal axis. *J Clin Psychopharmacol*, **22**, 109–14.

Sobrinho LG (1993). The psychogenic effects of prolactin. *Acta Endocrinol*, **29** (Suppl. 1), 38–40.

Tuomisto J and Mannisto P (1985). Neurotransmitter regulation of anterior pituitary hormones. *Pharmocol Rev*, **37**, 249–301.

Veldhuis JD and Johnson ML (1988). Operating characteristics of the hypothalamo-pituitary-gonadal axis in men: circadian, ultradian, and pulsatile release of prolactin and its temporal coupling with luteinizing hormone. *J Clin Endocrinol Metab*, **67**, 116–23.

Wang PS, Walker AM, Tsuang MT, *et al.* (2002). Dopamine antagonists and the development of breast cancer. *Arch Gen Psychiatry*, **59**, 1147–54.

Welsch CW and Nagasawa H (1977). Prolactin and murine mammary tumorigenesis: a review. *Cancer Res*, **37**, 951–63.

Wieck A and Haddad PM (2003). Antipsychotic-induced hyperprolactinaemia in women: pathophysiology, severity and consequences. Selective literature review. *Br J Psychiatry*, **182**, 199–204.

Windgassen K, Wesselmann U, and Schulze Monking H (1996). Galactorrhoea and hyperprolactinaemia in schizophrenic patients on neuroleptics: frequency and etiology. *Neuropsychobiology*, **33**, 142–6.

Wirshing DA, Pierre JM, Marder SR, *et al.* (2002). Sexual side-effects of novel antipsychotic medications. *Schizophr Res*, **56**, 25–30.

Wistedt B, Wiles D, and Kolakowska T (1981). Slow decline of plasma drug and prolactin levels after discontinuation of chronic treatments with depot neuroleptics. *Lancet*, **1**, 1163.

Wudarsky M, Nicolson R, Hamburger SD, *et al.* (1999). Elevated prolactin in paediatric patients on typical and atypical antipsychotics. *J Child Adoles Psychop*, **9**, 239–45.

Zelaschi NM, Delucchi GA, and Rodriguez JL (1996). High plasma prolactin levels after long-term neuroleptic treatment. *Biol Psychiatry*, **39**, 900–1.

Chapter 6

Adverse syndromes associated with lithium

Karine A N Macritchie and Allan H Young

Background

Lithium was discovered in 1817 by the Swedish Chemist, Johann Arfwedson. Initially, it was used in the treatment of gout, epilepsy, urinary calculi and rheumatoid arthritis (Shoemaker 1891) and was considered an active agent in 'artificial mineral waters' (Tichbourne and James 1883). By the end of the nineteenth century, its role in recurrent affective disorders predominated (Friedrich 1999; Cookson 1998). Records from that period make little mention of adverse effects associated with lithium, although Shoemaker (1891) commented on its diuretic effects. However, in the 1940s, reports of deaths and cases of severe toxicity related to its use in low-sodium salt preparations led to its withdrawal from the market.

Its rehabilitation into modern psychiatry followed the successful treatment of 'psychotic excitement' (Cade 1949). At first the use of lithium and the research which supported it was driven by a small group of academic enthusiasts (Coppen 1996). Fifty years later, lithium remains a mainstay of acute and prophylactic treatment for bipolar disorder (Sachs *et al.* 2000). It is reported to have specific anti-suicidal effects (Thies-Flechtner *et al.* 1996). In addition, it is extensively used in augmentation of antidepressant treatment (Austin *et al.* 1991). Other psychiatric applications include prophylaxis against affective and schizoaffective psychoses in the post-partum period (Stewart *et al.* 1991), the augmentation of clozapine therapy (Boshes *et al.* 2001), aggressive behaviour (Sheard *et al.* 1976) and recurrent mood swings and self-injurious behaviour in the learning disabled (Spreat *et al.* 1989). Lithium is also prescribed in other fields of medicine, for example, conditions of chronic pain such as orofacial neuralgia (Feinmann and Peatfield 1993).

Lithium has a narrow therapeutic index and a number of unwanted side effects, which are frequent reasons for non-compliance (McCreadie and Morrison 1985). Perhaps the most problematic adverse effects are a number of specific syndromes, namely acute toxicity, diabetes insipidus, renal impairment, hypothyroidism and 'rebound' mania. Before considering these in detail it is helpful to briefly review the pharmacological effects of lithium, including its pharmacokinetics.

The pharmacological effects of lithium

Numerous studies have demonstrated the effects of lithium in animal models and in man (Table 6.1), but its therapeutic mechanism remains uncertain.

Pharmacokinetics

Lithium is administered orally. It is produced in the form of its carbonate and citrate salts: lithium citrate may be obtained in liquid preparations. It is absorbed completely from the small intestine within eight hours. Peak levels are achieved at 2–4 hours. Slow release preparations are also available and produce later, lower peak concentrations. It circulates freely and is not plasma-protein bound. Preparations vary widely in bioavailability.

Drug monitoring, in the form of 12-hour standard serum lithium measurement, is necessary for safe and efficacious treatment, as the gap between therapeutic and toxic concentrations is small: in some cases there maybe a degree of overlap. Therapeutic serum concentrations for monotherapy in affective disorders range from 0.4 to 1.2 mEq/L. Dosage requirements vary significantly between patients and over time, for instance renal clearance gradually decreases with age (Vestergaard and Schou 1984), necessitating periodic dose reduction in long-term treatment.

Lithium concentration in the cerebrospinal fluid has been reported to be 40 per cent of plasma levels (Terhaag et al. 1978). Others report less marked differences in adults but similar findings in children (Moore et al. 2002). Lithium is, almost exclusively, eliminated by the kidney. The half-life of a single dose is between 12–27 hours (Amidsen 1975).

Following commencement of treatment, serum assays should be carried out after five days and, if necessary, the dose adjusted. Lithium equilibrates between extracellular and intracellular spaces over more than a week. Levels should be checked at least fortnightly for the first month, two monthly for the next six months and at least every six months thereafter. Should toxic symptoms occur, levels should be tested immediately.

Lithium toxicity

Clinical features

Lithium intoxication manifests a variety of symptoms depending on its degree: these may be subtle (Table 6.2). Symptom severity is generally

Table 6.1 Pharmacological effects of lithium

	Comments	Reference
Effects in neurotransmitters		
5-Hydroxytrypamine (5-HT)	Enhances brain serotonergic activity/function. Increases uptake of serotonin, levels of the metabolite 5-HIAA and 5-HT$_2$ receptor expression	Blier and De Montigny 1985, Treiser et al. 1981, Price et al. 1990, McCance et al. 1989, Carli et al. 1997, Shiah and Yatham 2000, Goodwin and Jamison 1990
Dopamine (DA)	Variable effects on concentrations in different regions. Decreases release and synthesis. Increases uptake, uptake sites and affinity. Increases D$_2$ receptor mRNA levels. Increases DA metabolite, DOPAC levels	Otero-Losada and Rubio 1985, Friedman and Gershon 1973, Dunigan and Shamoo 1995, Carli et al. 1997, Kameda et al. 2001, Dziedzicka-Wasylewska et al. 1996, Stefanini et al. 1976, Baptista et al. 1993
Noradrenaline (NA)	Variable effects on concentrations in different regions. Increases turnover rates. Decreases release and vesicular storage capacity	Katz et al. 1968, Colburn et al. 1967, Ahluwalia and Singhal 1984, Greenspan et al. 1970, Slotkin et al. 1980, Wood and Goodwin 1987
Gaba-aminobutyric acid (GABA)	Increases levels in both acute and short-term treatment. Chronic treatment increases binding of GABA B receptors, single treatment increases GABA A binding	Antonelli et al. 2000, Vargas et al. 1998, Motohashi 1992
Acetylcholine	Increases concentration and synthesis. Increases the binding of ligands to muscarinic receptors in the striatum	Jope 1979, Lerer and Stanley 1985, Tollefson and Senogles 1982
Effects in second messengers		
Inositol	Decreases intracellular inositol. Inhibits inositol monophosphatase	Hallcher and Sherman 1980, Berridge and Irvine 1989, Moscovich et al. 1990
IP$_3$	Increases accumulation intracellularly via postsynaptic stimulation of NMDA receptors	Hokin et al. 1996
Arachidonic acid	Decreases arachidonic acid turnover	Chang et al. 1996, Rintala et al. 1999

Table 6.1 (continued) Pharmacological effects of lithium

	Comments	Reference
cAMP	Decreased synthesis via competition for the magnesium dependent GTP binding proteins. Decreased levels via decreased activation of PKC	Goldberg 1988, Chen et al. 2000
Protein kinase 2	Decreased expression, activation and levels of membrane associated PKC 2	Friedman et al. 1993, Manji and Lenox 1999, Bitran et al. 1995, Wang et al. 2001, Wang and Friedman 1989, Manji and Rapaport 2001
GSK	Inhibits GSK-3 via competition for low affinity Mg^{+2} sites	Klein and Melton 1996, Stambolic et al. 1996, Ryves and Harwood 2001
MARKS	Decreased expression in hippocampus	Lenox et al. 1998
Glutamate	Increases extracellular glutamate via inhibiting presynaptic glutamate uptake	Dixon and Hokin 1998
Effects in ion channels		
Na^+/K^+	Increases the resting potential to normal control levels (depolarizes)	Hokin-Neaverson and Jefferson 1989, Thiruvengadam 2001, Johnston et al. 1980
Ca^{2+}	Induces Ca^{2+} influx	Gende 2000
Effects on HPA parameters		
HPA axis	Normalises HPA axis via increasing GR and MR receptor mRNA. Increased ACTH and cortisol response to CRH stimulation	Semba et al. 2000
Effects in nerve cells		
BDNF	Increases expression	Mai et al. 2002
Pro-apoptotic proteins	Decreased expression (p53, BAX)	Chuang et al. 2002
Anti-apoptotic proteins	Increased expression (Bcl-2)	Yuan et al. 2001, Manji et al. 2001

Table 6.2 Signs and symptoms of lithium toxicity

Mild toxicity
Nausea
Diarrhoea
Blurred vision
Polyuria
Light headedness
Fine resting tremor
Muscle weakness
Drowsiness

Moderate toxicity
Increasing confusion
Blackouts
Fasciculation
Increased deep tendon reflexes
Myoclonic twitches
Choreoathetoid movements
Incontinence
Hypernatraemia

Severe toxicity
Coma
Convulsions
Cardiac dysrhythmias including SA block
Cerebellar signs
Sinus and junctional bradycardia
First degree heart block
Hypotension
Hypertension (relatively rare occurrence)
Renal failure: oliguria, fluid retention and uraemia

proportional to serum levels, but toxicity may occur at levels within the therapeutic range (Spiers and Hirsch 1978; Bell *et al.* 1993). Conversely, in acute overdoses, although serum concentrations may be very high, intracellular concentrations may be non-toxic and the patient may initially present asymptomatically. Hansen and Amidsen (1978) devised guidelines where mild intoxication could be expected at serum lithium levels of 1.5–2.5 mmol/L, serious toxicity at 2.5–3.5 mmol/L and life-threatening toxicity at levels greater than >3.5 mmol/L. However, serum concentration should not be the only guide to the severity of lithium poisoning. Observation of the progression of symptoms over time is of great importance.

The symptoms and signs of lithium toxicity are listed in Table 6.2. Mild neurological effects such as tremor, fatigue and muscle weakness occur in non-toxic conditions, but more severe neurological symptoms indicate serious toxicity. Toxic effects on the basal ganglia may produce parkinsonism or chorea. Confusion may progress to impaired consciousness, seizures, coma and death. Neurological symptoms occasionally persist, usually in the form of cerebellar symptoms (Schou 1984): when they do persist, there may be some improvement over the following year. Although the persistence of neurological sequelae is unpredictable, the most severe and long-lasting cases of acute toxicity are probably at greater risk (Sheean 1991). Intoxication may induce failure of thermoregulatory mechanisms (Granoff and Davis 1978; Follezou and Bleisel 1985), possibly through the effects of lithium on hypothalamic inositol (Belmaker *et al.* 1998). Lithium-induced peripheral neuropathy (Pamphlett and Mackenzie 1982), myopathy (Julien *et al.* 1979) and leucopenia (Green and Dunn 1988) have been reported.

Electrocardiographic changes such as T wave flattening and inversion occur in 30 per cent of patients at therapeutic levels and may be benign (Levenson and Dwight 2000). However, cardiac intoxication may produce transient ST segment depression or inverted T waves in the lateral chest leads (Hansen and Amidsen 1978) and sinus node dysfunction leading to loss of consciousness (Hagman *et al.* 1979; Palileo *et al.* 1983) presumably through the effect of lithium on membrane conduction. Renal excretion of lithium is greatly diminished in lithium intoxication (Hansen and Amidsen 1978) and acute renal failure may occur.

Incidence

A recent study found that 6.8 per cent of over 2000 patients admitted to a psychiatric hospital had serum levels of 1.5 mmol/L or higher. Most were noted to have these levels at the time of admission, although some developed during their stay. Interestingly, only 27.8 per cent had symptoms and signs of toxicity (Webb *et al.* 2001). Mortality figures from lithium toxicity vary widely. Sheean (1991) quotes a mortality rate of 15 per cent in acute lithium toxicity. A recent study investigating the efficacy of haemodialysis, examined 205 cases of lithium toxicity whose management was discussed with a Poisons Control Centre. Twelve were acute overdoses in lithium naive patients, 174 were 'acute on chronic' cases and 19 were termed 'chronic poisonings'. There were two deaths, one in the 'acute on chronic' group, the other in the 'chronic poisonings' group (Bailey and McGuigan 2000). Hansen and Amidsen (1978) reported on 23 cases of lithium intoxication, 21 of whom developed intoxication during maintenance therapy on lithium doses that had remained steady for months or years: two patients in this group died.

Similarly, Oakley *et al.* (2002), in a review of 97 cases of intoxication found 28 with severe neurotoxicity. Twenty-six occurred during chronic therapeutic administration of lithium with no apparent precipitating overdose. Thus there is no room for complacency in cases of chronic treatment when toxicity may be insidious but severe.

Pharmacological basis

Unknown.

Differential diagnosis

The differential diagnosis for lithium intoxication includes multifactorial delirium, serotonin syndrome and any physical illness with similar presenting symptoms.

Management

Advice may be obtained from local poisons advice services. Prescribed lithium should be withdrawn when the diagnosis of lithium toxicity is established. If the diagnosis remains uncertain it may be sufficient to halve the dose, if it seems clinically judicious to do so. While recovery is in progress, it may be safer to use a benzodiazepine for treatment of psychiatric illness.

In the unconscious patient, airway protection and adequate ventilation is the priority. Hypovolaemia, potentially precipitating pre-renal failure, should be corrected. Convulsions are treated with intravenous or rectal diazepam, and with intubation if they persist. Those with mild symptoms should be observed, with attention to adequate hydration and electrolyte balance. Cardiac monitoring is indicated in the symptomatic patient.

Patients should be observed for at least 24 hours. Measurement of serum lithium concentration is undertaken immediately and then repeated 6–12 hourly (Sadosty et al. 1999). Overdoses using sustained release tablets should be approached with special caution: patients should be observed over 48 hours.

Gastric lavage should be considered. Sustained release tablets may be problematic as they do not disintegrate in the stomach and may block the lavage tube. Activated charcoal does not absorb lithium. Whole bowel irrigation (e.g. with polyethylene glycol) may be helpful, but evidence for its use is confined to a few case reports.

Haemodialysis is the established treatment for severe lithium intoxication. Lithium is readily dialysed because of its small atomic weight and lack of protein binding. Although no controlled studies exist on methods of renal clearance during intoxication, it is considered to offer higher levels of lithium clearance than alternative treatments such as peritoneal dialysis (Okusa and Crystal 1994). Forced diuresis is contraindicated.

Haemodialysis should be instituted at serum levels above 3 mmol/L, in cases of coma or shock or where conservative measures fail after 24 hours. Serum lithium levels during haemodialysis may mirror progress, but should be interpreted with caution due to the possibility of ongoing absorption of lithium from the gastrointestinal tract and delayed release of lithium from intracellular stores (Sellers *et al.* 1982). Rebound increases may occur on stopping dialysis. Clinical improvement lags behind lithium clearance.

An episode of lithium toxicity does not preclude its further use. However its reintroduction should be carefully considered. Following the acute episode, a review of its precipitants should be undertaken and the patient's concerns and wishes ascertained. In general, lithium may be reintroduced when the patient is asymptomatic and serum levels have reached the lower end of the therapeutic range.

Risk factors

Oakley *et al.* (2002) identified nephrogenic diabetes insipidus, age (over 50 years), thyroid dysfunction and impaired creatinine clearance as risk factors for toxicity. Pre-existing brain injury and intercurrent physical illness, especially those associated with hypovoluminaemia and sodium depletion are thought to predispose to lithium intoxication. Patients with hypertension, diabetes, congestive cardiac failure and chronic renal failure are considered to be at increased risk (Toxbase 2003).

Drug interactions are another frequent precipitant of lithium toxicity. Medications predisposing to hyponatraemia, for example frusemide, thiazide diuretics and antidepressants, may reduce lithium clearance. Non-steroidal anti-inflammatory drugs such as indomethacin and diclofenac may have a similar effect. ACE Inhibitors are also implicated (Correa and Eiser 1992). The concomitant prescription of antipsychotics, particularly phenothiazines, may result in lithium toxicity, especially in the elderly. Several case reports document encephalopathy, sometimes with persistent dyskinesias or cerebellar syndrome, induced by lithium and haloperidol (Normann *et al.* 1998; Gille *et al.* 1997; Sandyk and Hurwitz 1983). The serotonin syndrome has been described with the co-administration of lithium and paroxetine or venlafaxine (Fagiolini *et al.* 2001; Mekler and Woggon 1997). In the past, lithium was withdrawn prior to ECT following reports of persistent neurotoxicity (Small *et al.* 1980). However, more recent re-evaluation of this practice (Mukherjee 1993) supports continuation at a reduced dose.

Prevention

Clinician, patient and family should be aware of signs of toxicity, the potential risks of drug interactions and intercurrent illness. Patients who develop signs of gastroenteritis should be advised to ensure adequate fluid intake and to seek medical advice. A lithium level should be taken, and a lithium dose reduction may be necessary for the duration of the episode. Chronic treatment and increasing age also require more vigilance.

Diabetes insipidus

Clinical features

Changes in renal function associated with lithium therapy may be glomerular or tubular. Tubular dysfunction, affecting water reabsorption, is the more common occurrence, sometimes resulting in frank diabetes insipidus. Glomerular dysfunction, which can lead to irreversible renal failure, occurs more rarely although its precise incidence is controversial.

The characteristic features of diabetes insipidus are polyuria and polydipsia, symptoms that may disturb work and sleep. Patients may compensate with an excessive fluid intake. When severe, the syndrome may progress to marked dehydration with its associated risk of lithium toxicity and encephalopathy. There have been several published accounts of deaths resulting from lithium toxicity in this context and many milder cases of toxicity have been reported (Bendz and Aurell 1999).

Incidence

Diabetes insipidus is the most common renal complication of lithium therapy. Reviews of studies investigating its incidence are undermined by variations in methods of diagnosis and diagnostic criteria: thus, one such review found an incidence ranging from 15–87 per cent (Boton *et al.* 1987). Bendz *et al.* (1994) found prevalence rates of 12 per cent in patients on lithium therapy for at least fifteen years using the DDAVP test (see below).

Pharmacological basis of lithium-induced diabetes insipidus

The functioning unit of the kidney is the nephron (Fig. 6.1). In the proximal tubule, 60–80 per cent of water and sodium is reabsorbed from the glomerular filtrate with potassium, bicarbonate, glucose and amino acids. Aldosterone and antidiuretic hormone (ADH) influence the reabsorption of water and sodium in the distal and collecting tubules. Lithium has a number of important effects on nephron function (see Fig. 6.1). Some of these effects may induce diabetes insipidus.

Nephrogenic diabetes insipidus results from a failure of urine concentration in the collecting ducts. Water is absorbed from the distal tubule and the

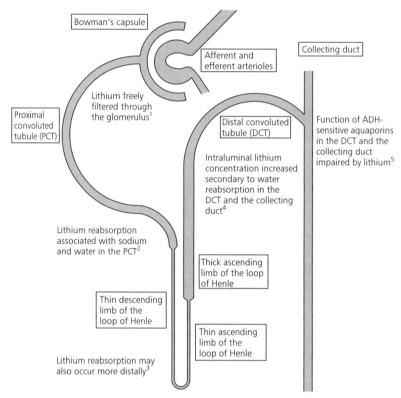

Fig. 6.1 The effect of lithium on nephron function. [1]Bendz and Aurell 1999; [2]Hayslett et al. 1979; [3]Atherton et al. 1991, Unwin et al. 1994; [4]Hayslett and Kashgarian 1979, Marples et al. 1995; [5]Christinasen et al. 1985, Dousa 1974, Marples et al. 1995.

collecting duct of the nephron through channels in luminal cell membranes termed aquaporins. Aquaporins are sensitive to the action of ADH, which enhances water absorption. In nephrogenic diabetes insipidus, the channels are impermeable to water despite adequate secretion of antidiuretic hormone. In neurogenic diabetes insipidus, there is inadequate production of antidiuretic hormone by the pituitary gland.

Lithium-induced diabetes insipidus is thought to be predominantly nephrogenic in origin (Bendz and Aurell 1999), although case reports of the neurogenic form exist (Posner and Mokrzycki 1996). Once filtered through the glomerulus, lithium is reabsorbed, predominantly in the proximal tubules and the loop of Henle (Hayslett and Kashgarian 1979). As water is reabsorbed in the distal tubule and collecting duct, the concentration of intraluminal lithium increases. Lithium may reduce ADH sensitivity through adenyl cyclase and cyclic adenosine monophosphate systems, within the cells lining the tubules (Christiansen *et al.* 1985; Dousa 1974). However, other mechanisms may play a role, such as the down-regulation of aquaporin gene expression (Marples *et al.* 1995). Initially, lithium-induced diabetes insipidus is reversible on withdrawal, but it may eventually become irreversible, an indication of structural damage (Gitlin 1997; Markowitz *et al.* 2000).

Differential diagnosis

The differential diagnosis of lithium-induced nephrogenic diabetes insipidus comprises idiopathic diabetes insipidus, hypokalaemia, hypercalcaemia and chronic pyelonephritis. Iatrogenic causes include glibenclamide, cimetidine, fluvoxamine and antipsychotic medications. Neurogenic causes include ischaemia, trauma and neoplasia. The possibility of psychogenic polydipsia should be considered.

Two important tests for confirming the diagnosis of diabetes insipidus are the water deprivation test and the desmopressin (DDAVP) test. In the former, the patient is deprived of fluid over several hours and blood and urine specimens are collected for osmolality measurement. A rising plasma osmolality and failure to concentrate urine under these circumstances are consistent with diabetes insipidus. The desmopressin test, which immediately follows the water deprivation period, is performed by the administration of DDAVP. A rising plasma osmolality and failure to concentrate urine despite the administration of DDAVP and increasing plasma osmolality specifies that the diabetes insipidus is nephrogenic in origin (Smith *et al.* 1998). Clearly patients should be carefully observed for excessive fluid loss during the procedure.

Management

In mild, reversible cases, simple dose reduction or once daily dosing may provide adequate treatment. Alternative strategies include combination therapy or lithium substitution.

In severe cases of acute diabetes insipidus, referral to a renal physician is required. The initial priority is the restoration of water and electrolyte imbalance. The potential for lithium toxicity, neurological impairment and encephalopathy should be recognized.

In severe cases, with suitable precautions, thiazide diuretics may enhance lithium reabsorption in the proximal tubule, thereby reducing the concentration of lithium more distally (Lippmann *et al.* 1981). It should be noted, however, that the British National Formulary warns against prescribing lithium and thiazides together (British National Formulary 2002). Kosten and Forrest (1986) reported successful treatment using the potassium-sparing diuretic amiloride: clearly, there is a risk of hyperkalaemia, therefore electrolytes should be monitored closely. In refractory cases, hydrochlorothiazide may be used. If amiloride or hydrochlorothiazide are used, the dose of lithium should be reduced.

Risk factors

The risk of diabetes insipidus increases with duration of treatment, the requirement for polypharmacy and frequent admissions to hospital (Bendz *et al.* 1994). Lithium-induced polyuria is reportedly less frequent in once daily dosing (Bowen *et al.* 1991).

Prevention

Prevention of lithium-induced diabetes insipidus is not always possible. Patients should be warned about the condition and should remain vigilant for symptoms, especially thirst. The lowest therapeutic dose of lithium should be employed. Urine production should be monitored once yearly. If 24-hour urine volumes exceed four litres, then a change in treatment should be considered.

Renal impairment

Clinical features

Glomerular function is assessed by estimation of glomerular filtration rate (GFR). In health, it remains constant due to regulatory intra-renal mechanisms. Damage or loss of glomeruli results in a fall in GFR, potentially compromising waste elimination and fluid/electrolyte homeostasis. Renal impairment may progress to acute or chronic renal failure. Glomerular filtration rates can be measured in several ways. Serum creatinine is a crude measure of GFR as the linear relationship is skewed by muscle mass, extra-renal excretion of creatinine and other factors. GFR may fall substantially (up to 60 per cent) with almost no change in serum levels. Creatinine clearance and [51][Chromium] Ethylenediamine tetra-acetic acid clearance provide more accurate measurements.

Review of the literature concerning lithium-induced glomerular impairment is hindered by variations in patient characteristics and study methodology. Differences in duration of treatment, serum lithium concentrations, the method of assessment of glomerular function and study structure further frustrate comparison.

Given these limitations, it would appear that generally, lithium treatment is not associated with clinically significant decreases in glomerular filtration rates. In review of early studies (from 1979 to 1986) comprising over one thousand subjects on chronic lithium therapy, Boton *et al.* (1987) estimated that glomerular filtration rates were normal in 85 per cent of patients; the remaining 15 per cent showed only mild reduction in GFR.

Subsequent studies have been reviewed by Gitlin (1997) and will be considered briefly here. Most studies concurred with the optimistic findings of the previous review (Conte *et al.* 1989; Coskunol *et al.* 1997). However, Bendz *et al.* (1994) examined 142 patients in receipt of lithium therapy for at least 15 years. In comparison with control subjects, 21 per cent of patients had significantly reduced GFRs associated with higher urine volumes. Interestingly, this group of patients had previously been studied after six years of therapy: a smaller proportion (7 per cent) had a reduced GFR at that point, suggesting that prevalence of deterioration in glomerular rate (albeit to a clinically insignificant degree) increased with time. Gitlin also reviewed four longitudinal studies demonstrating decreased creatinine clearances or increased serum creatinine over time (Jorkasky *et al.* 1988; Hetmar *et al.* 1991; Kallner and Peterson 1995; Nilsson and Axelsson 1989). However, when the effects of ageing on creatinine were considered (Hetmar *et al.* 1991; Kallner and Peterson 1995) the difference in glomerular function was minimal. Regarding the effects of lithium discontinuation, Gitlin concluded that the bulk of the evidence supported no significant change in glomerular function (Vestergaard and Amidsen 1981; Hetmar *et al.* 1991; Bucht and Wahlin 1980; Bendz *et al.* 1996).

Turning to pathological studies, renal biopsies from patients on lithium therapy show chronic interstitial or tubulointerstitial nephropathy, but on the whole there is relative preservation of glomeruli (for example Hansen *et al.* 1979; Albrecht *et al.* 1980; Aurell *et al.* 1981). Furthermore the changes that are observed should be interpreted with caution as they are also found in non-lithium treated psychiatric patients (Walker *et al.* 1982).

Despite these encouraging findings from both physiological and pathological studies, more recent reports warn that lithium nephropathy inducing progressive renal failure does occur and may be under-recognized (Chugh and Yager 1997; Markowitz *et al.* 2000; Presne *et al.* 2002). This includes biopsy data indicating glomerular involvement in a selected group of patients (Markowitz *et al.* 2000). As considerable uncertainty remains regarding the prevalence of renal impairment, clinicians should remain alert to the potential for renal failure in patients on lithium treatment.

Acute renal failure, which may occur in the context of lithium toxicity, may present with acute oliguria, fluid retention and uraemia with associated anorexia, nausea and vomiting. Chronic renal failure may be asymptomatic in the early phases with insidious onset of thirst, polyuria, proteinuria and hypertension.

Pharmacological basis

Unknown.

Differential diagnosis

In addition to causes of pre-renal and post-renal failure, the differential diagnosis of renal insufficiency in context of lithium treatment includes chronic pyelonephritis, chronic effects of NSAIDS and other forms of drug intoxication, diabetes mellitus and sickle cell disease.

Management

In acute renal failure, a nephrology opinion should be sought. Lithium should be stopped and alternative treatment instituted. If treatment is required for bipolar patients, consider sodium valproate or olanzapine, although doses of both may be reduced in cases of chronic renal failure.

Risk factors

Risk factors for renal failure associated with lithium include long duration of therapy, concomitant use of other medications, episodes of lithium intoxication and pre-existing somatic disorders. A once-daily dosing regimen is thought to lessen nephrotoxic effects (Bowen *et al.* 1991).

Prevention

Before commencing lithium, a routine analysis of renal function should be undertaken including measurement of serum electrolytes, creatinine, and urine analysis plus blood urea nitrogen (see Table 6.3). During treatment, lithium levels should be carefully monitored and kept at the most optimal low level. Episodes of lithium toxicity should, of course, be avoided. Where possible, once daily dosing is recommended. Serum creatinine levels should be checked at least six monthly. Climbing serum creatinine levels, or levels greater than 140 mmol/L are significant.

Thyroid dysfunction

It is widely recognized that lithium affects thyroid function, most commonly precipitating hypothyroidism or goitre. However, there is also an association with hyperthyroidism and thyroiditis.

Clinical features

Lithium most commonly causes goitre and hypothyroidism. The lithium-induced goitre is usually smooth and uniformly enlarged. Symptoms of

Table 6.3 General measures on commencing lithium treatment

Establishment of diagnosis, the need for treatment and risk factors for side effects

Psychiatric, medical and family history and current/past medications

Consider comorbid disease (including substance misuse)

Exclude organic aetiology

History or family history of renal, thyroid, cardiac or neurological illness

Physical examination including blood pressure, baseline weight and examination of thyroid

FBC

Electrolytes, urea and creatinine, urinalysis and urine microscopy

Thyroid function tests and antithyroid antibodies

ECG if over 40 years of age

For women, plans for pregnancy

Consider other treatments

Alternative or adjunctive agents, psychotherapy, psychoeducation, occupational therapy
  and social support

Discussion with patient and family regarding diagnosis and treatment:

- The nature of psychiatric treatment
- The requirement for lithium
- The need for blood monitoring
- Anticipated side effects and their management
- Toxic effects and the need for urgent treatment
- For women, teratogenicity and the advisability of planned pregnancy

Danger periods

- Commencing new medications, (including 'over the counter' preparations)
- Abrupt withdrawal
- Coexisting or new physical illnesses especially dehydration
- Dietary change

Provide factsheets and use 'lithium cards'
Commencing lithium

Start at a low dose (e.g. Priadel 400 mg; less in the elderly)

Build up slowly

Measure lithium levels after five days then weekly until satisfactory
  blood levels are achieved

Review for efficacy and side effects at least monthly for first six months

Serum lithium levels every two months for first six months

Initial thyroid function tests (TSH) at three months

Ongoing monitoring

Assess efficacy and acceptability of treatment: is there established benefit?

Ask about side effects. Consider the use of questionnaires

Specifically, ask about thirst and symptoms of thyroid dysfunction

After first six months, perform serum lithium levels at least three monthly

Monitor thyroid function (TSH) six monthly

Monitor renal function: Urea, electrolytes and creatinine six monthly

NB Creatinine clearance and urinalysis are more sensitive measures of renal function than
  the monitoring of urea and creatinine only

24 hour urine volumes and serum/urine osmolality assessments six to twelve monthly,
  if indicated

Increased vigilance as patients age or with physical illnesses/new medications hypothyroidism may be subtle in mild cases, but include fatigue, cold intolerance, weight gain, deafness, goitre, dry skin and hair, menstrual irregularity and menorrhagia, poor libido, constipation, myalgia and arthralgia. Psychiatric symptoms such as memory disturbance, depression and psychosis may also occur.

Hypothyroidism is graded depending on thyroid function tests and the presence of symptoms. Overt hypothyroidism is defined by the presence of clinical symptoms and a low free thyroxine index or free thyroxine despite a high thyroid stimulating hormone (TSH) level. In subclinical hypothyroidism, a normal thyroxine level is found but serum thyroid stimulating hormone is raised. Symptomless thyroiditis is characterized by the presence of antithyroid antibodies, but normal thyroid function tests: it may later lead to overt hypothyroidism (Gordin and Lamberg 1981).

Subclinical hypothyroidism, biochemically defined above, can be accompanied by clinical symptoms associated with an underactive thyroid. In addition, alterations in lipid metabolism, cardiac function and menstrual cycle have been described with psychiatric symptoms such as lethargy, poor concentration and memory (for review, see Kleiner et al. 1999).

Rarely, lithium precipitates hyperthyroidism, which is evident in weight loss, increased appetite, restlessness, malaise, muscle weakness and tremor, choreoathetosis, breathlessness, palpitations, heat intolerance, vomiting and diarrhoea, menstrual disturbances, gynaecomastia and restlessness.

Incidence

Estimates of lithium-induced overt hypothyroidism in patients receiving long-term lithium treatment vary widely, from no cases of symptomatic illness to a 42 per cent incidence after fifteen years (Yassa et al. 1988; Bocchetta et al. 1991; Kirov 1998; Joffe and Levitt 1993; Stancer and Forbath 1989). A further 20 per cent develop subclinical hypothyroidism and up to 50 per cent develop goitres (Perrild et al. 1990). Unsurprisingly, antithyroid antibodies indicate increased risk of thyroid dysfunction: 50 per cent of lithium-treated patients with antithyroid antibodies have subclinical hypothyroidism (Bocchetta et al. 1991).

Thyroid dysfunction appears to occur relatively early in treatment. Vincent et al. (1993) reported that 74 per cent of cases of hypothyroidism developed in the first 2 years of treatment. Kirov (1998) found that 35 per cent of cases developed in the first two years and Yassa et al. (1988) reported that most cases occurred within the first four years. Increased rates of lithium-induced thyrotoxicosis have been reported in the literature (McDermott et al. 1986; Barclay et al. 1994; Kirov 1998) but definitive studies on incidence are required.

Pharmacological basis

Lithium is concentrated in the thyroid and has many effects on the HPT axis, summarized by Lazarus (1998). Amongst many, possible mechanisms include the modulation of TRH receptor expression (Sattin *et al.* 2002), reduction of iodine uptake in the thyroid (Burrow *et al.* 1971), inhibition of thyroid hormone secretion (Spaulding *et al.* 1972) and enhancement of peripheral conversion of thyroxine to the more active tri-iodothyronine (Terao *et al.* 1995). Reduction in thyroid hormone secretion and the compensatory increase in TSH release may precipitate goitre formation.

Other endocrine systems are also affected. For instance, elevated parathyroid hormone levels, mild hypercalcaemia and hypermagnesaemia are associated with long-term lithium use. Parathyroid adenomas and hyperplasia have been reported (Abdullah *et al.* 1999). These are often reversible on withdrawal, but surgical intervention may be necessary.

Differential diagnosis

Goitre may occur at puberty or in pregnancy, Grave's disease or Hashimoto's thyroiditis. It may be mistakenly diagnosed in the presence of a cyst, tumour, sarcoidosis or tuberculosis. The differential diagnosis of acquired hypothyroidism includes euthyroid sick syndrome, non-thyroidal illness, iodine deficiency, antithyroid drugs such as carbamazepine and phenytoin, autoimmune thyroiditis, post surgery or irradiation, neoplasia and hypopituitarism or peripheral resistance to thyroid hormone.

Management

In hypothyroidism, other possible reasons for abnormal thyroid tests should be considered (see above) before commencing treatment. Overt hypothyroidism should be treated with thyroxine. The use of thyroxine in subclinical hypothyroidism is controversial (Kleiner *et al.* 1999), but has been advocated where serum TSH levels are greater than 5–10 mU/L in the presence of symptoms, or greater than 10 mU/L in the asymptomatic. As thyroxine may aggravate angina or cardiac dysrhythmias, cardiac function should be assessed. When in doubt, a specialist endocrinology opinion should be sought.

Euthyroid or hypothyroid goitre tend to resolve on lithium withdrawal or the use of supplementary thyroxine.

Risk factors

Female sex, age greater than forty, the presence of thyroid autoantibodies and rapid cycling disorder are thought to be risk factors for hypothyroidism

(Cowdry *et al.* 1983; Emerson *et al.* 1973; Kirov 1998; Bauer *et al.* 1990) in addition to a family history of thyroid disease.

Prevention

All patients should be screened for thyroid dysfunction before and periodically during treatment, even if they are asymptomatic (see Table 6.3). Past medical history and family history should be ascertained. Laboratory tests should include thyroid stimulating hormone, thyroxine and anti-thyroglobulin measurements. TSH should be measured 3 months after initiation of treatment and then every six to twelve months. An elevated TSH level should be followed by measurement of free thyroxine (or the free thyroxine index).

Rebound mania and depression after withdrawal

Clinical features

Abrupt discontinuation of lithium prophylaxis may precipitate early manic recurrence and depressive episodes (Mander and Loudon 1988; Suppes *et al.* 1991). Goodwin (1994) suggested that this phenomenon may negate the benefits of treatment altogether and in consequence, lithium prophylaxis should be maintained for at least 24 months before an overall advantage is conferred. However, Schou (1993) disputed the existence of lithium rebound mania. He highlighted methodological weaknesses in several discontinuation studies, in particular the need to verify remission at the time of cessation. These criticisms are not applicable to all studies: in particular, Mander and Loudon (1988) conducted a scientifically rigorous study with convincing results.

It would appear that there is an earlier and greater risk of mania than of depression (Suppes *et al.* 1991). Mander and Loudon (1988) recorded a manic recurrence rate of 50 per cent in a group of 14 bipolar patients on lithium prophylaxis, beginning 13–19 days after cessation of treatment (mean 15 days). In a meta-analysis of bipolar (I) patients stopping lithium prophylaxis abruptly, an overall risk of recurrence of 50 per cent was found within five months of stopping treatment. Recurrence of mania was particularly rapid, with 50 per cent of episodes occurring within three months. It occurred in 25 per cent of patients within three months. There was a 22 per cent risk of suffering recurrence of depression within twelve months. The risk of depressive, but not manic, recurrence is also found in bipolar II patients (Faedda *et al.* 1993). Lithium discontinuation may result in the development of resistance to treatment (Post *et al.* 1992; Bauer 1994; Maj *et al.* 1995), although this possibility remains controversial and subject to dispute (Coryell *et al.* 1998).

To our knowledge, abrupt withdrawal of lithium has not been clearly associated with a physical withdrawal syndrome (Jefferson 2000).

Pharmacological basis

It has been postulated that the precipitation of mania on abrupt lithium withdrawal may result from a neurophysiological 'rebound' phenomenon (Lenox *et al.* 1998), but the basis of this 'rebound' phenomenon remains uncertain. It is not yet clear whether alternative bipolar prophylactic treatments also precipitate mania, although preliminary evidence indicates that carbamazepine may not (Macritchie and Hunt 2000). As sodium valproate is the most frequently prescribed mood stabilizer in the United States and is increasingly used in Europe, further, more methodologically rigorous investigation of the existence of anticonvulsant 'rebound' mania is required.

Differential diagnosis

The main differential diagnosis is that of recurrence of the index illness. In addition, delirium has been reported on cessation of lithium treatment (Wilkinson 1979).

Management

There are no specific case reports that can guide us, however, clinical experience and extrapolation from what is known about discontinuation symptoms with other drugs, especially antidepressants (see Chapter 10), suggests that the symptoms are rapidly reversed by restarting lithium. Alternatively rebound mania can be treated with an antipsychotic drug or rebound depression with an antidepressant. However one should consider the possibility of antidepressants inducing a manic switch or rapid cycling.

Risk factors for 'rebound' mania

Risk factors include abrupt discontinuation and bipolar I disorder. Intuitively, those who have suffered 'rebound' mania in the past seem at risk of repetition. It is unclear whether some lithium-responding patients are consistently unaffected by its withdrawal. It is possible that a subgroup exists of patients who are particularly susceptible to manic recurrence on cessation of lithium treatment. A small number of patients in the studies reviewed by Suppes *et al.* (1991) appear to have suffered a particularly early recurrence, within one week of withdrawal.

Prevention

Patients should be made aware of that abrupt discontinuation of treatment carries a high risk of manic recurrence. Gradual discontinuation of treatment (over four weeks) may lead to a lower rate of recurrence (Faedda *et al.* 1993).

Other adverse effects

Central nervous system

Fine tremor is one of the most frequent non-toxic side effects, reported in 34 per cent (Ghose 1977). It may be treated by dose reduction, split daily doses or the use of slow-release preparations or beta-blockers. It may be exacerbated by the use of tricyclic antidepressants. Extra-pyramidal side effects occur when lithium is used in combination with antipsychotics or in long-term treatment.

Cognitive impairment may occur. Ghose (1977) reported memory problems in 52 per cent of patients on long-term lithium treatment. Studies of healthy volunteers show decreases in ability to memorize, concentrate and learn (Judd 1979; Stip *et al.* 2000).

Skin

Skin complaints of various forms occur in lithium treatment. Carter (1972) first reported the association between lithium and psoriasis. Lithium-induced psoriasis is resistant to treatment but resolves after its discontinuation (Krahn and Goldberg 1994). In bipolar patients with psoriasis, alternative agents such as valproate or carbamazepine may be preferable.

Other cutaneous side effects include the exacerbation of acne, maculopapular and urticarial eruptions, warts, folliculitis, lupus-like syndrome, nail pigmentation and exfoliative dermatitis.

Hair loss has been reported, mainly in females (Mortimer and Dawber 1984). It occurs most frequently six months after commencement of lithium. Hair loss may be associated with hypothyroidism. Others report changes in hair texture (McCreadie and Farmer 1985).

Weight gain

Weight gain is a well-recognized adverse effect of lithium, although the underlying mechanism is unclear. On average, a weight gain of 10 kg in 6–10 years has been reported (Pijl and Meinders 1996). It is dose-related, more common in women, and in those who are already overweight (Ackermann and Nolan 1998; Pijl and Meinders 1996). It is a common cause of non-compliance. Patients should be aware of the potential for weight gain before commencing treatment. Options for treatment include dose reduction, implementing a weight loss programme or switching to another medication.

Conclusion

After fifty years, lithium remains a frequently prescribed, efficacious treatment, especially in affective disorders. Its mechanism of action continues to

Table 6.4 Adverse syndromes associated with lithium

1 Lithium is an efficacious treatment, especially in affective disorders, but has troublesome side effects and a narrow herapeutic index.
2 Lithium intoxication may occur at therapeutic serum levels and varies in presentation: it demands vigilance and immediate action.
3 Nephrogenic diabetes insipidus occurs frequently; glomerular impairment occurs less frequently, but its precise incidence is a matter of ongoing debate.
4 Hypothyroidism and goitre are the most frequent forms of thyroid dysfunction. The treatment of subclinical hypothyroidism is controversial, but may result in functional improvements.
5 'Rebound' mania and depression occurs on abrupt withdrawal of treatment and may negate the benefits of treatment altogether.
6 Other common side effects at therapeutic levels include tremor, cognitive impairment, skin disorders and weight gain. Many may be ameliorated using simple measures. All may affect quality of life and compliance and should be addressed sympathetically.
7 Patient education regarding diagnosis, need for treatment, anticipated side effects and toxic effects is of prime importance.
8 The elderly, children and those with concomitant illness require special care in the institution and ongoing provision of lithium therapy.

challenge psychopharmacologists. In clinical practice, decisions to initiate and maintain treatment must be based on careful consideration of the individual's pattern of illness, risk factors, adverse effects and benefits of treatment (see Table 6.4). Adverse syndromes associated with lithium can lead to permanent impairment (e.g. renal failure) and be potentially life threatening (e.g. lithium toxicity). Poor compliance, which is intimately linked to adverse effects, may negate the benefits of lithium treatment entirely due to the occurrence of 'rebound' mania. Appropriate prescribing, vigilance and regular review are the tenets of successful management.

Acknowledgements

The authors wish to thank Dr Alastair Durie, Wellcome Centre for the History of Medicine, University of Glasgow, for his help in researching the use of lithium in the nineteenth century, Ms Lindsey Ferrie for constructing Table 6.1, Mr Peter Gallagher for help in constructing Fig. 6.1 and Ms Anne Maule for assistance in preparing the manuscript.

Summary: Lithium toxicity

Definition	Lithium poisoning: this may be mild, moderate or severe. It may result in reversible or irreversible adverse effects outlined in Table 6.2 and in the text. It may occur in several contexts. It may occur acutely in the lithium-naive or during chronic treatment, perhaps due to a change in dose or the introduction of new medication.
	Chronic toxicity is insidious but potentially severe and occurs during long-term therapy.
Incidence	One study found that 6.8% of 2,210 patients admitted to a psychiatric hospital had serum levels of 1.5 mmol/L or higher; 27.8% had symptoms or signs of toxicity (Webb *et al.* 2001).
Drugs causing syndrome	Lithium. Possible drug interactions predisposing to toxicity include medications causing hyponatraemia e.g. frusemide, thiazide diuretics and some antidepressants through reduction in lithium clearance. Others include non-steroidal anti-inflammatory drugs, ACE inhibitors and antipsychotics, especially phenothiazines.
	Encephalopathy has been reported when lithium is co-prescribed with haloperidol.
Key symptoms	Mild, moderate and severe symptoms of lithium toxicity are outlined in Table 6.2. Mild neurological effects (tremor, fatigue and muscle weakness) and ECG. changes such as T wave flattening may occur in non-toxic conditions.
	NB Observation of symptom progression over time is of extreme importance. Serum lithium concentrations should not be used as the sole guide to the severity of poisoning. See text.
Pharmacological mechanism	Essentially unknown.
Investigations to confirm diagnosis	Lithium levels (but see text for warning regarding their interpretation).
	Renal function tests
	ECG
	Neurological examination and investigation.
	If delirious or unconscious, consider other contributory factors and investigate accordingly. E.g. consider neuroimaging.
Lithium overdose	Observe for at least 24 hours (or at least 48 hours if sustained release preparation used).
	Measure lithium level immediately and then repeatedly at 6–12 hour periods, depending on clinical presentation.

	Gastric lavage should be considered NB Sustained release tablets may block tube.
	Obtain advice from the Local Poisons Unit.
	Withdraw prescribed lithium if diagnosis established
	Consider using benzodiazepine during withdrawal period
Mild toxicity	Observe with attention to adequate hydration and electrolyte balance.
	Monitor cardiac function.
More severe toxicity	Haemodialysis is the treatment for severe lithium intoxication. Institute if levels are above 3 mmol/L, in cases of coma or shock, or if conservative measures have failed after 24 hours.
	See text for advice on lithium monitoring during dialysis.
	NB Forced diuresis is contraindicated.
	If unconscious, protect airway and ensure adequate ventilation.
	Correct hypovolaemia.
	Treat convulsions with intravenous or rectal diazepam or intubation
Further reading	Bailey B and McGuigan M (2000). Comparison of patients hemodialyzed for lithium poisoning and those for whom dialysis was recommended by PCC but not done: what lesson can we learn? *Clinical Nephrology* **54**, 388–92.
	Hansen HE and Amidsen A (1978). Lithium intoxication. *Quarterly Journal of Medicine* **47**, 123–44.
	Oakley PW, Whyte IM and Carter CL (2002). Lithium toxicity: an iatrogenic problem in susceptible individuals. *Australian and New Zealand Journal of Psychiatry* **35**, 833–40.
	Toxbase http://www.spib.axl.co.uk/Factsheets/14871-Factsheet.htm

Summary: Diabetes insipidus

Definition	Failure of antidiuretic hormone dependent urine concentration by the kidney resulting in the persistent excretion of excessive quantities of urine of low specific gravity. Neurogenic diabetes insipidus results from an inadequate production of antidiuretic hormone by the

	pituitary gland. In nephrogenic diabetes insipidus, there is a failure of urine concentration in the collecting ducts of the nephron.
Incidence	Estimation of incidence undermined by variations in methods of diagnosis. Estimates range from 15–87%.
Drugs causing syndrome	Lithium
Key symptoms	Polyuria, polydipsia
	Marked dehydration
	Associated risk of lithium toxicity and encephalopathy.
Pharmacological mechanism	Lithium-induced diabetes insipidus predominantly nephrogenic in origin. Possible mechanisms include a reduction in ADH sensitivity through adenyl cyclase and cyclic adenosine monophosphate systems within the tubular cells and down-regulation of aquaporin gene expression.
Investigation to confirm diagnosis	Water deprivation test and the desmopressin test
Management	Mild, reversible cases, can be treated with lithium dose reduction, combination therapy or lithium substitution. In severe cases, referral to renal physician is mandatory for restoration of water and electrolyte imbalance.
	Thiazide diuretics may be efficacious, but should be used under expert guidance only.
Further reading	Bendz A and Aurell M (1999). Drug-induced diabetes insipidus: incidence, prevention and management. *Drug Safety* **21**, 449–56.

Summary: Renal impairment

Definition	Deterioration in glomerular filtration rate through damage to or loss of glomeruli, potentially compromising fluid/electrolyte homeostasis and elimination of waste.
Incidence	Considerable uncertainty remains regarding its incidence (see text).
Key psychotropic drugs causing syndrome	Lithium especially in combination with other medications that may result in lithium toxicity.
Key symptoms and features	
Acute renal failure	(e.g. in acute lithium toxicity): acute oliguria, fluid retention, uraemia associated with nausea, vomiting and anorexia.

Chronic renal failure	May be asymptomatic in the early phases with insidious onset of thirst, polyuria, proteinuria and hypertension.
Pharmacological mechanism	The mechanism of renal cell death is essentially unknown.
Investigation to confirm diagnosis	Serum urea and creatinine (crude measure of glomerular filtration rate)
	Creatinine clearance
	Nephrology referral for further investigations.
Management	Seek nephrology opinion, especially in acute renal failure.
	Institute alternative treatment e.g. valproate or olanzapine for bipolar patients.
Further reading	Boton R, Gavina M, and Battle DC (1987). Prevalence, pathogenesis, and treatment of renal dysfunction associated with chronic lithium therapy. *American Journal of Kidney Disease* **10**, 329–345.
	Gitlin M (1997). Lithium and the kidney: an updated review. *Drug Safety* **20**, 231–243.
	Markowitz GS, Kambham N, Maruyama S, *et al.* (2000). Membranous glomerulopathy with Bowman's capsular and tubular basement membrane deposits. *Clinical Nephrology* **54**, 478–486.
	Lithium nephrotoxicity: a progressive combined glomerular and tubulointerstitial nephropathy. *Journal of the American Society of Nephrology* **11**, 1439–1448.

Summary: Thyroid dysfunction

Definition	Hypothyroidism, in the overt form, is defined by the presence of clinical symptoms and a low serum free thyroxine index or free thyroxine despite high TSH levels. Subclinical hypothyroidism: a normal thyroxine level, but increased TSH.
	Goitre (thyroid enlargement).
	See text for other rarer forms of lithium-associated thyroid dysfunction.
Incidence	Variation in figures for incidence.
	Lithium-induced clinical hypothyroidism: 0–42% after 15 years of treatment.
	20% develop subclinical hypothyroidism.
	Goitres: up to 50%.
Drugs causing syndrome	Lithium.

Key symptoms	Lithium-induced goitre is usually smooth and uniformly enlarged.
	Symptoms of hypothyroidism may be subtle in mild cases:
	Fatigue, cold intolerance, weight gain, deafness, goitre, dry skin, menstrual irregularity and menorrhagia, poor libido, constipation, myalgia and arthralgia. Depression and rarely, psychosis.
Pharmacological mechanism	Many proposed mechanisms, including modulation of TRH receptor expression, reduction of iodine reuptake and inhibition of thyroid hormone secretion.
Investigation to confirm diagnosis	Thyroid function tests including thyroid stimulating hormone, free thyroxine index or free thyroxine.
	Anti-thyroglobulin measurement.
	If thyroid enlargement is multinodular or there is a single nodule then it may require thyroid imaging.
Management	Overt hypothyroidism requires treatment with thyroxine.
	Thyroxine prescription in subclinical hypothyroidism controversial.
	If other medical complications (e.g. angina, dysrhythmias) then refer to endocrinologist.
	Euthyroid or hypothyroid goitres tend to resolve on lithium withdrawal or use of supplementary thyroxine.
Further reading	Lazarus JH (1998). The effects of lithium therapy on thyroid and thyrotropin-releasing hormone. *Thyroid* **8**, 909–913.
	Kleiner J, Altshuler L, Hendrick V, *et al*. (1999). Lithium-induced subclinical hypothyroidism: review of the literature and guidelines for treatment. *Journal of Clinical Psychiatry* **60**, 249–255.

Summary: Rebound mania and depression after withdrawal

Definition	Recurrence of episode of mania or depression following withdrawal of lithium prophylaxis.
Incidence	Estimates vary (see text).
	In one meta-analysis, overall risk of 50% recurrence of any episode within 5 months of stopping treatment in bipolar I patients. Recurrence of mania particularly rapid: 50% within three months of cessation.
Drugs causing syndrome	Lithium. Unclear whether anticonvulsant mood stabilizers exhibit similar effects.

Key symptoms	As above. Physical withdrawal syndrome not reported.
Pharmacological mechanism	Pharmacological basis remains unknown.
Investigation to confirm diagnosis	Clinical examination is the mainstay of diagnostic confirmation in these cases.
Management	Preventative: gradual withdrawal, if necessary.
	Patient education re. increased risk of manic depression on abrupt cessation.
Further reading	Goodwin G (1994). Recurrence of mania after lithium withdrawal. Implications for the use of lithium in the treatment of bipolar affective disorder. *British Journal of Psychiatry* **164**, 149–152.
	Mander AJ and Loudon JB (1988). Rapid recurrence of mania following abrupt discontinuation of lithium. *Lancet* **2**, 15–17.
	Suppes T, Baldessarini RJ, Faedda GL *et al.* (1991). Risk of recurrence following discontinuation of lithium treatment in bipolar disorder. *Archives of General Psychiatry* **48**, 1082–1088.

References

Abdullah H, Bliss R, Guinea AI, *et al.* (1999). Pathology and outcome of surgical treatment for lithium-associated hyperparathyroidism. *Br J Surg*, **86**, 91–3.

Ackermann S and Nolan LJ (1998). Bodyweight gain induced by psychtropic drugs: incidence, mechanisms and management. *CNS Drugs*, **9**, 135–51.

Ahluwalia P and Singhal RL (1984). Comparison of the changes in central catecholamine systems following short and long term lithium treatment and the consequences of lithium withdrawal. *Neuropsychobiology*, **12**, 217–23.

Albrecht J, Kampf D, and Muller-Oerlinghausen B (1980). Renal function and biopsy in patients on lithium-therapy. *Pharmakopsychiatrica Neuropsychopharmakologica*, **13** (4), 228–34.

Amidsen A (1975). Monitoring lithium treatment through determination of lithium concentration. *Dan Med Bull*, **22**, 277–91.

Antonelli T, Ferioli V, Lo Gallo G, *et al.* (2000). Differential effects of acute and short-term lithium administration on dialysate glutamate and GABA levels in the frontal cortex of the conscious rat. *Synapse*, **38**, 355–62.

Atherton JC, Doyle A, Gee A, *et al.* (1991). Lithium clearance: modification by the loop of Henle in man. *J Physiol*, **437**, 377–91.

Aurell M, Svalander C, Wallin L, *et al.* (1981). Renal function and biopsy findings in patients on long-term lithium treatment. *Kidney Int*, **20**, 663–70.

Austin M-P, Souza FGM, and Goodwin GM (1991). Lithium augmentation in antidepressant resistant patients. A quantitative analysis. *Br J Psychiatry*, **159**, 510–14.

Bailey B and McGuigan M (2000). Comparison of patients hemodialyzed for lithium poisoning and those for whom dialysis was recommended by PCC but not done: what lesson can we learn? *Clin Nephrol*, **54**, 388–92.

Baptista T, Teneud L, Contreras Q, *et al.* (1993). Effects of acute and chronic lithium treatment on amphetamine-induced dopamine increase in the nucleus accumbens and prefrontal cortex in rats as studied by microdialysis. *J Neural Transm*, **94**, 75–89.

Barclay ML, Brownlie BE, Turner JG, *et al.* (1994). Lithium associated thyrotoxicosis: a report of 14 cases, with statistical analysis of incidence. *Clin Endocrinol*, **40**, 759–64.

Bauer MS, Whybrow PC, and Winokur A (1990). Rapid cycling bipolar affective disorder. I. Association with grade I hypothyroidism. *Arch Gen Psychiatry*, **47**, 427–32.

Bauer M (1994). Refractoriness induced by lithium discontinuation despite adequate serum lithium levels. *Am J Psychiatry*, **151** (10), 1522.

Bell AJ, Cole A, Eccleston D, *et al.* (1993). Lithium neurotoxicity at normal therapeutic levels. *Br J Psychiatry*, **162**, 689–92.

Belmaker RH, Agam G, van Calker D, *et al.* (1998). Behavioral reversal of lithium effects by four inositol isomers correlates perfectly with biochemical effects on the PI cycle: depletion by chronic lithium of brain inositol is specific to hypothalamus, and inositol levels may be abnormal in postmortem brain from bipolar patients. *Neuropsychopharmacology*, **19**, 220–32.

Bendz H, Aurell M, Balldin J, *et al.* (1994). Kidney damage in long-term lithium patients: a cross-sectional study of patients with 15 years or more on lithium. *Nephrol Dial Transplant*, **9**, 250–4.

Bendz A and Aurell M (1999). Drug-induced diabetes insipidus: incidence, prevention and management. *Drug Saf*, **21**, 449–56.

Bendz H, Sjodin I, and Aurell M (1996). Renal function on and off lithium in patients treated with lithium for 15 years or more. A controlled, prospective lithium-withdrawal study. *Nephrol Dial Transplant*, **11**, 57–60.

Berridge MJ and Irvine RF (1989). Inositol phosphates and cell signalling. *Nature*, **341**, 197–205.

Bitran JA, Manji HK, Potter WZ, *et al.* (1995). Down-regulation of PKC alpha by lithium *in vitro*. *Psychopharmacol Bull*, **31**, 449–52.

Blier P and de Montigny C (1985). Short-term lithium administration enhances serotonergic neurotransmission: electrophysiological evidence in rat CNS. *Eur J Pharmacol*, **113**, 69–77.

Bocchetta A, Bernardi F, Bedditzi M, *et al.* (1991). Thyroid abnormalities during lithium treatment. *Acta Psychiatr Scand*, **83**, 193–8.

Boshes RA, Manschreck TC, Desrosiers J, *et al.* (2001). Initiation of clozapine therapy in a patient with pre-existing leukopenia: a discussion of the rationale of current treatment options. *Ann Clin Psychiatry*, **13**, 233–7.

Boton R, Gavina M, and Battle DC (1987). Prevalence, pathogenesis, and treatment of renal dysfunction associated with chronic lithium therapy. *Am J Kidney Dis*, **10**, 329–45.

Bowen RC, Grof P, and Grof E (1991). Less frequent lithium administration and lower urine volume. *Am J Psychiatry*, **148**, 189–92.

British National Formulary (2002). *Section 423 Antimanic Drugs: Interactions*. No 44, September, 189. London: British Medical Association.

Bucht G and Wahlin A (1980). Renal concentrating capacity in long-term lithium treatment and after withdrawal of lithium. *Acta Med Scand*, **207**, 309–14.

Burrow GN, Burke WR, Himmelhoch JM, *et al.* (1971). Effect of lithium on thyroid function. *J Clin Endocrinol*, **32**, 647–52.

Cade JFJ (1949). Lithium salts in the treatment of psychotic excitement. *Med J Australia*, **36**, 349–52.

Carli M, Morissette M, Herbert C, *et al.* (1997). Effects of a chronic lithium treatment on central dopamine neurotransporters. *Biochem Pharmacol*, **54**, 391–7.

Carter TN (1972). The relationship of lithium carbonate to psoriasis. *Psychosomatics*, **13**, 325–7.

Chang MC, Grange E, Rabin O, *et al.* (1996). Lithium decreases turnover of arachidonate in several brain phospholipids. *Neurosci Lett*, **220**, 171–4.

Chen G, Masana MI, and Manji HK (2000). Lithium regulates PKC-mediated intracellular cross-talk and gene expression in the CNS *in vivo. Bipolar Disord*, **2** (3 pt 2), 217–36.

Christiansen S, Kusano E, Yusufi ANK, *et al.* (1985). Pathogenesis of nephrogenic diabetes insipidus due to chronic administration of lithium in rats. *J Clin Invest*, **75**, 1869–79.

Chuang DM, Cheng RW, Chalecka-Franaszek E, *et al.* (2002). Neuroprotective effects of lithium in cultured cells and animal models of diseases. *Bipolar Disord*, **4**, 129–36.

Chugh S and Yager H (1997). End-stage renal disease after treatment with lithium. *J Clin Psychopharmacol*, **17**, 495–7.

Colburn RW, Goodwin FK, Bunney WE, *et al.* (1967). Effect of lithium on the uptake of noradrenaline by synaptosomes. *Nature*, **215**, 1395–7.

Conte G, Vazzola A, and Sacchetti E (1989). Renal function in chronic lithium-treated patients. *Acta Psychiatr Scand*, **79**, 503–4.

Cookson J (1998). Mania, bipolar disorder and treatment. In *Seminars in General Adult Psychiatry Volume 1*, G Stein and G Wilkinson (ed.). Gaskell: London.

Coppen A (1996). Biological psychiatry in Britain. In *The Psychopharmacologists. Interviews by Dr David Healy*, pp. 265–86. Altman, Chapman and Hall: New York.

Correa F and Eiser A (1992). Angiotensin converting enzyme inhibitors and lithium toxicity. *Am J Med*, **93**, 108–9.

Coryell W, Solomon D, Leon AC, *et al.* (1998). Lithium discontinuation and subsequent effectiveness. *Am J Psychiatry*, **155**, 895–8.

Cokunol H, Vahip S, Dorhout Mees E, *et al.* (1997). Renal side-effects of long-term lithium treatment. *J Affect Disorders*, **43**, 5–10.

Cowdry RW, Wehr TA, Zis AP, *et al.* (1983). Thyroid abnormalities associated with rapid-cycling bipolar illness. *Arch Gen Psychiatry*, **40**, 414–20.

Dixon JF and Hokin LE (1998). Lithium acutely inhibits and chronically up-regulates and stabilizes glutamate uptake by presynaptic nerve endings in mouse cerebral cortex. *Proc Nat Acad Sci USA*, **94**, 8363–8.

Dousa TP (1974). Interaction of lithium with vasopressin-sensitive cyclic AMP system of the human renal medulla. *Endocrinology*, **9** (S), 1359–66.

Dunigan CD and Shamoo AE (1995). Li + stimulates ATP-regulated dopamine uptake in PC12 cells. *Neuroscience*, **65**, 1–4.

Dziedzicka-Wasylewska M, Mackowiak M, Fijar K, *et al.* (1996). Adaptive changes in the rat dopaminergic transmission following repeated lithium administration. *J Neural Transm*, **103**, 765–76.

Emerson CH, Dyson WL, and Utiger RD (1973). Serum thyrotropin and thyroxine concentrations in patients receiving lithium carbonate. *J Clin Endocrinol Metab*, **36**, 338–46.

Faedda GL, Tondo L, Baldessarinini RJ, *et al.* (1993). Outcome after rapid vs gradual discontinuation of lithium treatment in bipolar disorders. *Arch Gen Psychiatry*, **50**, 448–55.

Fagiolini A, Buysse DJ, Frank E, *et al.* (2001). Tolerability of combined treatment with lithium and paroxetine in patients with bipolar disorder and depression. *J Clin Psychopharmacol*, **21**, 474–8.

Feinmann C and Peatfield R (1993). Orofacial neuralgia. Diagnosis and treatment guidelines. *Drugs*, **46**, 263–8.

Follezou J and Bleisel J (1985). Reduction of temperature and lithium poisoning. *New Engl J Med*, **313**, 1609.

Friedman E and Gershon S (1973). Effects of lithium on brain dopamine. *Nature*, **243**, 520–1.

Friedman E, Haou Yan W, Levinson D, *et al.* (1993). Altered platelet protein kinase C activity in bipolar affective disorder, manic episode. *Biol Psychiatry*, **33**, 520–5.

Friedrich MJ (1999). Lithium: proving its mettle for 50 years. *JAMA*, **281**, 2271–3.

Gende OA (2000). Lithium opens store-operated channels in human platelets. *Biochem Biophys Res Commun*, **267**, 546–50.

Ghose K (1977). Lithium salts: therapeutic and unwanted effects. *Br J Hosp Med*, **18**, 578–83.

Gille M, Ghariani S, Pieret F, *et al.* (1997). Acute encephalomyopathy and persistent cerebellar syndrome after lithium salt and haloperidol poisoning. *Revue Neurologique* (Paris), **153**, 268–70.

Gitlin M (1997). Lithium and the kidney: an updated review. *Drug Saf*, **20**, 231–43.

Goldberg H, Clayman P, and Skorecki K (1988). Mechanism of Li inhibition of vasopressin-sensitive adenylate cyclase in cultured renal epithelial cells. *Am J Physiol*, **255** (5 pt 2), F995–1002.

Goodwin FK and Jamison KR (1990). *Manic-depressive Illness*. Oxford University Press: New York.

Goodwin G (1994). Recurrence of mania after lithium withdrawal. Implications for the use of lithium in the treatment of bipolar affective disorder. *Br J Psychiatry*, **164**, 149–52.

Gordin A and Lamberg BA (1981). Spontaneous hypothyroidism in symptomless auto-immune thyroiditis. A long-term follow-up study. *Clin Endocrinol*, **15**, 537–43.

Granoff AL and Davis JM (1978). Heat illness syndrome and lithium intoxication. *J Clin Psychiatry*, **39**, 103–7.

Green ST and Dunn FG (1988). Severe leucopenia in fatal lithium poisoning. *BMJ*, **290**, 517.

Greenspan K, Aronoff MS, and Bogdanski DF (1970). Effects of lithium carbonate on turnover and metabolism of norepinephrine in the rat brain—correlation to gross behavioural effects. *Pharmacology*, **3**, 129–36.

Hagman A, Arnman K, and Ryden L (1979). Syncope caused by lithium treatment. *Acta Med Scand*, **205**, 467–71.

Hallcher LM and Sherman WR (1980). The effects of lithium ion and other agents on the activity of myo-inositol-1-phosphatase from bovine brain. *J Biol Chem*, **255**, 10896–901.

Hansen HE and Amidsen A (1978). Lithium intoxication. *Q J Med*, **47**, 123–44.

Hansen HE, Hestbech J, Sorensen JL, *et al.* (1979). Chronic interstitial nephropathy in patients on long-term lithium treatment. *Q J Med*, **48**, 577–91.

Hayslett JO and Kashgarian M (1979). A micropuncture study of the renal handling of lithium. *Pflugers Arch*, **380**, 159–63.

Hetmar O, Povlsen UJ, Ladefoged J, *et al.* (1991). Lithium: long-term effects on the kidney. A prospective follow-up study ten years after kidney biopsy. *Br J Psychiatry*, **158**, 153–8.

Hokin LE, Dixon JF, and Los GV (1996). A novel action of lithium: Stimulation of glutamate release and inositol 1,4,5 triphosphate accumulation via activation of the N-Metyl D-Aspartate receptor in monkey and mouse cerebral cortex slices. *Adv Enzyme Regu*, **36**, 229–44.

Hokin-Neaverson M and Jefferson JW (1989). Deficient erythrocyte Na, K-ATPase in different affective states in bipolar affective disorder and normalization by lithium therapy. *Neuropsychobiology*, **22**, 18–25.

Jefferson JW (2000). Lithium. In MNG Dukes and JK Aronson (ed.) *Meyler's Side Effects of Drugs*, 14th edn. Elsevier Science: Amsterdam.

Joffe RT and Levitt AJ (1993). The thyroid and depression. In *The Thyroid Axis and Psychiatric Illness*, RT Joffe and AJ Levitt (ed.), American Psychiatric Press: Washington, DC.

Johnston BB, Naylor GJ, Dick EG, *et al.* (1980). Prediction of course of bipolar manic-depressive illness treated with lithium. *Psychol Med*, **10**, 329–34.

Jope RS (1979). Effects of lithium treatment *in vitro* and *in vivo* on acetylcholine metabolism in rat brain. *J Neurochem*, **33**, 487–95.

Jorkasky DK, Amsterdam JD, Oler J, *et al.* (1988). Lithium-induced renal disease: a prospective study. *Clin Nephrol*, **30**, 293–302.

Judd LL (1979). Effect of lithium on mood, cognition, and personality function in normal subjects. *Arch Gen Psychiatry*, **20**, 36 (8 Spec No), 860–6.

Julien J, Valient JM, Lagueny A, *et al.* (1979). Myopathy and cerebellar syndrome during acute poisoning with lithium carbonate. *Muscle Nerve*, **2**, 240.

Kallner G and Peterson U (1995). Renal, thyroid and parathyroid function during lithium treatment: laboratory tests in 207 people treated for 1–30 years. *Acta Psychiatr Scand*, **91**, 48–51.

Kameda K, Miura J, Suzuki K, *et al.* (2001). Effects of lithium on dopamine D_2 receptor expression in the rat brain striatum. *J Neural Transm*, **108**, 321–34.

Katz RI, Chase TN, and Kopin IJ (1968). Evoked release of norepinephrine and serotonin from brain slices: inhibition by lithium. *Science*, **162**, 466–7.

Kirov G (1998). Thyroid disorders in lithium-treated patients. *J Affec Disorders*, **50**, 33–40.

Klein PS and Melton DA (1996). A molecular mechanism for the effect of lithium on development. *Proc Nat Acad Sci USA*, **93**, 8455–9.

Kleiner J, Altshuler L, Hendrick V, *et al.* (1999). Lithium-induced subclinical hypothyroidism: review of the literature and guidelines for treatment. *J Clin Psychiatry*, **60**, 249–55.

Kosten TN and Forrest JN (1986). Treatment of severe lithium-induced polyuria with amiloride. *Am J Psychiatry*, **143**, 1563–8.

Krahn LE and Goldberg RL (1994). Psychotropic medications and the skin. In *Psychotropic Drug Use in the Medically Ill*, vol. 21, PA Silver (ed.), pp. 90–106. S Karger AG: Basel.

Lazarus JH (1998). The effects of lithium therapy on thyroid and thyrotropin-releasing hormone. *Thyroid*, **8**, 909–13.

Lenox RH, McNamara RK, Papke RL, *et al.* (1998). Neurobiology of lithium: an update. *J Clin Psychiatry*, **59** (Suppl. 6), 37–47.

Lerer B and Stanley M (1985). Effect of chronic lithium on cholinergically mediated responses and 3H-QNB binding in rat brain. *Brain Res*, **244**, 211–19.

Levenson JL and Dwight M (2000). Cardiology. In *Psychiatric Care of the Medical Patient*, A Stoudemire, BS Fogel, and DB Greenberg (ed.), p. 724. Oxford University Press: New York.

Lippmann S, Wagemaker H, and Tucker D (1981). A practical approach to management of lithium concurrent with hyponatremia, diuretic therapy and/or chronic renal failure. *J Clin Psychiatry*, **42**, 304–6.

McCance SL, Cohen PR, and Cowen PJ (1989). Lithium increases 5-HT-mediated prolactin release. *Psychopharmacology*, **99**, 276–81.

McCreadie RG and Farmer JG (1985). Lithium and hair texture. *Acta Psychiatr Scand*, **72**, 387–8.

McCreadie RG and Morrison DP (1985). The impact of lithium in South-West Scotland: I. Demographic and clinical findings. *Br J Psychiatry*, **146**, 70–4.

McDermott MT, Burman KD, Hofeldt FD, *et al.* (1986). Lithium-associated thyrotoxicosis. *Am J Med*, **80**, 1245–8.

Macritchie KAN and Hunt NJ (2000). Does 'rebound mania' occur after stopping carbamazepine? A pilot study. *J Psychopharmacol*, **14**, 266–8.

Mai L, Jope RS, and Li X (2002). BDNF-mediated signal transduction is modulated by GSK3B and mood stabilizing agents. *J Neurochem*, **82**, 75–83.

Maj M, Pirozzi R, and Magliano L (1995). Nonresponse to reinstituted lithium prophylaxis in previously responsive bipolar patients: prevalence and predictors. *Am J Psychiatry*, **152**, 1810–11.

Mander AJ and Loudon JB (1988). Rapid recurrence of mania following abrupt discontinuation of lithium. *Lancet*, **2**, 15–17.

Manji HK and Lenox RH (1999). Ziskind-Somerfeld Research Award. Protein kinase C signalling in the brain: molecular transduction of mood stabilization in the treatment of manic-depressive illness. *Biol Psychiatry*, **46**, 1328–51.

Manji HK, Moore GJ, and Chen G (2001). Bipolar disorder: leads from molecular and cellular mechanisms of action of mood stabilizers. *Br J Psychiatry*, (Suppl. 41), 107–19.

Manji HK and Rapaport MH (2001). The effects of lithium on *ex vivo* cytokine production. *Biol Psychiatry*, **50**, 217–24.

Markowitz GS, Radhakrishnan J, Kambham N, *et al.* (2000). Lithium nephrotoxicity: a progressive combined glomerular and tubulointerstitial nephropathy. *J Am Soc Nephrol*, **11**, 1439–48.

Marples D, Christensen S, Ilso Christensen E, *et al.* (1995). Lithium induced down-regulation of aquaporin–2 expression in rat kidney medulla. *J Clin Invest*, **95**, 1838–45.

Mekler G and Woggon B (1997). A case of serotonin syndrome caused by venlafaxine and lithium. *Pharmacopsychiatry*, **30**, 272–3.

Moore CM, Demopulos CM, Henry ME, *et al*. (2002). Brain-to-serum lithium ratio and age: an *in vivo* magnetic resonance spectroscopy study. *Am J Psychiatry*, **159**, 1240–2.

Mortimer PS and Dawber RP (1984). Hair loss and lithium. *Int J Dermatol*, **23**, 603–4.

Moscovich DG, Belmaker RH, Agam G, *et al*. (1990). Inositol-1-phosphatase in red blood cells of manic-depressive patients before and during treatment with lithium. *Biol Psychiatry*, **27**, 552–5.

Motohashi N (1992). GABA receptor alterations after chronic lithium administration. Comparison with carbamazepine and sodium valproate. *Progress in Neuropsychopharmacol Biol Psychiatry*, **16**, 571–9.

Mukherjee S (1993). Combined ECT and lithium therapy. *Convuls Ther*, **9**, 274–84.

Nilsson A and Axelsson R (1989). Effects of long-term lithium treatment on thyroid and renal function (serum creatinine and maximal urine osmolality)—a prospective study in psychiatric patients. *Curr Therapeut Res*, **46**, 85–102.

Normann C, Brandt C, Berger M, *et al*. (1998). Delirium and persistent dyskinesia induced by a lithium-neuroleptic interaction. *Pharmacopsychiatry*, **31**, 201–4.

Oakley PW, Whyte IM, and Carter CL (2002). Lithium toxicity: an iatrogenic problem in susceptible individuals. *Aust NZ J Psychiatry*, **35**, 833–40.

Okusa MD and Crystal LJT (1994). Clinical manifestations and management of acute lithium intoxication. *Am J Med*, **97**, 383–9.

Otero-Losada ME and Rubio MC (1985). Striatal dopamine and motor activity changes observed shortly after lithium administration. *N-S Arch Pharmacol*, **330**, 169–74.

Palileo EV, Coehlo A, Westveer S, *et al*. (1983). Persistent sinus node dysfunction secondary to lithium therapy. *Am Heart J*, **106**, 1443–4.

Pamphlett RS and Mackenzie RA (1982). Severe peripheral neuropathy due to lithium intoxication. *J Neurol Neurosurg Psychiatry*, **45**, 656.

Perrild H, Hegedus L, Baastrup PC, *et al*. (1990). Thyroid function and ultrasonically determined thyroid size in patients receiving long-term lithium treatment. *Am J Psychiatry*, **147** (11), 1518–21.

Pijl H and Meinders AE (1996). Bodyweight change as an adverse effect of drug treatment: mechanism and management. *Drug Saf*, **14**, 329–42.

Posner L and Mokrzycki MH (1996). Transient central diabetes insipidus in the setting of underlying chronic nephrogenic diabetes insipidus associated with lithium use. *Am J Nephrol*, **16**, 339–43.

Post RM, Leverich GS, Altshuler L, *et al*. (1992). Lithium-discontinuation-induced refractoriness: preliminary observations. *Am J Psychiatry*, **149**, 1727–9.

Presne C, Fakhouri F, Kenouch S, *et al*. (2002). Progressive renal failure caused by lithium nephropathy. *Presse Medi*, **31**, 828–33.

Price LH, Charney DS, Delgado PL, *et al*. (1990). Lithium and serotonin function: implications for the serotonin hypothesis of depression. *Psychopharmacology*, **100**, 3–12.

Rintala J, Seemann R, Chandrasekaran K, *et al*. (1999). An arachidonic acid-specific 85 kDA cytosolic phospholipase A2 is a target for chronic lithium in rat brain. *Neuroreport*, **10**, 3887–90.

Ryves WJ and Harwood AJ (2001). Lithium inhibits glycogen synthase kinase-3 by competition for magnesium. *Biochem Biophys Res Commun*, **280**, 720–5.

Sachs GS, Printz DJ, Kahn DA, *et al.* (2000). The Expert Consensus Guideline Series: Medication Treatment of Bipolar Disorder 2000. *Postgraduate Medicine* April Spec. no. 1–104.

Sadosty AT, Groleau GA, and Atcherson MM (1999). The use of lithium levels in the emergency department. *J Emerg Med*, **17**, 887–91.

Sandyk R and Hurwitz MD (1983). Toxic irreversible encephalopathy induced by lithium carbonate and haloperidol. A report of 2 cases. *SAMJ*, **64**, 875–6.

Sattin A, Senanayake SS, and Pekary AE (2002). Lithium modulates expression of TRH receptors and TRH-related peptides in rat brain. *Neuroscience*, **115**, 263–73.

Schou M (1984). Long-lasting neurological sequelae after lithium intoxication. *Acta Psychiatr Scand*, **70**, 594–602.

Schou M (1993). Is there a lithium withdrawal syndrome? An examination of the evidence. *Br J Psychiatry*, **163**, 514–18.

Sellers J, Tyrer P, Whiteley A, *et al.* (1982). Neurotoxic effects of lithium with delayed rise in serum lithium levels. *Br J Psychiatry*, **140**, 623–5.

Semba J, Wantanabe H, Suhara T, *et al.* (2000). Chronic lithium chloride injection increases glucocorticoid receptor but not mineralocorticoid receptor mRNA expression in rat brain. *Neurosci Res*, **38**, 313–19.

Sheard MH, Marini JL, Bridges CI, *et al.* (1976). The effect of lithium on impulsive aggressive behaviour in man. *Am J Psychiatry*, **133**, 1409–13.

Sheean GL (1991). Lithium neurotoxicity. *Clin Exp Neurol*, **28**, 112–27.

Shiah I-S and Yatham LN (2000). Serotonin in mania and in the mechanism of action of mood stabilizers: a review of clinical studies. *Bipolar Disorders*, **2**, 77–92.

Shoemaker JV (1891). Lithium. In *Materia Medica and Therapeutics with Especial Reference to the Clinical Application of Drugs. Volume II of a Treatise on Materia Medica, Pharmacology and Therapeutics*, FA Davis (ed.), p. 728. FA Davis: Philadelphia and London.

Slotkin TA, Seidler FJ, Whitmore WL, *et al.* (1980). Release of [3H] norepinephrine from synaptic vesicles isolated from rat brain after the intracisternal administration of [3H] norepinephrine: influence of nucleotides, ions and drugs, and destabilization of transmitter storage caused by acute and chronic lithium administration. *Neuroscience*, **5**, 753–62.

Small JG, Kellams JJ, Milstein V, *et al.* (1980). Complications with electroconvulsive treatment combined with lithium. *Biol Psychiatry*, **15**, 103–12.

Smith, AF, Beckett GJ, Walker GJ, *et al.* (1998). Renal disease. Tests of tubular function P57. In *Lecture Notes in Clinical Biochemistry*, 6th edn, AF Smith, GJ Beckett, GJ Walker *et al.* Blackwell Science: Edinburgh.

Spaulding SW, Burrow GN, Bermudez F, *et al.* (1972). The inhibitory effect of lithium on thyroid hormone release in both euthyroid and thyrotoxic patients. *J Clin Endocrinol Metab*, **35**, 905–11.

Spreat S, Behar D, Reneski B, *et al.* (1989). Lithium carbonate for aggression in mentally retarded persons. *Compr Psychiatry*, **30**, 505–11.

Spiers J and Hirsch SR (1978). Severe lithium toxicity with 'normal' serum concentrations. *BMJ*, **281**, 815–16.

Stambolic V, Ruel L, and Woodgett JR (1996). Lithium inhibits glycogen synthesis kinase-3 activity and mimics wingless signalling in intact cells. *Curr Biol*, **6**, 1664–8.

Stancer HC and Forbath N (1989). Hyperparathyroidism, hypothyroidism, and impaired renal function after 10 to 20 years of lithium treatment. *Arch Intern Med*, **149**, 1042–5.

Stefanini E, Argiolas A, Gessa GL, *et al.* (1976). Effect of lithium on dopamine uptake by brain synaptosomes. *J Neurochem*, **27**, 1237–9.

Stewart DE, Klompenhouwer JL, Kendell RE, *et al.* (1991). Prophylactic lithium in puerperal psychosis. The experience of three centres. *Br J Psychiatry*, **158**, 393–7.

Stip E, Dufresne J, Lussier I, *et al.* (2000). A double-blind, placebo-controlled study of the effects of lithium on cognition in healthy subjects: mild and selective effects on learning. *J Affect Disorders*, **60**, 147–57.

Suppes T, Baldessarini RJ, Faedda GL, *et al.* (1991). Risk of recurrence following discontinuation of lithium treatment in bipolar disorder. *Arch Gen Psychiatry*, **48**, 1082–8.

Terao T, Oga T, Nozaki S, *et al.* (1995). Possible inhibitory effect of lithium on peripheral conversion of thyroxine tri-iodothyronine-A prospective study. *Int Clin Psychopharmacol*, **10**, 103–5.

Terhaag B, Scherber A, Schaps P, *et al.* (1978). The distribution of lithium into cerebrospinal fluid, brain tissue and bile in man. *Int J Clin Pharmacol Biopharmacol*, **16**, 333–5.

Thies-Flechtner K, Muller-Oerlinghausen B, Seibert W, *et al.* (1996). Effect of prophylactic treatment on suicide risk in patients with major affective disorders. Data from a randomized prospective trial. *Pharmacopsychiatry*, **29**, 103–7.

Thiruvengadam A (2001). Effect of lithium and sodium valproate ions on resting membrane potentials in neurons: an hypothesis. *J Affect Disorders*, **65**, 95–9.

Tichbourne CRC and James P (1883). *The Mineral Waters of Europe: Including a Short Description of Artificial Mineral Waters. Chemistry of Purgative Waters.* Balliere, Tindall and Cox: London.

Tollefson GD and Senogles SE (1982). A cholinergic role in the mechanism of lithium in mania. *Biol Psychiatry*, **18**, 467–79.

Treiser SL, Cascio CS, O'Donohue TL, *et al.* (1981). Lithium increases serotonin release and decreases serotonin receptors in the hippocampus. *Science*, **213**, 1529–31.

Unwin RJ, Walter SJ, and Shirley DG (1994). Lithium reabsorption in perfused loops of Henle: effects of perfusion rate and bumetanide. *Am J Physiol*, **266** (5 Pt 2), F806–12.

Vargas C, Tannhauser M, and Barros HMT (1998). Dissimilar effects of lithium and valproic acid on GABA and glutamate concentrations in rat cerebrospinal fluid. *Gen Pharmacol*, **30**, 601–4.

Vestergaard P and Amidsen A (1981). Lithium treatment and kidney function. *Acta Psychiatr Scand*, **63**, 333–45.

Vestergaard P and Schou M (1984). The effect of age on lithium dosage requirements. *Pharmacopsychiatry*, **17**, 199–201.

Vincent A, Baruch P, and Vincent P (1993). Early onset of lithium-associated hypothyroidism. *J Psychiatry Neurosc*, **18**, 74–7.

Walker RG, Bennett WM, Davies BM, *et al.* (1982). Structural and functional effects of long-term lithium therapy. *Kidney Int*, (Suppl. 11), S13–19.

Wang HY and Friedman E (1989). Lithium inhibition of protein kinase C activation-induced serotonin release. *Psychopharmacology*, **99**, 213–18.

Wang HY, Johnson GP, and Friedman E (2001). Lithium treatment inhibits protein kinase C translocation in rat brain cortex. *Psychopharmacology*, **158**, 80–6.

Webb AL, Solomon DA, and Ryan CE (2001). Lithium levels and toxicity among hospitalised patients. *Psychiatr Serv*, **52** (2), 229–31.

Wilkinson DG (1979). Difficulty in stopping lithium prophylaxis. *BMJ*, **27**, 1(6158), 235–6.

Wood AJ and Goodwin GM (1987). A review of the biochemical and neuropharmacological actions of lithium. *Psychol Med*, **17**, 579–600.

Yassa R, Saunders A, Nastase C, *et al*. (1988). Lithium-induced thyroid disorders: a prevalence study. *J Clin Psychiatry*, **49**, 14–16.

Yuan PX, Huang LD, Jiang YM, *et al*. (2001). The mood stabilizer valproic acid activates mitogen-activated protein kinases and promotes neurite growth. *J Biol Chem*, **276**, 31674–83.

Website reference

Toxbase http://www.spib.axl.co.uk/Factsheets/14871-Factsheet.htm

Chapter 7

Sexual dysfunction

David S Baldwin, Andrew G Mayers, and
Anna Lambert

Many psychotropic drugs can cause sexual dysfunction. This includes antide-pressants, antipsychotics and mood stabilizers. Research into this area is compli-cated by confounding factors including individual variation in what constitutes normal sexual functioning, age, the impact of the underlying psychiatric illness and the presence of comorbid conditions such as physical health problems and alcohol and substance misuse. Nevertheless, existing research indicates that drug-related sexual dysfunction is common but that its prevalence and impact on patients is often underestimated by clinical staff.

Clinical features

The human sexual response cycle is divided into four phases, described below. Disorders of the sexual response can occur at one or more phase.

1 *Desire.* Typically this consists of fantasies about, and the desire to have, sexual activity.

2 *Excitement.* The subjective sense of sexual pleasure and accompanying physiological changes, namely penile tumescence and erection in men, and pelvic congestion, swelling of the external genitalia, and vaginal lubrica-tion and expansion in women.

3 *Orgasm.* Sexual pleasure peaks, with release of sexual tension and rhythmic contraction of the perineal muscles and reproductive organs. In men, the sensation of ejaculatory inevitability is followed by ejaculation of semen. In women, contractions of the outer third of the vaginal wall occur.

4 *Resolution.* The sense of muscular relaxation and general well-being. Men are physiologically refractory to erection and orgasm for a variable period, whereas women may sometimes be able to respond to further stimulation.

The two main classifications of sexual dysfunction are those provided by the World Health Organization and the American Psychiatric Association. The tenth edition of the *International Classification of Mental and Behavioural*

Disorders (ICD-10) uses the term 'sexual dysfunction' to cover the ways in which an individual is unable to participate in a sexual relationship as he or she would wish (World Health Organization 1992). The disturbance must occur frequently, and persist for at least six months. The fourth edition of the *Diagnostic and Statistical Manual of Mental Disorders* (DSM-IV) describes sexual dysfunction as a disturbance in sexual desire and in the psychophysiological changes that characterize the normal sexual response cycle, that causes marked personal distress and interpersonal difficulty (American Psychiatric Association 1994).

In DSM-IV, sexual dysfunction can be categorized further into various subtypes including substance-induced sexual dysfunction. Sexual dysfunction is specified according to the aspect of the sexual response cycle that is affected. DSM-IV notes that the clinical presentation resembles other forms of sexual dysfunction, but the full criteria for these disorders need not be met.

It has been argued that the categorical approach to sexual dysfunction adopted by the ICD-10 and DSM-IV simply serves 'to obscure the varied and often unique ways in which individuals and couples present with sexual problems' (Bancroft 1989).

Sexual dysfunction and psychiatric drugs

Conventional antipsychotic drugs

Treatment-emergent sexual problems have been called 'the unspoken side effect of antipsychotics' (Peuskens *et al.* 1998). In a recent questionnaire survey of patient satisfaction with antipsychotic drug treatment, 43 per cent of 202 respondents reported sexual dysfunction (Wallace 2001). Another survey suggested that health professionals underestimate the sexual and menstrual adverse effects of antipsychotics (Hellewell 1998).

A survey of psychosexual arousability in 63 male patients on depot neuroleptics found that the response to imagined or audio-erotic erotic stimuli was surprisingly unimpaired, although physical sexual dysfunction was common (Wesby *et al.* 1996). Erectile failure often occurs during phenothiazine treatment; in one study, 38 per cent of men had difficulty in achieving and 42 per cent in maintaining erection (Ghadirian *et al.* 1982). In contrast certain antipsychotic drugs, including chlorpromazine and thioridazine, can prevent detumescence and cause painful prolonged erection of the penis or clitoris. Approximately 20 per cent of cases of drug-induced priapism are due to antipsychotic drugs; the risk seems independent of dosage or duration of treatment (Patel *et al.* 1996). Drug-induced priapism results from alpha-adrenergic blockade combined with anticholinergic activity.

Ejaculatory problems are common with conventional antipsychotic drugs. Total inhibition of ejaculation is most common (Mitchell and Popkin 1983*a*) but reduced ejaculatory volume (Ghadirian *et al.* 1982) and 'retrograde' ejaculation are not unusual. Spontaneous ejaculation without sexual stimulation can occur with antipsychotic drugs, but is rare (Keitner and Selub 1993). Antipsychotic drug treatment is often associated with qualitative changes in orgasm. For example, painful orgasm has been reported during treatment with thioridazine, trifluoperazine and haloperidol (Baldwin and Birtwistle 1997).

Atypical antipsychotic drugs

There is conflicting data as to whether the atypical antipsychotics are associated with less sexual dysfunction than the conventional agents. An early comparison of the effects of clozapine and haloperidol in 153 schizophrenic patients found that there were no significant differences in the effects on sexual function (Hummer *et al.* 1999). In a comparative study of schizophrenic men treated with clozapine or conventional antipsychotic drugs, clozapine was associated with significantly better sexual functioning, as assessed by frequency of orgasm, enjoyment of sex and sexual satisfaction. It was argued that the efficacy of clozapine in relieving positive, negative and cognitive symptoms may also have favourable effects on interpersonal relationships and sexual health (Aizenberg *et al.* 2001).

It is uncertain whether differences exist between the atypical antipsychotics in their propensity to cause sexual side effects. In a randomized controlled trial of olanzapine and risperidone, sexual dysfunction was significantly less common in male patients treated with olanzapine (2.8 per cent) than with risperidone (11.5 per cent) (Tran *et al.* 1997). Quetiapine treatment is not associated with hyperprolactinaemia, which may be an advantage in preserving sexual function. A recent retrospective cross-sectional study indicated that sexual dysfunction is less common with quetiapine (18.2 per cent, mean dose 360.5 mg/day) than with haloperidol (38.1 per cent, 10.6 mg/day), olanzapine (35.3 per cent, 13.5 mg/day) or risperidone (43.2 per cent, 5.3 mg/day) (Bobes *et al.* 2001). Both amisulpride and risperidone can cause substantial rises in prolactin levels. An analysis of treatment studies found similar overall rates of all forms of endocrine disorder with amisulpride and risperidone (4 per cent vs 6 per cent), but the rate of erectile failure was significantly lower with amisulpride (1 per cent vs 5 per cent) (Coulouvrat and Dondey-Nouvel 1999).

There are case reports of retrograde ejaculation and priapism with clozapine, risperidone and olanzapine (Compton *et al.* 2000; Diermenjian *et al.* 1998; Emes and Milson 1994; Rosen and Hanno 1992; Songer and Barclay 2001). A case report has described the development of priapism following an overdosage of quetiapine (Pais and Ayvazian 2001). Furthermore, during the clinical trial programme with sertindole, 20 per cent of men reported at least one episode of abnormal ejaculation (Jones, personal communication, 1997).

Mood-stabilizing drugs

Given the use of lithium in long-term treatment, there have been surprisingly few investigations of its effects on sexual function. In a comparison of sexual function in 24 male lithium-treated patients with varying mood disorders with a control population of surgical outpatients, there were no major differences between groups in the overall prevalence of sexual dysfunction, in either men or women. Dissatisfaction with sexual function was significantly more common in the psychiatric patients, but similar numbers of patients reported beneficial and detrimental changes in sexual function (Kristensen and Jorgensen 1987). An uncontrolled investigation of sexual function in 104 euthymic bipolar patients found that only 14 per cent of those receiving lithium monotherapy reported sexual difficulties, compared to 49 per cent of those receiving combination treatment with lithium and benzodiazepines; furthermore there was no relationship between lithium levels and sexual function (Ghadirian *et al.* 1992). Similar findings were seen in another uncontrolled evaluation, of sexual function in 35 men with bipolar or schizoaffective disorders who were currently euthymic and receiving lithium monotherapy, which also found low levels of sexual dissatisfaction, and again no relationship between lithium level and sexual difficulties (Aizenberg *et al.* 1996).

The effects of anticonvulsant drugs on sexual function has been investigated more extensively, perhaps because of the association between epilepsy and altered sexual activity: predominantly retrospective studies indicate that sexual dysfunction is seen in 14–66 per cent of patients with recurrent epileptiform seizures.

Newer anticonvulsants may have fewer adverse effects on sexual function than older antiepilieptics, although case reports have suggested gabapentin treatment may be associated with sexual dysfunction (Labbate and Rubey 1999; Brannon and Rolland 2000; Grant and Oh 2002). A small case series ($n = 3$) suggests that substitution with lamotrigine may be beneficial in patients who develop sexual dysfunction with gabapentin (Husain *et al.* 2000).

Antidepressant drugs

Treatment-emergent sexual dysfunction can occur with tricyclic antidepressants (TCAs), selective serotonin reuptake inhibitors (SSRIs) and monoamine oxidase inhibitors (MAOIs). Some antidepressants (bupropion, mirtazapine, moclobemide, nefazodone, reboxetine) may be associated with a relatively lower incidence of sexual dysfunction but most data for these newer drugs come from reviews of clinical trial adverse event databases or work with healthy volunteers (Baldwin 2001).

Few data have been published on sexual dysfunction occurring with TCAs, although anorgasmia was common in a study of clomipramine in patients with obsessive-compulsive disorder (Monteiro *et al.* 1987). The majority of studies have assessed sexual dysfunction with SSRIs, but it is difficult to interpret these findings, as the study design varies considerably. For example, fluoxetine had both the highest (75 per cent) and the lowest (8 per cent) reported prevalence of treatment-emergent sexual dysfunction, one figure being derived from specific questioning about abnormal ejaculation (Patterson 1993), the other from spontaneous reports of orgasmic problems (Zajecka *et al.* 1991). Comparative studies of SSRIs have generally found no significant differences between drugs, but one study reported more sexual dysfunction with sertraline than fluvoxamine (Nemeroff *et al.* 1995).

Bupropion may be associated with a low incidence of sexual adverse effects, being significantly superior to sertraline in one study (Croft *et al.* 1999) and to SSRIs in another (Modell *et al.* 1997). A comparative study with nefazodone and sertraline found nefazodone (a 5-HT$_2$ antagonist) to be significantly superior to sertraline on some measures of sexual function (Feiger *et al.* 1996). An analysis of the clinical trial database for mirtazapine indicated that it may be associated with less sexual dysfunction than other antidepressants (Montgomery 1995). However the findings of a recent 24-week double-blind randomized controlled trial in primary care depressed patients found there were no differences in the degree of improvement of sexual dysfunction during treatment with mirtazapine or paroxetine (Wade *et al.* 2003).

The findings of a randomized controlled trial comparing moclobemide (a reversible inhibitor of monoamine oxidase type A) with the TCA doxepin, together with a study in healthy volunteers, and the findings of post-marketing surveillance studies all suggest that moclobemide is relatively free of adverse effects on sexual function (Baldwin 2001). Finally, a recent report from a placebo-controlled randomized controlled trial indicates that reboxetine and the SSRI fluoxetine may differ in their effects on sexual function. Using the Rush Sexual Inventory, RSI reboxetine treatment was found to be associated with a significantly greater improvement in sexual satisfaction than was seen with fluoxetine; by contrast, fluoxetine treatment was associated with significantly worse sexual function than that seen with placebo (Clayton *et al.* 2003).

Prolonged painful penile erection is a long-recognized but rare side effect of a number of antidepressants (reviewed by Mitchell and Popkin 1983*b*; Gitlin 1994). Case reports have implicated most SSRIs (citalopram, fluoxetine, paroxetine and sertraline); and bupropion, nefazodone and phenelzine. Most reports, however, describe the development of priapism with trazodone, either alone or in combination with other psychotropic drugs. The results of a placebo-controlled psychophysiological investigation in healthy volunteers indicate that trazodone significantly increases nocturnal penile erectile activity, whereas imipramine does not; furthermore, trazodone significantly prolongs the detumescence phase of erection (Saenz de Tejada *et al.* 1991). The mechanism of priapism with trazodone is thought similar to that with conventional antipsychotic drugs (i.e. through the blockade of muscarinic and α_1-receptors), but the mechanism associated with SSRIs is unclear. Although occasional case reports have indicated that trazodone might facilitate erection in men with erectile failure, a double-blind randomized placebo-controlled fixed-dose (50 mg) crossover study found that trazodone was no more efficacious than placebo in improving erections and sexual function (Costabile and Spevak 1999). Priapism of the clitoris during antidepressant treatment is probably uncommon, but has been described as a side effect of citalopram (Berk and Acton 1997), nefazodone (Brodie-Meijer *et al.* 1999) and trazodone (Pescatori *et al.* 1993).

Pharmacological mechanisms

Detailed accounts of the physiological mechanisms underlying normal sexual behaviour have been provided by various authors including Shiloh *et al.* (1999) and Rotella (2002). Most evidence is derived from studies in animal models: clearly human sexual behaviour is much more complex, and affected by biological, personal, interpersonal, and sociocultural factors. With regard to biological factors, hormones and dopamine and serotonin pathways play a crucial role in sexual response. Other transmitters that are involved include noradrenaline, acetylcholine, and gamma-aminobutytic acid.

Given this complexity, and the fact that most psychotropic drugs interact with multiple receptors, it is not surprising that many drugs can affect sexual functioning. Furthermore it is apparent that there are various mechanisms by which drugs can cause sexual dysfunction. Non-specific drug effects such as sedation may also be relevant. This section concentrates on some specific mechanisms that may explain sexual dysfunction with psychotropic drugs but the fact that a combination of mechanisms may be involved should be kept in mind. Mechanisms relevant to problems with penile erection and ejaculation are dealt with separately as the physiology is well understood.

Hyperprolactinaemia

It is still uncertain whether the unwanted sexual effects of antipsychotic drugs arise mainly from direct pharmacological effects (e.g. dopamine receptor antagonism) or through hyperprolactinaemia secondary to blockade of dopamine 2 (D_2) receptors at the pituitary gland. Evidence that hyperprolactinaemia can cause sexual dysfunction is provided by studies of patients with prolactin-secreting tumours. In these patients hypeprolactinaemia can result in loss of sexual desire, erectile failure and reduced spermatogenesis in men; and altered ovarian cyclic function, amenorrhea, reduced sexual desire, and hirsutism in women (Petty 1999).

Chronic hyperprolactinaemia suppresses all aspects of sexual behaviour, this effect is independent of steroid activity, as it occurs in men in whom serum testosterone levels remain unchanged. Sexual dysfunction associated with hyperprolactinaemia is not due to direct alterations in dopaminergic activity, as hyperprolactinaemia does not affect the enhanced sexual behaviour seen after administration of dopaminergic agonists. It may instead occur indirectly, as prolactin enhances the inhibitory effects of gamma-aminobutyric acid and opioid activity.

Conventional antipsychotic drugs can certainly increase prolactin levels to a range associated with sexual dysfunction in non-psychiatric patients, so hyperprolactinaemia probably explains some of the sexual dysfunction seen during antipsychotic drug treatment. In an early small study in male schizophrenic patients, those with erectile failure had higher prolactin levels than patients without sexual problems (Arato et al. 1979). A subsequent investigation found that elevated prolactin levels were associated with sexual dysfunction in men and menstrual disturbances in women (Ghadirian et al. 1982). A recent study of sexual function in patients taking conventional neuroleptics found that hyperprolactinaemia was the probable main cause of sexual dysfunction in women, whereas in men, sexual dysfunction occurred with normal and elevated prolactin levels (Smith et al. 2002).

As already discussed, there is conflicting data as to whether the atypical and conventional antipsychotics differ in their propensity to cause sexual dysfunction. However the fact that some atypical antipsychotics are prolactin-sparing provides a theoretical reason as to why some of these drugs may be expected to be associated with lower rates of sexual dysfunction.

Decreased gonadal hormones

Sexual activity in most male animals declines gradually after castration, but testosterone replacement allows activity to continue. Testosterone also helps maintain normal dopaminergic activity in limbic structures, especially the nucleus accumbens: levels of dopamine and its major metabolite decrease following castration, and increase with testosterone replacement. Oestrogen and progesterone are essential to maintain female sexual behaviour, as no pharmacological agent has been shown to enhance sexual behaviour in the absence of oestrogen. In rodents, sexual activity ceases immediately after ovariectomy, but oestrogen replacement will reinstate sexual behaviour.

Hyperprolactinaemia can cause reduced testosterone levels in men and reduced oestrogen levels in women. Although hyperprolactinaemia can cause sexual dysfunction when gonadal hormones levels are normal, the occurrence of secondary gonadal hypoactivity provides a further mechanism by which prolactin-raising antipsychotics may cause sexual dysfunction.

Traditional anticonvulsant treatment (phenytoin, carbamazepine) has been found to be associated with reduced levels of circulating free testosterone in male patients in some (e.g. Toone *et al.* 1983; Macphee *et al.* 1988; Heroz *et al.* 1991; Wheeler *et al.* 1991; Brunet *et al.* 1995; Isojarvi *et al.* 1995) but not all studies (e.g. Rodin *et al.* 1987; Duncan *et al.* 1999). The low levels of free testosterone may result from induction of sex hormone binding globulin synthetase or through enhanced conversion of testosterone to oestradiol through induction of the aromatase enzyme.

Effects on dopamine transmission

Dopamine may affect sexual behaviour directly, or may act indirectly, through other neurotransmitter systems. The net effects of enhanced dopaminergic activity are sexual arousal. Dopamine probably affects sexual behaviour through central and peripheral mechanisms, as dopaminergic agonists (e.g. bromocriptine, levodopa) can induce penile erection in spinally transected rats. Decreased dopaminergic activity also enhances prolactin secretion.

Loss of sexual interest during treatment with phenothiazines or butyrophenones probably results from the combined effects of dopamine receptor antagonism, secondary hyperprolactinaemia and other adverse effects such as sedation, depression, extra-pyramidal side effects and weight gain (Baldwin and Birtwistle 1997) .

Effects on serotonin transmission

In general serotonergic neurotransmission inhibits male and female sexual behaviour, probably through stimulation of postsynaptic $5\text{-}HT_{2A}$ and $5\text{-}HT_{2C}$ receptors in the venteromedial nucleus. In animal models, compounds that block $5\text{-}HT_2$ receptors (e.g. cyproheptadine) facilitate sexual behaviour. Sexual dysfunction with selective serotonin re-uptake inhibitors (principally delayed ejaculation in men and anorgasmia in women) probably results from increased availability of serotonin at $5\text{-}HT_{2A}$ and $5\text{-}HT_{2C}$ receptors.

Some atypical antipsychotic drugs (e.g. quetiapine) have a notable affinity for $5\text{-}HT_2$ receptors; as $5\text{-}HT_2$ antagonists can facilitate sexual behaviour, antipsychotic drugs with this effect might be expected to cause relatively fewer sexual side effects. This provides a further theoretical mechanism by which certain atypical antipsychotics may have less capacity to cause sexual dysfunction than conventional agents. Further research is needed to determine whether this difference is convincingly apparent in clinical practice.

Compounds with 5-HT$_3$ antagonist properties (e.g. ondansetron) stimulate receptivity in animal models, so it is reasonable to assume that activation of 5-HT$_3$ receptors also inhibits sexual behaviour. The antidepressant drug mirtazapine possesses 5-HT$_2$ and 5-HT$_3$ antagonist properties, and may cause relatively less adverse effects on sexual function than drugs without this property.

Mechanisms relevant to penile erection and ejaculation

For erection to occur, the corpora cavernosa have to be filled with arterial blood. The supplying arterial vessels are innervated predominantly by adrenergic fibres, and have alpha-1 and alpha-2 adrenergic receptors; the vessels are also affected by cyclic guanine monophosphate (cGMP) activity. Stimulation of alpha-1 receptors induces vasoconstriction, whereas stimulation of alpha-2 receptors or enhanced cGMP activity facilitates vasodilatation. In the flaccid state, arterial vessels supplying the corpora cavernosa are relatively vasoconstricted due to predominant alpha-1 tonus. In addition, enhanced central cholinergic activity stimulates alpha-1 activity, leading to suppressed erection.

Enhanced alpha-1 activity also contracts the sphincter between the urethra and urinary bladder; in the non-erect penis, alpha-1 tonus is insufficient to fully constrict the sphincter, thereby enabling micturition. During erection however, the sphincter is fully constricted preventing the passage of urine into the urethra and the passage of semen into the bladder. Erection occurs when alpha-2 or cGMP activity predominates over alpha-1 activity, facilitating vasodilatation of the corpora cavernosa. In humans, spontaneous erections can be induced by administration of selective (e.g. phentolamine) or non-selective (e.g. trazodone) alpha-1 blockers. Drugs that block both alpha-1 and muscarinic receptors (e.g. chlorpromazine, thioridazine) can also induce spontaneous erections and priapism (prolonged painful penile erection).

The smooth muscle of the corpora cavernosa is rich in phosphodiesterase (PDE) enzymes, the most important being PDE5, which exists in at least three different forms. Sexual stimulation releases nitric oxide from neuronal fibres and endothelial tissue, with subsequent activation of soluble guanylyl cyclase, which converts GTP to cGMP. As intracellular phosphodiesterase enzymes degrade cGMP, inhibition of PDE5 enhances cGMP activity, leading to decreased smooth muscle tonus and vasodilatation, resulting in penile erection. The PDE5 inhibitor drugs sildenafil and vardenafil are efficacious in relieving sexual dysfunction.

Like erection, ejaculation is regulated by central and peripheral mechanisms. Normal anterograde ejaculation occurs when the sphincter between the bladder and urethra is fully constricted. Synchronized rhythmic contractions of the vas deferens result in the passage of sperm from the testis into the urethra, the vas being innervated by sympathetic nerves under the primary control of alpha-1 activity. Retrograde ejaculation (i.e. the passage of semen into the bladder) results typically from surgical procedures or prescribed medication. The drugs that can cause retrograde ejaculation (e.g. thioridazine, chlorpromazine, clomipramine) all possess alpha-1 blocking activity. Retrograde ejaculation can sometimes be reversed by sympathomimetic drugs (e.g. ephedrine) or drugs with anticholinergic or antihistaminic properties, although the mechanism for this is not understood fully.

Differential diagnosis

It is often hard to discern the cause of sexual dysfunction. Whilst sexual difficulties are often reported during treatment with psychotropic drugs, most patients will not have undergone an assessment of sexual function and satisfaction prior to starting treatment. The most important differential diagnosis is from continuing psychiatric illness and coexistent physical ill health: sexual dysfunction is associated with peripheral vascular disease, and a range of neurological conditions and endocrine disorders, and careful enquiry about medical conditions, together with physical examination, may be helpful.

Sexual dysfunction is highly prevalent in the general population. A detailed and systematic review (Dunn *et al.* 2002) has produced some clear findings. First, the prevalence of erectile dysfunction increases with age, such that around 15 per cent of 50-year old men experience the problem. Second, the prevalence of premature ejaculation is similar to that of erectile dysfunction, but with no clear age pattern. Third, vaginal dryness is probably the most common sexual problem, and increases with age, affecting around 25 per cent of women aged 60 years and older. Fourth, anorgasmia and dyspareunia are less common, with no clear age pattern, but together affecting around 10–20 per cent of women aged 60 years. Finally, the lack of consensus on definitions of sexual dysfunction hampers attempts to perform meaningful comparisons between studies (Dunn *et al.* 2002).

Many drugs used to treat physical illness have been associated with sexual side effects. Particular attention has been focused on antihypertensive drugs, but many other classes can cause sexual problems, including steroids, proton pump inhibitors, histamine antagonists and opiate analgesics. For this reason, a detailed drug history is required, which should also include the use of over-the-counter remedies and drugs of abuse, particularly alcohol.

DSM-IV provides guidance on determining whether the dysfunction is indeed substance-induced, by asking clinicians to consider whether symptoms had their onset whilst the patient received the substance or medication; whether symptoms resolved promptly after stopping the substance or medication; and whether there was a prior history of sexual dysfunction, not related to use of substances or medication.

Management

Sexual dysfunction should be assessed sensitively, and treatment tailored to individual needs and circumstances. Assessment of a patient who complains of sexual difficulties whilst taking a psychotropic drug involves the detailed evaluation of a range of factors. This includes an evaluation of sexual function before the development of mental health problems; the severity of the primary and any comorbid psychiatric disorders; the presence of comorbid physical illness; the range of currently prescribed psychotropic drugs and medications for physical illness; the use of over-the-counter remedies or illicit drugs; and the overall relationship with any sexual partner(s).

Several strategies may be beneficial in treatment, including:

- waiting for the development of tolerance
- reduction in dosage
- delaying drug intake until after sexual activity
- 'drug holidays'
- adjuvant treatments
- changing to a different psychotropic drug
- behavioural strategies to improve sexual technique
- individual psychotherapy
- couple therapy.

The role of psychological approaches is outside the scope of this chapter. The choice of a particular strategy is determined, among other factors, by considering the type and severity of the dysfunction, the nature of the psychiatric diagnosis, the current mental state of the patient, the potential risks of stopping treatment, the risk of untoward drug interactions, and the presence or absence of a sexual partner.

Augmentation or switching studies with antidepressants

Several studies have investigated whether SSRI-associated sexual dysfunction can be resolved by adding, or changing to, a different antidepressant. For example, a retrospective review of 16 patients who complained of sexual dysfunction during SSRI treatment found that 11 (69 per cent) rated their sexual function as much or very much improved when buspirone was added (Norden 1994).

Mirtazapine (which possesses 5-HT$_2$ antagonist properties) may be useful in some patients who develop sexual dysfunction with SSRIs. In a study of 20 patients with SSRI-associated sexual dysfunction who switched to mirtazapine, sexual function improved in 9 of 12 patients (75 per cent) who completed 6 weeks treatment, although 6 patients developed irritability and 9 reported sedation (Gelenberg *et al.* 1998). A second study in 11 patients who stopped SSRIs because of sexual problems found that mirtazapine treatment did not result in the re-emergence of sexual dysfunction (Koutouvidis *et al.* 1999). These observations are supported by findings in a group of 25 depressed outpatients, indicating that mirtazapine treatment had beneficial effects on sexual function (Boyarsky *et al.* 1999). In a complex double-blind re-exposure study, the antidepressant nefazodone (which has mixed SSRI and 5-HT$_2$ antagonist properties), caused less re-emergence of sexual dysfunction than sertraline, in patients who had previously developed sexual dysfunction during sertraline treatment (Ferguson *et al.* 2001).

The largest body of data is for bupropion, where the findings of one augmentation study, and two substitution studies, suggest that bupropion can ameliorate SSRI-induced sexual dysfunction (Baldwin 2001). However, not all data are consistent: a retrospective review in 27 patients found that sexual dysfunction occurred in 11 patients (41 per cent) when they were receiving combination bupropion-SSRI treatment, not significantly different to the rate (52 per cent) when they were taking either agent alone (Bodkin *et al.* 1997). A recent augmentation study with bupropion (150 mg/day) indicates that it can be usefully combined with venlafaxine, paroxetine or fluoxetine (Kennedy *et al.* 2002).

Drug holidays, involving brief interruptions of treatment, have been advocated as an approach to SSRI-induced sexual dysfunction (Rothschild 1995). However, this puts the patient at risk of discontinuation symptoms and possible relapse of depression: furthermore, a drug holiday is only possible with drugs with a short half-life and not with fluoxetine, where sexual side effects may not resolve until a few weeks after stopping treatment.

Many adjuvant compounds have been advocated for relieving sexual dysfunction associated with antidepressant or antipsychotic drug treatment, including amantadine, buspirone, cyproheptadine, dexamphetamine, gepirone, Ginko biloba, granisetron, mianserin, neostigmine, olanzapine, prostaglandin E (by intracavernosal injection) sildenafil, vardenafil and yohimbine. However, the results of placebo-controlled studies in this area have generally failed to distinguish between 'active' treatments and placebo; it is wise to be cautious when using unfamiliar treatments. A recent small ($n = 19$) placebo-controlled augmentation study with Ginkgo biloba found no difference between treatments in reversing sexual dysfunction associated with antidepressant treatment (Kang *et al.* 2002). Another placebo-controlled study found no significant advantage for mirtazapine, yohimbine or olanzapine in relieving sexual dysfunction in patients taking SSRIs (Michelson *et al.* 2000).

Phosphodiesterase-5 inhibitors

It seems likely that PDE5 inhibitors like sildenafil or vardenafil may come to have a role in relieving sexual dysfunction associated with psychotropic drugs. In a subgroup of 136 depressed patients included within the placebo-controlled clinical trial database, 76 per cent described improvements with sildenafil, compared to 18 per cent of the group who received placebo (Price 1999). In an open study, sildenafil was effective in 10 of 14 patients with antidepressant drug-induced sexual dysfunction (Fava *et al.* 1998). The benefits of sildenafil may also apply to patients with schizophrenia, as a case report has described successful treatment of reduced sexual desire and erectile failure in a schizophrenic man receiving antipsychotic drugs (Benatov *et al.* 1999). A double-blind placebo-controlled study in 160 men with erectile dysfunction and comorbid minor depression found that response of erectile problems to sildenafil treatment was associated with a significant reduction in depressive symptoms (Seidman *et al.* 2001). A more recent randomized controlled trial found that sildenafil was efficacious in treating erectile dysfunction in antidepressant-treated remitted depressed patients (Nurnberg *et al.* 2003).

Risk factors and prevention

Few studies have identified risk factors for the development of sexual dysfunction during treatment with psychotropic drugs. A prospective naturalistic study in secondary care settings in Spain ($n = 1022$) identified a range of risk factors for reported sexual dysfunction with antidepressants, including male gender; older age and longer duration of treatment. Sexual dysfunction was significantly more common during treatment with SSRIs (range, 58–73 per cent) or venlafaxine (67 per cent), than with mirtazapine (24 per cent) or nefazodone (8 per cent) (Montejo *et al.* 2001).

A cross-sectional naturalistic study in US primary care settings ($n = 1101$) found that reported sexual dysfunction with antidepressants was significantly more common with a number of demographic and socio-economic variables, including increasing age (overall trend, significantly so in those aged 50–59 years); being married; lower academic achievement; and lack of full-time employment outside the home. Other risk factors were comorbid physical illness; concomitant medication; previous sexual dysfunction; little perceived importance of sexual functioning; and history of little or no sexual enjoyment. Sexual dysfunction was significantly more common during treatment with SSRIs, mirtazapine, or venlafaxine (range, 36–43 per cent) than with bupropion (25 per cent) or nefazodone (28 per cent). There was no evidence that higher doses were associated with greater risk of reported sexual dysfunction (Clayton *et al.* 2002).

In a prospective comparative study in psychiatric outpatients taking conventional antipsychotic drugs ($n = 101$), general practice attenders ($n = 57$) and sexual dysfunction clinic attenders ($n = 55$) male gender and older age (in women) were risk factors for sexual dysfunction. Among the male psychiatric patients, risk factors for differing types of sexual problem were greater reported depression (poor libido, erectile and orgasmic dysfunction); dose of medication (erectile dysfunction); anticholinergic effects (erectile dysfunction); and antiadrenergic effects (abnormal ejaculation). In female patients, risk factors for sexual dysfunction were dose of medication (reduced arousal); depression (poor libido, reduced arousal, orgasmic problems) and hyperprolactinaemia (poor libido, reduced arousal) (Smith *et al.* 2002).

Theoretically, these observational studies suggest some prevention of sexual dysfunction during psychotropic drug treatment might therefore be possible through the preferential use of antidepressants other than SSRIs, and antipsychotics that do not cause hyperprolactinaemia. However, the risk of developing sexual dysfunction during treatment is only one consideration among many, when making treatment decisions for patients with psychiatric illness.

Summary: Sexual dysfunction associated with psychotropic drugs

Definition	A disturbance in sexual desire and in the psychophysiological changes that characterize the normal sexual response cycle, that causes marked personal distress and interpersonal difficulty (DSM-IV definition).
Incidence	Unclear, as often difficult to distinguish features of illness from effects of treatment. The incidence of treatment-emergent sexual dysfunction reported in randomized controlled trials probably underestimates the extent of sexual adverse effects. Around 50% of patients report sexual dysfunction whilst taking antidepressants; a similar proportion describe problems during treatment with antipsychotic drugs.
Drugs causing problem	Tricyclic antidepressants
	Selective serotonin re-uptake inhibitors

	Conventional antipsychotic drugs
	Some atypical antipsychotic drugs
	Many non-psychiatric drugs can cause sexual dysfunction e.g. antihypertensives.
Key symptoms	Lack or loss of sexual desire
	Difficulty achieving penile erection
	Difficulty achieving vaginal lubrication
	Difficulty maintaining penile erection
	Premature ejaculation
	Delayed or inhibited orgasm
Pharmacological mechanism	Results from direct pharmacological properties (e.g. increased availability of serotonin at $5\text{-}HT_2$ receptors, antagonism at D_2 receptors) and indirect effects (e.g. development of hyperprolactinaemia, drowsiness).
Investigations to confirm diagnosis	Limited role. Comprehensive history and examination most relevant. Prolactin levels may be helpful in patients taking antipsychotic drugs. More complex investigations (e.g. nerve conduction studies, plethysmography) are used only rarely, in specialist clinics. Rating scale assessments may be useful in evaluating change with treatment.
Management	Wait for the development of tolerance
	Reduction in dosage
	Delaying drug intake until after sexual activity
	'Drug holidays' (e.g. with short acting SSRIs)
	Adjuvant treatments (e.g. sildenafil)
	Changing to a different psychotropic drug (e.g. mirtazapine and bupropion appear to be associated with lower rates of sexual dysfunction than many antidepressants)
	Behavioural strategies to improve sexual technique
	Individual psychotherapy
	Couple therapy
Further reading	Angst J (1998). Sexual problems in healthy and depressed persons. *International Clinical Psychopharmacology*, **13** (Suppl. 6), S1–S4.
	Baldwin DS (2001). Depression and sexual dysfunction. *British Medical Bulletin*, **57**, 81–99.
	Cutler AJ (2003). Sexual dysfunction and antipsychotic treatment. *Psychoneuroendocrinology*, **28**, 69–82.

References

Aizenberg D, Sigler M, Zemishlany Z, *et al.* (1996). Lithium and male sexual function in affective patients. *Clin Neuropharmacol*, **19**, 515–19.

Aizenberg D, Modai I, Landa A, *et al.* (2001). Comparison of sexual dysfunction in male schizophrenic patients maintained on treatment with classical antipsychotics versus clozapine. *J Clin Psychiatry*, **62**, 541–4.

American Psychiatric Assocation (1994). *Diagnostic and Statistical Manual of Mental Disorders*, 4th edn. APA: Washington, DC.

Angst J (1998). Sexual problems in healthy and depressed patients. *Int Clin Psychopharmacol*, **13** (Suppl. 6), S1–S3.

Arato M, Erdos A, and Polgar M (1979). Endocrinological changes in patients with sexual dysfunction under long-term neuroleptic treatment. *Pharmakopsychiatrie Neuro-psychopharmakologie*, **12**, 426–31.

Baldwin DS and Birtwistle J (1997). Schizophrenia, antipsychotic drugs and sexual function. *Prim Care Psychiatry*, **3**, 115–23.

Baldwin DS (2001). Depression and sexual dysfunction. *Br Med Bull*, **57**, 81–99.

Bancroft J (1989). *Human Sexuality and Its Problems*, 2nd edn. Churchill Livingstone: Edinburgh.

Benatov R, Reznik I, and Zemishlany Z (1999). Sildenafil citrate (Viagra) treatment of sexual dysfunction in a schizophrenic patient. *Eur Psychiatry*, **14**, 353–5.

Berk M and Acton M (1997). Citalopram-associated clitoral priapism: a case series. *Int Clin Psychopharmacol*, **12**, 121–2.

Bobes J, Rejas J, Garcia M, *et al.* (2001). *Frequency and management of sexual dysfunction with antipsychotic drugs in schizophrenic patients: results from the EIRE study.* American Psychiatric Association: New Orleans, LA.

Bodkin JA, Lasser RA, Wines JD, *et al.* (1997). Combining serotonin reuptake inhibitors and bupropion in partial responders to antidepressant monotherapy. *J Clin Psychiatry*, **58**, 137–45.

Boyarsky BK, Haque W, Rouleau MR, *et al.* (1999). Sexual functioning in depressed outpatients taking mirtazapine. *Depress Anxiety*, **9**, 175–9.

Brannon GE and Rolland PD (2000). norgasmia in a patient with bipolar disorder type 1 treated with gabapentin. *J Clin Psychopharmacol*, **20**, 379–81.

Brodie-Meijer CC, Diemont WL, and Buijs PJ (1999). Nefazodone-induced clitoral priapism. *Int Clin Psychopharmacol*, **14**, 257–8.

Brunet M, Rodamilans M, Martinez-Osaba MJ, *et al.* (1995). Effects of long-term antiepileptic therapy on the catabolism of testosterone. *Pharmacol Toxicol*, **76**, 371–5.

Clayton AH, Pradko JF, Croft HA, *et al.* (2002). Prevalence of sexual dysfunction among newer antidepressants. *J Clin Psychiatry*, **63**, 4, 357–66.

Clayton AH, Zajecka J, Ferguson JM, *et al.* (2003). Lack of sexual dysfunction with the selective noradrenaline reuptake inhibitor reboxetine during treatment for major depressive disorder. *Int Clin Psychopharmacol*, **18**, 151–6.

Compton MT, Saldivia A, and Berry SA (2000). Recurrent priapism during treatment with clozapine and olanzapine. *Am J Psychiatry*, **157**, 659.

Costabile RA and Spevak M (1999). Oral trazodone is not effective therapy for erectile dysfunction: a double blind, placebo controlled trial. *J Urol*, **161**, 1819–22.

Coulouvrat C and Dodney-Nouvel L (1999). Safety of amisulpride (Solian): a review of 11 clinical studies. *Int Clin Psychopharmacol*, **14**, 209–18.

Croft H, Settle E, Jr Houser T, *et al.* (1999). A placebo-controlled comparison of the antidepressant efficacy and effects on sexual functioning of sustained-release bupropion and sertraline. *Clin Ther*, **21**, 643–58.

Cutler AJ (2003). Sexual dysfunction and antipsychotic treatment. *Psychoneuroendocrinol*, **28**, 69–82.

Deirmenjian JH, Erhart SM, Wirshing DA, *et al.* (1998). Olanzapine-induced reversible priapism: a case report. *J Clin Psychopharmacol*, **18**, 351–3.

Duncan S, Blacklaw J, Beastall GH, *et al.* (1999). Antiepileptic drug therapy and sexual function in men with epilepsy. *Epilepsia*, **40**, 197–204.

Dunn KM, Jordan K, Croft PR, *et al.* (2002). Systematic review of sexual problems: epidemiology and methodology. *J Sex Marital Ther*, **28**, 399–422.

Emes CE and Milson RC (1994). Risperidone-induced priapism. *Can J Psychiatry*, **39**, 315–16.

Fava M, Rankin MA, Alpert JE, *et al.* (1998). An open trial of sildenafil in antidepressant-induced sexual dysfunction. *Psychother Psychosom*, **67**, 328–31.

Feiger A, Kiev A, Shrivastava RK, *et al.* (1996). Nefazodone versus sertraline in outpatients with major depression: focus on efficacy, tolerability and effects on sexual function and satisfaction. *J Clin Psychiatry*, **57** (Suppl. 2), S53–62.

Ferguson JM, Shrivastava RK, Stahl SM, *et al.* (2001). Reemergence of sexual dysfunction in patients with major depressive disorder: double-blind comparison of nefazodone and sertraline. *J Clin Psychiatry*, **62**, 24–9.

Gelenberg AJ, Laukes C, McGahuey C, *et al.* (1998). Mirtazapine substitution in SSRI-induced sexual dysfunction (abstract). *Biol Psychiatry*, **43**, 104S.

Ghadirian AM, Chouinard G, and Annable L (1982). Sexual dysfunction and plasma prolactin levels in neuroleptic-treated schizophrenic outpatients. *J Nerv Ment Dis*, **170**, 8, 463–7.

Ghadirian AM, Annable L, and Belanger MC (1992). Lithium, benzodiazepines, and sexual function in bipolar patients. *Am J Psychiatry*, **149**, 801–5.

Gitlin MJ (1994). Psychotropic medications and their effects on sexual function: diagnosis, biology, and treatment approaches. *J Clin Psychiatry*, **55**, 406–13.

Grant AC and Oh H (2002). Gabapentin-induced anorgasmia in women. *Am J Psychiatry*, **159**, 1247.

Hellewell JSE (1998). Antipsychotic tolerability: the attitudes and perceptions of medical professionals, patients and caregivers towards the side effects of antipsychotic therapy (abstract). *Eur Neuropsychopharmacol*, **8** (Suppl.), S248.

Heroz AG, Levesque LA, Drislane FW, *et al.* (1991). Phenytoin-induced elevation of serum estradiol and reproductive dysfunction in men with epilepsy. *Epilepsia*, **32**, 550–3.

Hummer M, Kemmler G, Kurz M, *et al.* (1999). Sexual disturbances during clozapine and haloperidol treatment for schizophrenia. *Am J Psychiatry*, **156**, 631–3.

Husain AM, Carwile ST, Miller PP, *et al.* (2000). Improved sexual function in three men taking lamotrigine for epilepsy. *South Med J*, **93**, 335–6.

Isojarvi JI, Repo M, Pakarinen AJ, *et al.* (1995). Carbamazepine, phenytoin, sex hormones, and sexual function in men with epilepsy. *Epilepsia*, **36**, 366–70.

Kang B-J, Lee S-J, Kim M-D, *et al.* (2002). A placebo-controlled, double-blind trial of Ginko biloba for antidepressant-induced sexual dysfunction. *Human Psychopharm: Clin*, **17**, 279–84.

Keitner GI and Selub S (1993). Spontaneous ejaculations and neuroleptics. *J Clin Psychopharmacol*, **3**, 34–6.

Kennedy SH, McCann SM, Masellis M, *et al.* (2002). Combining bupropion SR with venlafaxine, paroxetine or fluoxetine: a preliminary report on pharmacokinetic, therapeutic and sexual dysfunction effects. *J Clin Psychiatry*, **63**, 181–6.

Koutouvidis N, Pratikakis M, and Fotiadou A (1999). The use of mirtazapine in a group of 11 patients following poor compliance to selective serotonin reuptake inhibitor treatment due to sexual dysfunction. *Int Clin Psychopharmacol*, **14**, 253–5.

Kristensen E and Jorgensen P (1987). Sexual function in lithium-treated manic-depressive patients. *Pharmacopsychiatry*, **20**, 165–7.

Labbate LA and Rubey RN (1999). Gabapentin-induced ejaculatory failure and anorgasmia. *Am J Psychiatry*, **156**, **6**, 972.

Macphee GJ, Larkin JG, Butler E, *et al.* (1988). Circulating hormones and pituitary responsiveness in young epileptic men receiving long-term antiepileptic medication. *Epilepsia*, **29**, 468–75.

Michelson D, Bancroft J, Targum S, *et al.* (2000). Female sexual dysfunction associated with antidepressant administration: a randomized, placebo-controlled study of pharmacologic intervention. *Am J Psychiatry*, **157**, 239–43.

Mitchell J and Popkin M (1983*a*). The pathophysiology of sexual dysfunction associated with antipsychotic drug therapy in males: A review. *Arch Sex Behav*, **12**, 173–83.

Mitchell JE and Popkin MK (1983*b*). Antidepressant drug therapy and sexual dysfunction in men: a review. *J Clin Psychopharmacol*, **3**, 76–9.

Modell JG, Katholi CR, Modell JD, *et al.* (1997). Comparative sexual side effects of bupropion, fluoxetine, paroxetine, and sertraline. *Clin Pharmacol Ther*, **61**, 476–87.

Monteiro WO, Noshirvani HF, Marks IM, *et al.* (1987). Anorgasmia from clomipramine in obsessive-compulsive disorder: a controlled trial. *Br J Psychiatry*, **151**, 107–12.

Montejo AL, Llorca G, Izquierdo JA, *et al.* (2001). Incidence of sexual dysfunction associated with antidepressant agents: a prospective multicenter study of 1022 outpatients. Spanish Working Group for the Study of Psychotropic-Related Sexual Dysfunction. *J Clin Psychiatry*, **62** (Suppl. 3), S10–21.

Montgomery SA (1995). Safety of mirtazapine: a review. *Int Clin Psychopharmacol*, **10** (Suppl. 4), S37–45.

Nemeroff CB, Ninan PT, Ballenger J, *et al.* (1995). Double-blind multicenter comparison of fluvoxamine versus sertraline in the treatment of depressed outpatients. *Depression*, **3**, 163–9.

Norden MJ (1994). Buspirone treatment of sexual dysfunction associated with selective serotonin reuptake inhibitors. *Depression*, **2**, 109–12.

Nurnberg HG, Hensley PL, Gelenberg AJ, *et al.* (2003). Treatment of antidepressant-associated sexual dysfunction with sildenafil: a randomized controlled trial. *J Am Med Assoc*, **289**, 56–64.

Pais VM and Ayvazian PJ (2001). Priapism from quetiapine overdose: first report and proposal of mechanism. *Urology*, **58**, 462.

Patel AG, Mukherji K, and Lee A (1996). Priapism associated with psychotropic drugs. *Br J Hosp Med*, **55**, 315–19.

Patterson WM (1993). Fluoxetine-induced sexual dysfunction. *J Clin Psychiatry*, **54**, 71.

Pescatori ES, Engelman JC, Davism G, *et al.* (1993). Priapism of the clitoris: a case report following trazodone use. *J Urol*, **149**, 1557–9.

Petty RG (1999). Prolactin and antipsychotic medications: Mechanism of action. *Schizophr Res*, **35** (Suppl.), S67–73.

Peuskens J, Sienaert P, and De Heft M (1998). Sexual dysfunction: The unspoken side effect of antipsychotics. *Eur Psychiatry*, **13** (Suppl. 1), S23–30.

Price D (1999). Sildenafil citrate (Viagra) in the treatment of erectile dysfunction in patients with common concomitant conditions. In H. Padma-Nathan (ed.), Selected Proceedings from the 8th World Meeting of the International Society for Impotence Research, Amsterdam, 24–28 August 1996. *Int J Clin Practice*, **102**, 21–3.

Rodin E, Subramanian MG, Schmaltz S, *et al.* (1987). Testosterone levels in adult male epileptic patients. *Neurology*, **37**, 706–8.

Rosen SI and Hanno PM (1992). Clozapine-induced priapism. *J Urol*, **148**, 876–7.

Rotella DP (2002). Phosphodiesterase 5 inhibitors: current status and potential applications. *Nat Rev Drug Discov*, **1**, 674–82.

Rothschild AJ (1995). Selective serotonin reuptake inhibitor-induced sexual dysfunction: efficacy of a drug holiday. *Am J Psychiatry*, **152**, 514–16.

Saenz de Tejada I, Ware JC, Blanco R, *et al.* (1991). Pathophysiology of prolonged penile erection associated with trazodone use. *J Urol*, **145**, 60–4.

Seidman SN, Roose SP, Menza MA, *et al.* (2001). Treatment of erectile dysfunction in men with depressive symptoms: results of a placebo-controlled trial with sildenafil citrate. *Am J Psychiatry*, **158**, 1623–30.

Shiloh R, Nutt D, and Weizman A (1999). *Atlas of Psychiatric Pharmacotherapy*. Martin Dunitz: London.

Smith SM, O'Keane V, and Murray R (2002). Sexual dysfunction in patients taking conventional antipsychotic medication. *Br J Psychiatry*, **181**, 49–55.

Songer DA and Barclay JC (2001). Olanzapine-induced priapism. *Am J Psychiatry*, **158**, 2087–8.

Toone BK, Wheeler M, Nanjee M, *et al.* (1983). Sex hormones, sexual activity and plasma anticonvulsant levels in male epileptics. *J Neurol Neurosurg Psychiatry*, **46**, 824–6.

Tran PV, Hamilton SH, Kuntz AJ, *et al.* (1997). Double-blind comparison of olanzapine versus risperidone in the treatment of schizophrenia and other psychotic disorders. *J Clin Psychopharmacol*, **17**, 407–18.

Wade A, Crawford GM, Angus M, *et al.* (2003). A randomized, double-blind, 24-week study comparing the efficacy and tolerability of mirtazapine and paroxetine in depressed patients in primary care. *Int Clin Psychopharmacol*, **18**, 133–41.

Wallace M (2001). Real progress – The patient's perspective. *Int Clin Psychopharmacol*, **16** (Suppl.), S21–4.

Wesby R, Bullmore E, Earle J, *et al.* (1996). A survey of psychosexual arousability in male patients on depot neuroleptic medication. *Eur Psychiatry*, **11**, 81–6.

Wheeler MJ, Toone BK, Dannatt A, *et al.* (1991). Metabolic clearance rate of testosterone in male epileptic patients on anti-convulsant therapy. *J Endocrinol,* **129**, 465–8.

World Health Organization (1992). *The ICD-10 Classification of Mental and Behavioural Disorders: Diagnostic criteria for research.* World Health Organization: Geneva.

Zajecka J, Fawcett J, Schaff M, *et al.* (1991). The role of serotonin in sexual dysfunction: fluoxetine-associated orgasm dysfunction. *J Clin Psychiatry,* **52**, 66–8.

Chapter 8

Diabetes mellitus

David M Taylor

Diabetes mellitus is a syndrome characterized by hyperglycaemia and brought about by a functional or absolute deficiency of insulin. Impaired glucose tolerance can also occur when blood sugar is above the upper limit of the normal range but below the threshold used to define diabetes. Diabetes can be divided in to Type I and Type II. In Type 1 diabetes, no insulin is produced by pancreatic islet cells and insulin replacement is essential. In Type 2 diabetes insulin production is reduced (but not absent), there is increased hepatic glucose production and reduced sensitivity to the action of insulin (insulin resistance). Antipsychotic medication is usually associated with Type II diabetes though Type I diabetes can occur.

Clinical features

Key features

Insulin regulates glucose, lipid, and protein metabolism. It promotes muscle uptake of glucose and inhibits hepatic glucose output. It also acts on adipose tissue to inhibit lipolysis and promotes amino acid transport and protein synthesis.

When insulin action is deficient muscle utilization of glucose is reduced and liver production increased, leading to hyperglycaemia. This may present as fatigue. Glucose may then be excreted in the urine leading to polyuria (an osmotic diuresis) and polydipsia. Severe insulin deficiency promotes increased lipolysis which may in turn lead to the production of ketones which are utilized as an energy source and may, via increased plasma osmolality, give rise to tissue dehydration and, because of their acidic nature, acidosis (diabetic ketoacidosis).

Type 1 diabetes, where insulin production ceases over a short period, usually presents with fatigue, polyuria, dehydration and, in some cases, ketoacidosis. In Type 2 diabetes where functional insulin deficiency develops over several years, symptoms may be absent or unnoticed for a prolonged period. Polyuria may develop in proportion to the degree of hyperglycaemia but ketoacidosis is rare because only low concentrations of insulin are required to suppress lipolysis.

Complications and prognosis

Left untreated, Type 1 diabetes is rapidly fatal and insulin replacement therapy is essential to maintain life. Type 2 diabetes may be controlled by diet alone or by diet and oral hypoglycaemic drugs of various types. Occasionally, insulin replacement is necessary.

In the medium to long term, complications arise largely as a result of damage to large and small blood vessels. The mechanism by which this occurs is complex but is essentially a result of adverse metabolic events in endothelial cells which occur as a result of hyperglycaemia and excess free fatty acids. The end result of these events – vasoconstriction, inflammation, thrombosis – is atherogenesis (see Hayden and Reaven (2000) and Beckman *et al.* (2002) for full discussion). Diabetes markedly increases the risk of atheroma-related events such as myocardial infarction, stroke, amputation and death. Damage to small blood vessels (diabetic microangiopathy) may lead to renal failure and blindness. Even non-diabetic, moderately elevated plasma glucose may be a continuous risk factor for myocardial infarction (Gerstein *et al.* 1999).

Diagnostic criteria

Several measures are used to define the presence of impaired glucose tolerance and diabetes mellitus. These include:

- 'random' plasma glucose (sampled at a random time without heed to food ingestion)
- fasting plasma glucose (sampled 12 hours after last food ingestion)
- oral glucose tolerance (plasma glucose after measured glucose ingestion) and
- plasma glycosylated haemoglobin (Hb_{A1C}), a glucose-haemoglobin complex reflecting average plasma glucose over several months.

Diabetes mellitus is diagnosed if random plasma glucose exceeds 11.1 mmol/L (200 mg/dL), if fasting plasma glucose exceeds 7.0 mmol/L (126 mg/dL), or if two hour plasma glucose exceeds 11.1 mmol in a 75 g oral glucose tolerance test (National Diabetes Data Group 1979). More recently, additional criteria have been put forward to define sub-threshold syndromes (Table 8.1) (Lebovitz 2001).

In the UK, Hb_{A1C} is sometimes used diagnostically. Diabetes is said to occur in those with random blood glucose above 14 mmol/L and/or Hb_{A1C} of greater than 9.0 per cent (Edwards and Bouchier 1991).

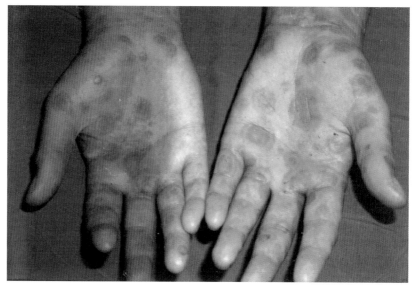

Plate 1 Typical target lesions on the hands in erythema multiforme minor (EMM). The targets have a central erythematous area surrounded by a paler ring and another erythematous ring. (See Chapter 15, p. 272.)

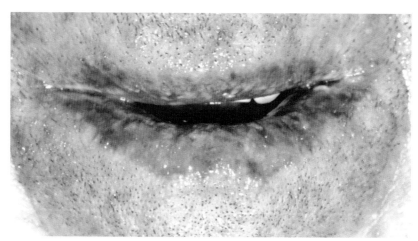

Plate 2 Mucosal involvement in Stevens–Johnson syndrome. (See Chapter 15, p. 273.)

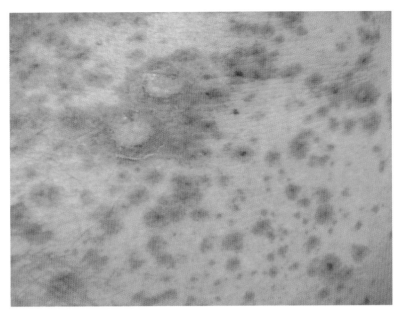

Plate 3 Extensive erythema with some epidermal attachment and target lesions becoming confluent on the trunk. (See Chapter 15, p. 273.)

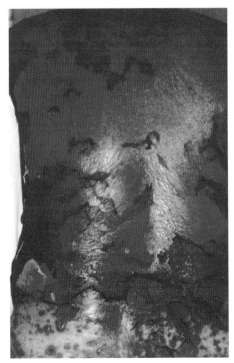

Plate 4 Toxic epidermal necrolysis due to carbamazepine treated successfully with IVIG. (See Chapter 15, p. 274.)

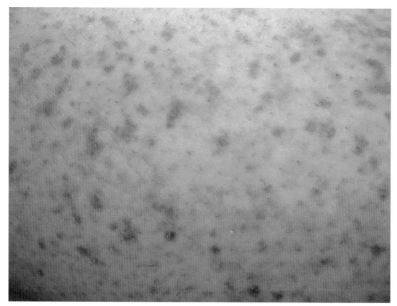

Plate 5 Typical non blanching palpable purpuric papules on the lower leg in vasculitis. (See Chapter 15, p. 279.)

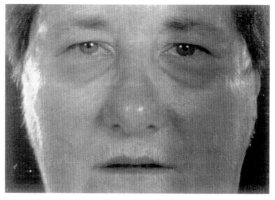

Plate 6 A patient with chlorpromazine induced pigmentation in sun exposed areas. (See Chapter 15, p. 281.)

Table 8.1 Suggested criteria for diabetes and sub-threshold syndromes (Lebovitz 2001)

Classification	Fasting plasma glucose (mmol/L)	Two hour plasma glucose after 75 g challenge (mmol/L)
Normal	<6.1	<7.8
Impaired glucose tolerance	–	≥7.8 and <11.1
Impaired fasting glucose	≥6.1 and <7.0	–
Diabetes mellitus	≥7.0	≥11.1

Psychosis and diabetes

Numerous reports dating back almost a century suggest that schizophrenia and other psychotic disorders are associated with relatively high incidences of diabetes and impaired glucose tolerance (e.g. Lorenz 1922; Braceland *et al.* 1946; Freeman 1946). The uniformity of findings strongly supports an association between psychotic disorder and impairment of glucose tolerance, but these early studies inevitably lack the rigorous diagnostic criteria expected today. Interestingly, more recent examinations have produced similar results.

For example, Mukherjee and co-workers (1996) showed the prevalence of diabetes in a cohort of Italian subjects with schizophrenia to be 15.8 per cent (as determined by fasting plasma glucose assay) but those who were taking no medication had higher rates of hyperglycaemia than those who were taking haloperidol. The expected prevalence in non-schizophrenic Italians was 2.1–3.2 per cent. A large database study (Dixon *et al.* 2000) conducted in the United States and including data on more than 20,000 people with schizophrenia, estimated the prevalence of diabetes (as reported in healthcare claims) to be 9.3 to 12.5 per cent. Corresponding rates of diabetes in the general population at that time were no higher than 6.3 per cent.

This association between psychotic disorder and diabetes may not be confined to schizophrenia. Cassidy and colleagues (1999) determined a diabetes prevalence of 9.9 per cent in a cohort of 345 inpatients diagnosed with bipolar affective disorder. This was in some contrast to the expected rate of 3.4 per cent reported for US citizens at that time.

Thus, there is a good deal of evidence strongly suggesting that psychotic disorders such as schizophrenia and bipolar disorder are associated with an increased risk of diabetes. The evidence, however, is not conclusive: diagnostic changes and the absence of carefully-matched cohort studies and longitudinal comparisons make firm conclusions premature. In addition to this, in many studies the influence of antipsychotic treatment, both current and past, cannot be discounted.

A recent study avoided the potential confounding effect of antipsychotic medication by studying first-episode, drug-naive patients with schizophrenia (Ryan *et al.* 2003). In this study 15.4 per cent of patients had impaired fasting glucose tolerance compared to none of a group of healthy controls matched for age, sex, various lifestyle and anthropometric measures. The patients had significantly higher fasting plasma levels of glucose and insulin than the controls. Although consistent with reports from the pre-neuroleptic era, the study is limited by the small number of subjects. Studies in newly diagnosed and untreated schizophrenia have also suggested a higher prevalence of Metabolic Syndrome than in age-matched controls (Ryan and Thakore 2002; Thakore *et al.* 2002). Metabolic syndrome (also know as Insulin Resistance Syndrome or Reaven's Syndrome) refers to a syndromal entity in which central obesity, hyperlipidaemia, hyperglycaemia, and hypertension are interdependent in some way (Reaven 1988; Reaven and Chen 1988; Lebovitz 2001).

The apparent increased prevalence of diabetes is psychotic disorders may reflect factors intrinsic to the underlying illness (e.g. shared genetic factors or hypercotisolaemia) or lifestyle factor that are associated with the psychiatric illness such as smoking (Wannamethee *et al.* 2001), poor diet and lack of exercise. These factors may act together in a multifactorial manner. A major problem in researching the effect of antipsychotics on glycaemic control is teasing apart the effects of drug, underlying illness and lifestyle.

Antipsychotics and diabetes

Conventional antipsychotics have long been suspected as being causally associated with hyperglycaemia and diabetes. For example, an observational study (Thonnard-Neuman 1968) found that the institutional prevalence of diabetes (fasting plasma glucose >130 mg/dL) increased from 4.2 per cent before the introduction of phenothiazines to 17.2 per cent twelve years later. Mean fasting glucose rose from 90 mg/dL to 189 mg/dL. When the 1966 cohort ($n = 528$) were categorized according to treatment, 27 per cent of those on phenothiazines were found to have diabetes compared with 8.6 per cent of those not receiving these drugs. Induction of diabetes appeared to be quite rapid: 42 per cent of those developing diabetes were diagnosed within a year of starting phenothiazines.

These observations were supported by further clinical evaluations (e.g. Keskiner *et al.* 1973) and animal experiments (e.g. Proakis *et al.* 1971) and the link between the use of antipsychotics (particularly phenothiazines) and diabetes was fairly well established. However, little attention was then paid to this adverse effect and, curiously, knowledge of it seems to have dissipated. For example, a standard textbook of pharmacology published in 1990 devotes only three lines to the association between antipsychotics and diabetes in a review of adverse effects spanning nine pages (Goodman-Gilman *et al.* 1990). The three lines read as follows: 'Chlorpromazine may also impair glucose tolerance and insulin release to a clinically appreciable degree in some "prediabetic" patients, however this effect is not known to occur with other neuroleptic agents'. More curious still is the fact that the British National Formulary (2002) does not mention at all the possible link between the conventional antipsychotics and hyperglycaemia or diabetes.

The emergence of an apparent association between the newer atypical antipsychotics and impairment of glucose tolerance (Mir and Taylor 2001; Henderson 2002) seems to have come as something of a surprise to clinicians in psychiatry. That it should have been a surprise is remarkable given the evidence relating to conventional drugs but understandable given the apparent dissipation of the knowledge of this effect.

Data relating to atypical antipsychotics and diabetes are derived from four main sources: case reports; studies of glucose tolerance; longitudinal studies and pharmaco–epidemiological studies of reported diabetes. These will be dealt with in turn.

Case reports

The value of case reports in determining relative or absolute rates of adverse effects is limited. The number of case reports appearing in the literature depends not only on the frequency of an adverse effect but also the extent to which a particular drug is used in practice, the novelty of the adverse effect, the expectation of an adverse event and the willingness of journal editors to publish reports of such events. Nonetheless, case reports are valuable in alerting clinicians to the possibility of adverse effects (for example, with thalidomide and teratogenicity) and in encouraging further, more cogent research.

Notwithstanding the reservations outlined above, case reports have advanced to some extent knowledge of the association between atypical antipsychotics and diabetes. Most atypicals have been reported to be linked to one or more aspects of impaired glucose tolerance. Clozapine has been associated with causing and worsening diabetes (Popli *et al.* 1997) and with ketoacidosis (Ai *et al.* 1998). An analysis of cases reported to the US Food and Drug Administration uncovered 25 deaths occurring as a result of diabetic ketoacidosis arising apparently as a result of clozapine treatment (Koller *et al.* 2001). In total there were 384 reports mentioning one or more aspect of impaired glucose tolerance.

Olanzapine has also been linked to hyperglycaemia (Ober *et al.* 1999), worsening of existing diabetes, *de novo* diabetes (Goldstein *et al.* 1999) and ketoacidosis (Lindenmayer and Patel 1999). An analysis of spontaneous reports to the FDA ($n = 237$) revealed fifteen deaths occurring as a result of ketoacidosis in patients taking olanzapine (Koller and Doraiswamy 2002). Interestingly, nearly three-quarters of all reports of hyperglycaemia occurred within six months of starting the drug.

Case reports relating to other atypicals are relatively few. As noted above, this may or may not be a reflection of a lower propensity for diabetes-related effects. Risperidone has been reported to be associated with new onset diabetes (Wirshing *et al.* 2001) and ketoacidosis (Croarkin *et al.* 2000). Quetiapine also has been linked to new-onset diabetes (Sobel *et al.* 1999; Procyshyn *et al.* 2000). There is also a report of hyperglycaemia occurring with ziprasidone (Yang and McNeely 2002) although this was in conjunction with pancreatitis and rhabdomyolysis. Overall, during the time period 1994–2001 there appeared in the world-wide literature the following number of case reports of diabetes (Cohen 2002):

- Clozapine 28
- Olanzapine 37
- Risperidone 4
- Quetiapine 3

Studies of glucose tolerance

Several researchers have sought to uncover the effect of different antipsychotics on glucose homeostasis by direct analysis of biochemical indicators of impaired glucose tolerance. These studies have the advantage of sensitive analysis but are usually compromised by small subject numbers.

Hägg and colleagues (1998) used plasma glucose measurement and oral glucose tolerance tests (OGTT) in patients taking either clozapine ($n = 60$) or depot antipsychotics ($n = 63$). In the clozapine group 12 per cent had diabetes mellitus (fasting glucose >6.7 mmol/L or 2 hour OGTT glucose >11.0 mmol/L) and 10 per cent impaired glucose tolerance (fasting glucose <6.7 mmol/L, 2 hour OGTT glucose between 7.8 and 11.0 mmol/L). Amongst those on depots, 6 per cent had diabetes and 3 per cent impaired glucose tolerance ($P > 0.05$ for both measures). Thus there was no statistically significant difference between treatments but the numerical difference is striking, especially since subjects in the clozapine group were significantly younger than those in the depot group.

A similar study was conducted by Newcomer and co-workers (2002) in patients taking a variety of antipsychotics ($n = 41$) and in untreated controls ($n = 38$). A complex statistical analysis suggested that olanzapine and clozapine were both associated with significantly higher levels of fasting plasma glucose and plasma glucose in a modified OGTT. With risperidone, these measures were significantly higher when compared with untreated controls but not compared with those on conventional antipsychotics. Using the homeostatic model assessment (HOMA) of insulin resistance, clozapine and olanzapine were shown to be associated with significantly higher measures of insulin resistance than conventional agents. Overall, clozapine and olanzapine were considered to have major effects on glucose homeostasis but risperidone and conventionals less so.

Longitudinal studies

Several longitudinal studies, mostly retrospective, have assessed the effect of antipsychotics on glucose control. Meyer (2002) compared the effects of olanzapine and risperidone (total sample $= 94$). After a year of treatment, olanzapine was associated with a rise in fasting plasma glucose of 10.8 mg/dL (0.9 mmol/L) whereas risperidone gave rise to only a $+ 0.7$ mg/dL change ($P = 0.03$). Olanzapine was also associated with a significantly greater rise in triglycerides and cholesterol.

In another retrospective analysis, Wirshing and colleagues (2002) compared relevant laboratory data for 215 patients receiving a variety of antipsychotics over $2\frac{1}{2}$ years. A significant rise in (random) plasma glucose was seen in patients given olanzapine ($+21$ per cent), clozapine ($+14$ per cent) and haloperidol ($+7$ per cent) but not in those receiving risperidone ($n = 49$), quetiapine ($n = 13$) or fluphenazine ($n = 41$). Olanzapine and clozapine were also associated with statistically significant rises in serum triglycerides, an effect previously identified as being closely associated with olanzapine treatment (Osser *et al.* 1999; Meyer 2002).

Other longitudinal studies have been conducted and reported. A 37-patient analysis of the effect of six weeks' treatment with ziprasidone (Kingsbury *et al.* 2001) showed that plasma glucose levels were unchanged but cholesterol and triglyceride levels fell. In contrast, a five year follow-up of 82 outpatients treated with clozapine (Henderson *et al.* 2000) found that 36.6 per cent of those patients were diagnosed with diabetes during the study period (67 per cent of patients experienced at least one episode of fasting plasma glucose above 7.0 mmol/L). Serum triglycerides were also significantly increased. Also of interest was the observation that weight gain continued for around 46 months in those patients before levelling off.

Pharmaco–epidemiological studies

The availability of computer database prescription or health insurance claims information has enabled better detection of adverse effects associated with drug treatment. Database studies have the advantage of the facility to include details of many thousands of patients, so allowing comparison of rates of reported adverse effects for different drugs. However, reported rates depend entirely upon detection and so there is usually a large margin of error, especially when adverse events have subtle or infrequent symptoms. This is especially relevant in drug-associated diabetes: only diabetes that is actually diagnosed will be reported and this may or may not represent a fixed proportion of the actual rate of diabetes.

Studies examining reported rates of diabetes are described in Table 8.2. The findings of these studies show some uniformity. Two studies (Sernyak *et al.* 2002; Kornegay *et al.* 2002) show that diabetes is more likely to be diagnosed in those taking in atypicals than in those taking conventional drugs. Four studies suggest that diabetes is more frequently diagnosed in patients taking olanzapine than in either those taking conventional drugs or those not taking antipsychotics (Sernyak *et al.* 2002; Kovo *et al.* 2002; Grogg *et al.* 2002; Gianfrancesco *et al.* 2002). In the same studies, risperidone is suggested to afford no increased risk of diabetes. Clozapine appears to be more frequently associated with diabetes than are conventional drugs (Sernyak *et al.* 2002; Gianfrancesco *et al.* 2002) but this not a consistent finding (Lund *et al.* 2001). Finally, conventional antipsychotics seems to confer an increased risk of diabetes compared with non-use (Grogg *et al.* 2002; Gianfrancesco *et al.* 2002).

Pharmacological basis

The mechanism by which antipsychotics cause diabetes mellitus is not known. The time course of this adverse effect is of interest: antipsychotic-related diabetes is essentially sub-acute rather than chronic, occurring after several weeks or months of treatment. Other observations include the acute (elevating) effect of antipsychotics on plasma insulin (Baptista *et al.* 1999; Melkersson *et al.* 1999, 2000) and the acute induction of insulin resistance (Newcomer *et al.* 2002). Elevation of serum insulin levels seems to be more profound in patients taking clozapine than in those taking conventional antipsychotics (Melkersson and Hulting 2001).

These observations suggest a prompt effect on insulin secretion, but it is not clear whether this effect is direct or indirect. The fact that hypoglycaemia is

Table 8.2 Studies comparing reported rates of diabetes with atypical antipsychotics

Reference	n	Outcomes	Comments
Lund et al. 2001	3013	Reported rates of diabetes Clozapine (n = 552) 4.0% Conventional antipsychotics (n = 2461) 3.4%	Difference not significantly different in whole group but patients aged 20–34 more likely to have diabetes if on clozapine Reports from Medicaid claims
Sernyak et al. 2002	38,632	Odds ratio of reported diabetes (P < 0.05 unless stated) Conventional 1.0 (set as comparison) Clozapine 1.25 Olanzapine 1.11 Quetiapine 1.31 Risperidone 1.05, P = 0.15	Those on atypicals 9% more likely to have diabetes than those on conventional drugs All atypicals confer increased risk of diabetes in those under 40 No 'untreated' comparison groups; odds ratio relative to conventionals
Koro et al. 2002	19,637	Odds ratio of reported diabetes (95% confidence interval) Olanzapine 5.8 (2.0–16.7) vs non-use 4.2 (1.5–12.2) vs conventionals Risperidone 2.2 (0.9–5.2) vs non-use 1.6 (0.7–3.8) vs conventionals	Incidence of reported diabetes in first 3 months of treatment less than 10/1000 patient years for all treatments
Kornegay et al. 2002	73,428	Odds ratio for reported diabetes (95% CI) Atypicals 4.7 (1.5–14.9) Conventional 1.7 (1.2–2.3) Any antipsychotic 1.7 (0.6–1.5)	Odds ratios are comparison against non-use in last year Analysis based on 424 cases of diabetes (0.5% of population)
Grogg et al. 2002	2608	Odds ratio for reported diabetes (95% CI) Olanzapine 4.29 (2.1–8.8) Risperidone 1.02 (0.35–3.0) High potency typical 1.95 (0.79–4.8) Low potency typical 4.97 (1.9–12.6)	Odds ratios are for comparison against untreated (before treatment with stated antipsychotic) Subjects with mood disorder, not schizophrenia
Gianfrancesco et al. 2002	4308	Odds ratio for reported diabetes (95% CI) Olanzapine 3.10 (1.62–5.9) Risperidone 0.88 (0.37–2.07) Clozapine 7.44 (0.60–34.75) High potency typical 2.13 (1.09–4.13) Low potency typical 3.46 (1.52–7.18)	Odds ratios are for comparison against untreated patients in same database Olanzapine showed dose-related risk of diabetes

not seen in response to drug-induced hyperinsulinaemia doses, however, suggest that increases in plasma insulin are secondary to drug-induced insulin resistance.

Insulin resistance may arise because of changes in any stage of the action of insulin. It has been suggested that antipsychotics inhibit in some way the action of insulin-sensitive glucose transporters in the cells of target tissues (Henderson 2002). Others have noted that studies of phenothiazines suggested that those drugs indirectly or directly decrease insulin secretion (Newcomer *et al.* 2002). It has also been proposed that antagonism of $5HT_{1A}$ receptors results in hyperglycaemia (Wirshing *et al.* 2002). Further research is clearly necessary. This is needed not only to discover the precise pharmacological processes involved, but also to explain some of the more unusual aspects of this adverse syndrome: that diabetes is induced relatively rapidly and that ketoacidosis occurs apparently more frequently than in non-iatrogenic Type 2 diabetes.

Differential diagnosis

Diabetes and hyperglycaemia are diagnosed definitively by blood analysis. Once this is done the clinician needs to consider other possible causes apart from antipsychotic medication. A minority of cases of hyperglycaemia and diabetes result from a recognisable pathological process or occur secondary to medical treatment. Examples of conditions that can lead to 'secondary diabetes' include liver disease (e.g. cirrhosis, hepatitis), pancreatic disease (e.g. pancreatitis, haemochromatosis, carcinoma) and endocrine disorders where there are excessive amounts of hormones antagonistic to insulin (e.g. acromegaly via excess growth hormone; hyperthyroidism via excess thyroid hormones; Cushing's syndrome via excess cortisol). Diabetes can also occur secondary to pregnancy (gestational diabetes). Several drugs, other than antipsychotics, can cause clinically-relevant elevations in plasma glucose. These include thiazide diuretics, corticosteroids, pentamidine and protease inhibitors. For most of these drugs the mechanism by which hyperglycaemia is induced is yet to be determined (Luna and Feinglos 2001). Most cases of hyperglycaemia and diabetes are primary, i.e. they do arise secondary to drug treatment or a recognized pathological process. Antipsychotic-induced diabetes is readily differentiated from other secondary diabetes but less easily separated primary diabetes.

If hyperglycaemia or diabetes appear within the first few months of starting an antipsychotic the close temporal link is a strong indicator that the drug is responsible. However, to make this link one needs pre-treatment measures of blood sugar and this is now recommended (Taylor *et al.* 2003). Where hyperglycaemia and/or ketoacidosis occur more than several months after the introduction of an antipsychotic, definitive diagnosis of drug-induced diabetes can probably only be made after withdrawal and re-challenge with the suspect drug. In practice it is unlikely that it will be appropriate to do this except in a few cases.

Management

There is no clear consensus on the management of antipsychotic-induced diabetes. In the review of Mir and Taylor (2001) outcomes of different management options were described. In patients developing hyperglycaemia on clozapine, those who remained on the drug required oral hypoglycaemics or insulin. In those who discontinued clozapine, half required continued hypoglycaemic treatment. In patients developing ketoacidosis on clozapine, four out of seven patients saw a resolution of symptoms on cessation of clozapine but three of these developed ketoacidosis on re-exposure. Outcomes were similar for olanzapine: those remaining on the drug required continued hypoglycaemic treatment whereas around a half of those who discontinued olanzapine required continued treatment.

These observations are closely reflected in analysis of reports to the US FDA (Koller *et al.* 2001; Koller and Doraiswarmy 2002). With clozapine, 46 of 384 patients (12 per cent) had 'improved glycaemic control' after dose reduction discontinuation. With olanzapine, 78 per cent had improved glycaemic control after withdrawal or dose reduction. Again, hyperglycaemia was reported to recur in almost all cases of the drug being re-challenged.

These observations suggest three options for the management of antipsychotic-related diabetes – continued use of the causative agent with active treatment of diabetes, switching from the causative agent to another antipsychotic, or complete withdrawal of antipsychotic treatment.

The last of these options is unlikely to be reasonable in a chronic illness such as schizophrenia. Continuing antipsychotic treatment with the causative agent is likely to be necessary only where clozapine is being used (other antipsychotics are unlikely to be as effective) but is not a safe option where ketoacidosis has occurred. Where hyperglycaemia occurs following olanzapine treatment switching may be the preferred option. Data reviewed in this chapter suggest that diabetes is less likely to occur with risperidone and high potency conventional antipsychotics. Thus switching to risperidone or haloperidol may be cautiously recommended, although it should be noted that studies demonstrating the safety of this strategy are absent.

In some cases the patient and team may feel that the benefits of remaining on the antipsychotic drug suspected of causing diabetes outweigh the risk of switching, and opt to continue the existing antipsychotic and treat the diabetes. This is more likely to be the case where the diabetes/hyperglycaemia is mild, it can be controlled by modification of lifestyle and/or oral hypoglycaemics (i.e. there is not a need for insulin), there is significant doubt about whether the drug is a causal factor and there are felt to be significant risk of psychotic relapse should the medication be changed. Modifiable risk factors for Type II diabetes include smoking, lack of physical activity and a diet with excessive fat and simple carbohydrate intake – all are therapeutic targets for prevention and treatment (Hu *et al.* 2001).

It is essential that the patient is actively involved in discussions about management options. If necessary the advice of the patient's GP or a diabetologist should be obtained. Whatever option is chosen, close monitoring of glucose parameters is essential. At the very least, random plasma glucose and Hb_{A1C} measurements should be undertaken at 3–6 monthly intervals. Ideally, monitoring should also incorporate fasting plasma glucose and OGTT at a similar frequency. Referral to a specialist for treatment of diabetes is strongly recommended.

Risk factors and prevention

The majority of reported cases of hyperglycaemia and ketoacidosis have occurred within six months of beginning treatment with the drug suspected as being the causative agent (Mir and Taylor 2001; Koller *et al.* 2001; Koller and Doraiswamy 2002). Certain patient groups may be at increased risk of antipsychotic-induced diabetes – these include males (Koller *et al.* 2001) and those of African descent (Ananth *et al.* 2001). Other risk factors include diagnosis of psychotic disorder, obesity, age (older patients more at risk), diet (high fat, low fibre), inactivity and family history of diabetes (Goran *et al.* 2003; Henderson 2002).

The risk of antipsychotic-related diabetes may be reduced by using drugs now established as being of relatively low risk of diabetes (risperidone, high potency conventionals) and/or by close monitoring of glucose parameters. All patients beginning treatment with any antipsychotic should have baseline measures of fasting plasma glucose (where possible) and Hb_{A1C} performed. These tests should be repeated every 3 months in patients taking clozapine and olanzapine, or every six months in patients receiving other antipsychotics.

Summary: Diabetes mellitus

Definition	Syndrome characterized by hyperglycaemia secondary to lack of, or decreased effectiveness of, insulin.
Incidence	Not clear. At least 1% with all antipsychotics; greater than 10% with some atypical drugs.

Drugs causing syndrome	Probably all antipsychotics. Clozapine and olanzapine appear to be associated with higher risk than other antipsychotics.
	Non-psychiatric drugs that impair glucose tolerance include thiazide diuretics, corticosteroids, pentamidine and protease inhibitors.
Key symptoms	May be symptomless in early stages. Thirst and polyuria usually develop. May present as diabetic ketoacidosis – nausea, vomiting, and dehydration.
Pharmacological mechanism	Induction of insulin resistance – exact mechanism unknown.
Investigation to confirm diagnosis	Fasting plasma glucose; oral glucose tolerance test; glycosylated haemoglobin.
Management	Withdraw causative agent where possible. Assess need for oral hypoglycaemic or insulin. Lifestyle changes to reduce impact of risk factors such as obesity, smoking, lack of exercise and inappropriate diet.
Further reading	Melkersson K, Hulting A-L, and Brismar KE (2000). Elevated levels of insulin, leptin and blood lipids in olanzapine-treated patients with schizophrenia or related psychoses. *Journal of Clinical Psychiatry*, **61**, 742–748.
	Newcomer JW, Haupt DW, Fucetola R *et al*. (2002). Abnormalities in glucose regulation druing antipsychotic treatment of schizophrenia. *Archives General Psychiatry*, **59**, 337–345.
	Sernyak MJ, Leslie DL, Alarcon RD, *et al*. (2002). Association of diabetes mellitus with sue of atypical neuroleptics in the treatment of schizophrenia. *American Journal Psychiatry*, **159**, 561–566.

References

Ai D, Roper TA, and Riley JA (1998). Diabetic ketoacidosis and clozapine. *Postgrad Med J*, **74**, 493–4.

Ananth J, Gunatilake S, Aquino S, *et al*. (2001). Are African American patients at a higher risk for olanzapine-induced glucose intolerance? *Psychopharmacology*, **157**, 324–5.

Baptista T, Alvarez L, Lacruz A, *et al*. (1999). Glucose tolerance and serum insulin levels in an animal model of obesity induced by sub-acute or chronic administration of antipsychotic drugs. *Neuro-Psychopharmacol Biol Psychiatry*, **23**, 277–87.

Beckman JA, Creager MA, and Libby P (2002). Diabetes and atherosclerosis – epidemiology, pathophysiology and management. *JAMA*, **287**, 2570–81.

Braceland Captain FJ, Meduna LJ, *et al*. (1946). Delayed action of insulin in schizophrenia. *Am J Psychiatry*, **102**, 108–9.

British National Formulary No. 44 (2003). British Medical Association and the Royal Pharmaceutical Society of Great Britain. London, UK.

Cassidy F, Ahearn E, and Carroll BJ (1999). Elevated frequency of diabetes mellitus in hospitalized manic-depressive patients. *Am J Psychiatry*, **156**, 1417–20.

Cohen D (2002). Atypical antipsychotics and new onset diabetes mellitus in literature. Poster presented at ECNP annual conference. October 5–9, 2002, Barcelona, Spain.

Croarkin PE, Jacobs KM, and Bain BK (2000). Diabetic ketoacidosis associated with risperidone treatment. *Psychosomatics*, **41**, 369.

Dixon L, Weiden P, Delahanty J, *et al.* (2000). Prevalence and correlates of diabetes in national schizophrenia samples. *Schizophr Bull*, **20**, 903–12.

Edwards CRW and Bouchier IAD (ed.) (1991). *Davidson's Principles and Practice of Medicine*. Churchill Livingstone: Edinburgh.

Freeman H (1946). Resistance to insulin in mentally disturbed soldiers. *Arch Neurol Psychiatry*, **56**, 74–7.

Gerstein HC, Pais P, Pogue J, *et al.* (1999). Relationship of glucose and insulin levels to the risk of myocardial infarction: a case-control study. *J Am Coll Cardiol*, **33**, 612–19.

Gianfrancesco FD, Grogg AL, Mahmoud RA, *et al.* (2002). Differential effects of risperidone, olanzapine, clozapine and conventional antipsychotics on type 2 diabetes: findings from a large health plan database. *J Clin Psychiatry*, **63**, 920–30.

Goldstein LE, Sporn J, Brown S, *et al.* (1999). New-onset diabetes mellitus and diabetic ketoacidosis associated with olanzapine treatment. *Psychosomatics*, **40**, 438–43.

Goodman-Gilman A, Rall TW, Nies AS, *et al.* (ed.) (1990). *The Pharmacological Basis of Therapeutics*, 8th edn. McGraw-Hill: New York, NY, USA.

Goran M, Ball G, and Cruz M (2003). Obesity and risk of type 2 diabetes and cardiovascular disease in children and adolescents. *J Clin Endocrinol Metab*, **88**, 1417–27.

Grogg A, Gianfrancesco F, Myers J, *et al.* (2002). Association of newly reported diabetes and antipsychotics in mood disorder patients: findings from a large health plan database. Poster presented at ECNP annual conference. October 5–9, 2002, Barcelona, Spain.

Hagg S, Joelsson L, Mjorndal T, *et al.* (1998). Prevalence of diabetes and impaired glucose tolerance in patients treated with clozapine compared with patients treated with conventional depot neuroleptic medications. *J Clin Psychiatry*, **59**, 294–9.

Hayden JM and Reaven PD (2000). Cardiovascular disease in diabetes mellitus type 2: a potential role for novel cardiovascular risk factors. *Curr Opin Lipidol*, **11**, 519–28.

Henderson DC (2002). Atypical antipsychotic-induced diabetes mellitus. How strong is the evidence. *CNS Drugs*, **16**, 77–89.

Henderson DC, Cagliero E, Gray C, *et al.* (2000). Clozapine, diabetes mellitus, weight gain and lipid and abnormalities: a five-year naturalistic study. *Am J Psychiatry*, **157**, 975–81.

Hu FB, Manson JE, Stampfer MJ, *et al.* (2001). Diet, lifestyle, and the risk of type 2 diabetes mellitus in women. *New Engl J Med*, **345**, 790–7.

Keskiner A, el-Toumi A, and Bousquet T (1973). Psychotropic drugs, diabetes and chronic mental patients. *Psychosomatics*, **14**, 176–81.

Kingsbury SJ, Fayek M, Trufasiu D, *et al.* (2001). The apparent effects of ziprasidone on plasma lipids and glucose. *J Clin Psychiatry*, **62**, 347–9.

Koller EA and Doraiswamy PM (2002). Olanzapine-associated diabetes mellitus. *Pharmacotherapy*, **22**, 841–52.

Koller E, Schnedier B, Bennett K, *et al.* (2001). Clozapine-associated diabetes. *Am J Med*, **111**, 716–23.

Koro CE, Fedder DO, L'Italien GJ, *et al.* (2002). Assessment of independent effect of olanzapine and risperidone on risk of diabetes among patients with schizophrenia: population-based nested case-control study. *BMJ*, **325**, 243–5.

Kornegay CJ, Vasilakis-Scaramozza C, and Jick H (2002). Incident diabetes associated with antipsychotic use in the United Kingdom general practice research database. *J Clin Psychiatry*, **63**, 758–62.

Lebovitz HE (2001). Diagnosis, classification, and pathogenesis of diabetes mellitus. *J Clin Psychiatry*, **62**, 5–9.

Lindenmayer J-P and Patel R (1999). Olanzapine-induced ketoacidosis with diabetes mellitus. *Am J Psychiatry*, **156**, 1471.

Lorenz W (1922). Sugar tolerance in dementia praecox and other mental disorders. *Arch Neurol Psychiatry*, **8**, 184–96.

Luna B and Feinglos MN (2001). Drug-induced hyperglycaemia. *JAMA*, **286**, 1945–8.

Lund BC, Perry PJ, Brooks JM, *et al.* (2001). Clozapine use in patients with schizophrenia and the risk of diabetes, hyperlipidaemia, and hypertension. *Arch Gen Psychiatry*, **58**, 1172–6.

Melkersson K, Hulting A-L, and Brismar KE (2000). Elevated levels of insulin, leptin and blood lipids in olanzapine-treated patients with schizophrenia or related psychoses. *J Clin Psychiatry*, **61**, 742–8.

Melkersson K and Hulting A-L (2001). Insulin and leptin levels in patients with schizophrenia or related psychoses – a comparison between different antipsychotic agents. *Psychopharmacology*, **154**, 205–12.

Melkersson KI, Hulting A-L, and Brismar KE (1999). Different influences of classical antipsychotics and clozapine on glucose-insulin homeostasis in patients with schizophrenia or related psychoses. *J Clin Psychiatry*, **60**, 783–91.

Meyer JM (2002). A retrospective comparison of weight, lipid and glucose changes between risperidone and olanzapine-treated inpatients: metabolic outcomes after 1 year. *J Clin Psychiatry*, **63**, 425–33.

Mir S and Taylor D (2001). Atypical antipsychotics and hyperglycaemia. *Int Clin Psychopharmacology*, **16**, 63–74.

Mukherjee S, Decina P, Bocola V, *et al.* (1996). Diabetes mellitus in schizophrenic patients. *Compr Psychiatry*, **37**, 68–73.

National Diabetes Data Group (1979). Classification and diagnosis of diabetes mellitus and other categories of glucose intolerance. *Diabetes*, **28**, 1039–57.

Newcomer JW, Haupt DW, Fucetola R, *et al.* (2002). Abnormalities in glucose regulation druing antipsychotic treatment of schizophrenia. *Arch Gen Psychiatry*, **59**, 337–45.

Ober SK, Hudak R, and Rusterholtz A (1999). Hyperglycaemia and olanzapine. *Am J Psychiatry*, **156**, 970.

Osser DN, Najarian DM, and Dufresne RL (1999). Olanzapine increases weight and serum triglyceride levels. *J Clin Psychiatry*, **60**, 767–70.

Proakis AG, Mennear JH, Miya TS, *et al.* (1971). Phenothiazine-induced hyperglycaemia: relation to CNS and adrenal effects. *Proc Soc Exp Biol Med*, **137**, 1385–8.

Popli AP, Konicki PE, Jurjus GJ, *et al.* (1997). Clozapine and associated diabetes mellitus. *J Clin Psychiatry*, **58**, 108–11.

Procyshyn RM, Pande S, and Tse G (2000). New-onset diabetes mellitus associated with quetiapine. *Can J Psychiatry*, **45**, 668–9.

Reaven GM (1988). Role of insulin resistance in human disease. *Diabetes*, **37**, 1595–607.

Reaven GM and Chen Y-D (1988). Role of abnormal free fatty acid metabolism in the development of non-insulin-dependent diabetes mellitus. *Am J Med*, **85**, 106–12.

Ryan MCM and Thakore JH (2002). Physical consequences of schizophrenia and its treatment: The metabolic syndrome. *Life Sci*, **71**, 239–57.

Ryan MC, Collins P, and Thakore JH (2003). Impaired fasting glucose tolerance in first-episode, drug-naive patients with schizophrenia. *Am J Psychiatry*, **160**, 284–9.

Sernyak MJ, Leslie DL, Alarcon RD, *et al.* (2002). Association of diabetes mellitus with use of atypical neuroleptics in the treatment of schizophrenia. *Am J Psychiatry*, **159**, 561–6.

Sobel M, Jaggers ED, and Franz MA (1999). New-onset diabetes mellitus associated with the initiation of quetiapine treatment. *J Clin Psychiatry*, **60**, 556–7.

Taylor D, Paton C, and Kerwin R (2003). *The Maudsley Prescribing Guidelines*, 7th edn. Martin Dunitz: London, UK.

Thakore JH, Mann JN, Vlahos I, *et al.* (2002). Increased visceral fat distribution in drug-naive and drug-free patients with schizophrenia. *Int J Obesity*, **26**, 137–41.

Thonnard-Neumann E (1968). Phenothiazines and diabetes in hospitalised women. *Am J Psychiatry*, **124**, 138–9.

Wannamethee SG, Shaper AG, and Perry IJ (2001). Smoking as a modifiable risk factor for type 2 diabetes in middle aged men. *Diabetes Care* **24**, 9, 1590–5.

Wirshing DA, Pierre JM, Eyeler J, *et al.* (2001). Risperidone-associated new-onset diabetes. *Biol Psychiatry*, **50**, 148–9.

Wirshing DA, Boyd JA, Meng LR, *et al.* (2002). The effects of novel antipsychotics on glucose and lipid levels. *J Clin Psychiatry*, **63**, 856–64.

Yang SH and McNeely MJ (2002). Rhabdomyolysis, pancreatitis, and hyperglycaemia and ziprasidone. *Am J Psychiatry*, **159**, 1435.

Chapter 9

Teratogenic syndromes

Angelika Wieck

Introduction

It can be estimated from general population studies that about 7 per cent of women of childbearing age have current symptoms of a moderate to severe mental illness or have recently recovered from an episode (Smith and Weissman 1992; Jablensky 2000). A proportion of these women will be treated with psychotropic medications that have the potential to cause congenital malformations. This is a significant clinical problem because a large number of pregnancies, about 50–60 per cent in the UK and the US, are unplanned and are typically only detected at about the time of the second missed period (Lo and Friedman 2002), when the child may already have been harmed. The rate of unplanned pregnancies in psychiatric patients is likely to be significantly higher.

Although most children exposed to psychotropic teratogens *in utero* will develop normally, the congenital malformations that are associated with some psychotropics can lead to a fatal outcome, serious disfigurement, or permanent functional impairment. Clinicians need to be aware of these risks and take them into account when managing women of childbearing age.

This chapter will focus on malformations associated with commonly used psychotropic agents, namely anticonvulsant syndrome and neural tube defects, both of which are associated with carbamazepine and valproate, and heart malformations which are associated with lithium. The neurodevelopment of children exposed to antiepileptic drugs *in utero* has also been included because it is an emerging issue. Before considering these specific syndromes, a brief review is provided of the following areas; (1) general principles in managing teratogenic risk, (2) the relationship between teratogenesis and *in utero* drug exposure, and (3) data sources and classification of teratogenic risk.

General principles in managing teratogenic risk

The psychiatrist and other mental health professionals have important roles in reducing the risk of an adverse outcome for the infant in women taking psychotropic drugs. First, women must be made aware of potential teratogenic side effects. A recent survey of patients treated with lithium indicated that this is not yet generally the case. In a knowledge test of lithium-related adverse effects, 40 per cent of women indicated that they did not think that pregnancy should be avoided during lithium treatment (Wieck *et al.* 1999). Doctors need to inform the patient about basic aspects of the type of defects which may occur, what is known about their relative risks compared to the general population, what the implications are for the infant and whether they can be diagnosed prenatally.

A second important aspect is to ensure that women know how to prevent unplanned pregnancies. If appropriate, this may involve education about menstrual cycle monitoring, advice on effective contraception, recognizing early signs of pregnancy, avoiding unprotected sexual intercourse and educating the partner. The patient needs to be instructed to contact their psychiatrist or family physician immediately if they get pregnant and have been taking a potentially teratogenic drug. Third, mental health professionals should contribute to educating patients about the role of lifestyle factors in intra-uterine development and that it can be compromised by obesity and nicotine and substance abuse.

Teratogens and intrauterine development

The term 'teratogen' derives from the Greek word *terato*, meaning monster. A teratogenic agent can be defined as a substance which is capable of inducing a permanent abnormality of structure or function in an organism exposed to it during embryonic or fetal life (Dicke 1978). The timing of exposure is of critical importance in determining the type and extent of abnormalities developing.

In the pre-embryonic phase of development (day 1–12) the conceptus is transported through the fallopian tube, implants into the uterine mucosa and forms the embryonic disc. Any teratogen administered during this time will have an 'all or nothing' effect, leading either to the death of the whole conceptus or causing only the death of some cells whose function is fully replaced by others.

In the embryonic phase (3–8 weeks of gestation) the main organ systems and body features are formed and teratogens may cause gross malformations. During the remainder of intrauterine development organs grow and develop functionally. Harmful agents administered during this time can cause growth retardation, structural abnormalities and organ dysfunction.

The timing of exposure to psychotropic drugs is of particular importance for the development of the cardiovascular and the central nervous system (CNS). A single heart tube forms by day 22, the septa by day 27–37, and the valves by day 35, i.e. 5 weeks after the first missed period. The development of the CNS begins on day 16–18 and the neural tube closes by day 30 (i.e. 2 weeks after the first missed period). Since the CNS develops more slowly than other organ systems, its structural and functional development continues to be particularly vulnerable to noxious substances up to the end of gestation.

Data sources and classifications of risk

Current data on the teratogenic effects of most psychotropic drugs come from a variety of sources and are in general unsatisfactory. When animal data exist these can point to a possible association, but the susceptibility between and even within species is so great that an extrapolation about the presence or degree of risk to humans cannot be made. In humans evidence consists of cases reported as part of post-marketing surveillance, published case reports, and more recently observations from studies that have enrolled pregnant women and monitored infant outcome. This approach has the advantage that the contribution of genetic and lifestyle factors can be assessed prospectively and that anatomical and functional anomalies can be studied in detail. The prospective studies of infant exposure to psychotropic medication published so far have been helpful in estimating the overall risk of all major congenital malformations for particular drugs compared to the background rate of 2–4 per cent in the general population (Nelson and Holmes 1989). However, the sample sizes are mostly too small to draw definite conclusions about specific defects.

In order to summarize available data on drug safety several countries have set up classification systems that allocate individual drugs to a level of teratogenic risk. The aim was to assist physicians prescribing for pregnant women. In 1979 the US Food and Drug Administration defined five risk categories for all drugs (see Table 9.1) and the allocated category must be displayed on their labels. Although widely used the system has given rise to increasing concerns including the oversimplification of evidence, the poor quality of data, the emphasis on risks and that the allocations to categories quickly becomes outdated (Hansen *et al.* 2002). In recognition of these considerations the FDA is now developing a new labeling system which distinguishes between information on risks and clinical advice and replaces letter categories with a narrative text of the available literature (Kennedy 2001). Several new prospective pregnancy registers have recently commenced in collaborating centers of Europe, Australia, Asia and the United States. Projects have focused particularly on psychotropic drugs such as old and new antipsychotics, most anti-epileptic drugs and some benzodiazepines.

Table 9.1 Food and Drug Administration pregnancy risk categories

Category	Definition
A	Adequate, well controlled studies in pregnant women have failed to demonstrate a risk to the developing fetus.
B	Either animal studies show a risk, but human studies do not; or, if no adequate studies have been conducted in pregnant women, then animal studies have not demonstrated a risk.
C	Human studies are lacking, and animal studies have either produced adverse effects or are also lacking. Therefore, the risk of medication exposure in the fetus cannot be ruled out. Medications should be used in pregnancy only when potential benefits outweigh potential risk.
D	Positive evidence of fetal risk has been demonstrated in humans. However, the potential benefits of use in pregnant women may outweigh the potential risks, thus decisions must be made on an individual basis.
X	The medication is contraindicated in women who are or may become pregnant. The fetal risk of medication exposure clearly outweighs any potential benefits to the mother.

Psychotropics and teratogenic potential

With rare exceptions all drugs administered to the mother are transferred across the placenta and reach the embryo and fetus. Among the antidepressant and antipsychotic drugs there are some agents that are regarded as probably safe to use in pregnancy on the basis of available pregnancy outcome data. In general more information exists for the older than for the newer agents.

Tricyclic antidepressant drugs are still allocated to the D category of the FDA classification as being associated with positive evidence of human fetal risk, although no such evidence exists and the available data suggest that they are probably safe. Most data are available for amitryptiline (Koren *et al.* 1998). All the available selective serotonin reuptake inhibitors have a FDA C-label although the relatively large database on fluoxetine of over 2000 cases of first trimester exposure and one prospective follow-up study of such children did not indicate increased risk for major congenital malformation or later neuro-developmental problems (Nulman *et al.* 1997).

Among the antipsychotic drugs most is known about phenothiazines. Altshuler *et al.* (1996) pooled data from retrospective and prospective studies of infant outcome after exposure to low potency phenothiazines in the first trimester. Although there was a small but significant increase in the rate of all congenital malformations among the exposed group ($N = 2,591$) than in the unexposed children ($N = 71,746$) there was no specific association with any anomaly. The high potency antipsychotics stelazine and haloperidol are also regarded as relatively safe in pregnancy (Altshuler *et al.* 1996).

Whereas there are relatively safe treatment options for psychotic and depressed women, the management of bipolar patients poses a dilemma because all commonly used mood stabilizers (i.e. lithium, carbamazepine, valproate) are associated with an increased risk of congenital abnormalities and some may lead to neurodevelopmental impairments.

The introduction of anti-epileptic drugs (AEDs) into the treatment of affective disorders is relatively recent and almost all data on the use of these compounds in pregnancy comes from studies of epileptic women. It has been known for some decades that congenital abnormalities are more common in infants of mothers treated with AEDs and recent studies have provided estimates of their incidence.

In a multi-center and prospective study from Japan the incidence of congenital malformation was 11.5 per cent in 638 live births of epileptic mothers treated with AEDs in the first trimester and 2.3 per cent in infants of non-medicated mothers with seizure disorders (Nakane *et al.* 1980). Two further multi-center prospective studies found the risk to be increased threefold in 885 exposed compared to 98 unexposed children (Kaneko *et al.* 1999), and 2.3-fold increased in 192 children exposed compared to 158 unexposed controls (Samren *et al.* 1997). Holmes *et al.* (2001) compared infant outcome in 98 untreated epileptic mothers, 223 mothers treated with one AED and 93 mothers treated with two or more AEDs and 508 controls. The odds ratio for the combined frequency of major congenital malformations (including growth retardation) was 2.8 for the group exposed to one AED and 4.2 in the group exposed to two or more AEDs. The finding that the rate was not increased in children of epileptic mothers unexposed to AEDs is consistent with more recent studies that maternal seizures do not make a large contribution to the congenital malformation rate (Robert *et al.* 2001). That polytherapy with two or more AEDs is associated with a greater risk of major malformations has been demonstrated in many other studies (Nakane *et al.* 1980; Tanganelli and Regesta 1992; Lindhout *et al.* 1992; Samren *et al.* 1997; Samren *et al.* 1999; Kaneko *et al.* 1999). A relationship between dose and the incidence of congenital malformations has been best demonstrated for valproate but less so with other drugs. Offspring of mothers using >1000 mg of valproate per day during pregnancy are at a significantly increased risk of major congenital malformations (Omtzigt *et al.* 1992).

In early descriptions of children exposed to AEDs *in utero* no specific patterns of birth defects were recognized. More recently syndromal patterns have been described as well as a specific association between the two anti-epileptics which are most commonly used in mood disorders – sodium valproate and carbamazepine – and neural tube defects. Some investigators have also presented evidence of impairments in psychomotor development in association with intrauterine exposure to AEDs. These have been included in this chapter because they may result from AED effects on the development of the brain in the second and third trimester.

Anticonvulsant syndrome

Clinical features

Hanson and Smith (1975) observed similarities in the anomalies of children born to mothers treated with phenytoin during pregnancy. These included orofacial clefts, growth retardation with a small head circumference, facial dysmorphisms, and cardiac defects. A characteristic feature was a distal digital hypoplasia with small nails. This pattern of anomalies became known as the fetal phenytoin syndrome.

In the 1980s a similar pattern of abnormalities was described for children after first trimester exposure to carbamazepine. Characteristics were upslanting palpebral fissures, epicanthal folds, short nose, long philtrum and distal digit hypoplasia and microcephaly (Jones *et al.* 1989). A dysmorphic syndrome was also defined by Di Liberti (1984) in children exposed to valproic acid characterized by facial dysmorphisms (inferior epicanthal folds, a flat nasal bridge, an upturned nasal tip, a thin vermilion border, a shallow philtrum and a downturned mouth), various finger and toe abnormalities (long, thin and overlapping with hyper-convex nails) and radial ray anomalies (for review see Robert *et al.* 2001). Because of the similarities in the features occurring with different agents some authors use the term anticonvulsant syndrome.

There are no reliable data yet for the incidence of these features in infants exposed to individual drugs.

Pharmacological basis

Unknown; may be due to the anti-folate action of AEDs.

Management

In exposed pregnancies sonographic assessments should screen for dysmorphic facial features and other associated defects, including microcephaly and heart defects. Orofacial clefts require intensive treatment after birth and possibly surgical corrections but other dysmorphic facial features tend to resolve as the children get older.

Risk factors and prevention

The general advice outlined at the start of this chapter is important, i.e. prior to prescribing women of childbearing age need to advised about the teratogenic risk of AEDs and the need for effective contraception. The clinician, ideally in discussion with the patient, should consider other treatment options. If therapy with an AED cannot be avoided in pregnancy, the patient should not be administered more than one drug from this class. Because of the relationship between the dose of sodium valproate and the malformation risk it is generally advised to avoid daily doses of valproate of 1000 mg or more (e.g. Royal College of Physicians of London 1997). The drug should be administered in several divided doses over the day to avoid high peak levels and serum concentrations should be measured regularly to avoid toxic levels. It is unclear whether folate intake in the three months before and after conception decreases the risk of anticonvulsant syndrome.

Neural tube defects

Clinical features

The major difference between the two AEDs which are commonly used as mood stabilizers – carbamazepine and sodium valproate – and other AEDs is that they have a specific association with neural tube defects.

Neural tube defects (NTDs) are among the most common human congenital malformations and are reported to occur in 0.06 per cent of live births in the United States (Nakano 1973). The primary defect in all NTD's is a failure of the neural tube to close and this can occur at any point along its formation within a small window of time (day 17 and 30 of gestation). Various forms and degrees of CNS abnormalities can result. Anencephaly is due to the failed closure of the proximal parts and is characterized by an absent cranial vault and cerebral hemispheres. The fetus has a deformed forehead, large ears and eyes and often otherwise normal facial features. If pregnancy is carried to term infants are either stillborn or die within a few days of birth.

Encephaloceles are occipital or frontal herniations of dura mater through a closure defect in the skull and skin. Varying amounts of brain tissue may be involved in the lesion. Isolated herniations of dura carry a good prognosis, whereas encephaloceles with microcephaly secondary to brain herniation have a very poor prognosis.

Open spinal cord defects include meningoceles or myelomeningoceles. Here a dural sac protrudes through an open vertebral arch and skin defect and may contain spinal cord tissue and nerve roots. The spinal cord often ends in this sac. The most common locations for these defects are the lumbar and lumbosacral regions (Ellenbogen 2002). Often the fetus also develops hydrocephalus and Chiari malformations. Milder forms of spina bifida are covered by skin with varying involvement of nervous tissues. There may be pointers to the underlying lesion in the form of cutaneous stigmata such as a hairy patch, a dimple, a haemangioma or a lipoma.

Spina bifida and anencephaly make up more than 95 per cent of neural tube defects. Fetuses with NTDs often have other malformations in the gastrointestinal tract, the heart and big vessels, the urogenital system and the lower extremities.

If children with spinal NTDs are born the neurological deficits are often severe. They depend on the spinal level and the amount of tissue involved and include motor and sensory deficits of the lower extremities, faecal and urinary incontinence and radicular pain.

Incidence

Matalon *et al.* (2002) analyzed data from prospective studies of carbamazepine exposure and pooled infant outcomes of a total of 1255 cases. They found that 0.5 per cent of offspring exposed to monotherapy and 0.67 per cent exposed to polytherapy had hydrocephalus and NTDs. This is consistent with Rosa (1991) who estimated the incidence of spinal NTDs in carbamazepine-exposed pregnancies as 1 per cent on the basis of a small number of cases pooled from published reports. In several studies the incidence of NTDs in children exposed to sodium valproate has been reported as 1–2 per cent (Lamner *et al.* 1987; Lindhout and Schmidt 1986).

Pharmacological basis

The formation of the neural plate, its growth and movements to form the neural tube in conjunction with surrounding tissues is a highly complicated process that most likely involves regulation by a multitude of genes. Strong candidates for an involvement are the 150 or so genes which regulate the metabolism and transport of folic acid (Finnell *et al.* 2003). This hypothsis is based on the finding that folate supplementation can reduce the incidence of NTDs and that both valproic acid and carbamazepine are folate antagonists.

Management

Prenatal investigations in women at risk of NTD pregnancies rely on ultrasound scanning and the measurement of serum markers. A woman at risk may be offered a scan at the end of the first trimester which can determine the gestational age and may show the absence of skull ossification as a sign of anencephaly. The diagnosis of NTDs is aided by the measurement of alpha-fetoprotein (AFP) in maternal serum (MS). The fetus has two major blood proteins, albumin and AFP. AFP enters amniotic fluid through fetal urination and gastrointestinal secretions and reaches the maternal circulation by transudation across the amnion and placenta. If a fetus has an open NTD, AFP rapidly diffuses from the exposed tissues into the amniotic fluid and maternal values rise into the abnormal range. MSAFP elevations can also be caused by other conditions and are not diagnostic of fetal NTDs.

If the MSAFP is elevated a non-targeted sonogram is performed to identify easily recognizable causes of false-positive results. If the cause is not explained the next step may be a targeted (level 2) scan carried out by an experienced examiner in weeks 18–23. Diagnosis of spinal NTD involves the systematic examination of each neural arch from the cervical to the sacral region. The extent of the lesion as well as the spinal level can be determined. With these procedures NTDs are detected in 90–100 per cent of cases (Goldstein and Caponigro 2001). Alternatively, the next step may be amniocentesis for the measurement of AFP and acetylcholinesterase levels in amniotic fluid. Acetylcholinesterase levels are elevated in the presence of NTDs and help differentiation from other causes of increased AFP levels. During a level 2 scan the infant may also be assessed for other structural abnormalities associated with AED exposure. If cardiac abnormalities are found a fetal echocardiogram may become necessary.

When a major congenital abnormality is diagnosed the patient and her partner will be advised about the benefits and disadvantages of management options by specialist staff in the obstetric department. Prenatal surgery for certain heart conditions and myelomeningocele is being pioneered in a few specialist and multidisciplinary fetal treatment centers, but is unavailable for most cases.

Depending on the severity and prognosis of the condition the mother and her partner may request a termination of pregnancy. Legal provisions for the termination of pregnancy in cases of severe fetal abnormalities vary widely between countries. In Great Britain it is available on request before viability at 24 weeks of gestation and beyond this time limit it is legally permitted if there is a 'substantial risk' that the child will be seriously handicapped after birth because of congenital abnormalities (The British Abortion Act 1967, amended in 1991). In the US, the time limit for abortion upon request varies between 13 and 28 weeks and only a few states have provisions for fetal malformations beyond these time limits (Beller and deProsse 1992).

The stress resulting from diagnostic procedures, the possible loss of pregnancy and the guilt some women may experience may lead to a deterioriation in the patient's mental state. Additional support from community mental health staff should be offered and the patient's mental state monitored closely.

The newborn child with myelomingocele requires intensive investigations. These include particularly an assessment of neurological and urological function, cerebral and cardiac ultrasound and orthopaedic evaluation. The surgical closure of the lesion is usually performed within a few days of birth. If a hydrocephalus is present a shunt can be placed at the same time or at a later date. The prognosis for survival and functioning depend on the severity of the initial defects.

Risk factors

The infant's risk to develop NTDs increases when a parent or previous sibling is affected by a NTD. Several maternal factors are associated with an increased prevalence of NTD including obesity, diabetes mellitus, a flu-like or febrile illness in the first trimester, lower socioeconomic status and diet, particularly excess vitamin A intake. There is also a significant geographic variation in the prevalence of NTD's. The British Isles, for example, have a higher rate than continental Europe (Frey and Hauser 2003). Similar variations have been seen within other countries and continents.

Prevention

There is no doubt that dietary folic acid supplements reduce the overall prevalence of NTD's. The evidence comes from studies of both high-risk pregnancies and first occurrences. In a double-blind trial by the Medical Research Council in the UK 1817 women with a previous pregnancy affected by a NTD were randomized to receive either 4 mg of folic acid, other vitamins, both or neither (MRC Vitamin Study Research Group 1991). There was a 72 per cent reduction of NTDs in the women receiving folic acid and no effect with other vitamins. Since then a number of randomized controlled trials have been published on the use of periconceptional folic acid intake to prevent first occurrences of NTD. In a recent systematic review of these trials Lumley *et al.* (2001) estimated that the vitamin reduces the relative NTD risk to 0.28. Since 1992 the Department of Health for the UK has recommended that all women of childbearing age should consume 0.4 mg folic acid daily in addition to their usual diet (Department of Health 1992). Women with a previous NTD pregnancy were advised to take 5 mg (preparations containing 4 mg as initially used in the MRC trial are not available). Supplements should be taken from three months before conception until 12 weeks of gestation. A similar recommendation has been made in the US (Centers for Disease Control 1992) although women with a previous NTD pregnancy are being advised to seek advice from their physician.

It is uncertain whether additional dietary folate intake protects children at risk from AED-induced NTDs. Hernandez-Diaz *et al.* (2000) reported that when pregnant women treated with AEDs also took a multivitamin supplement containing folic acid it did not reduce the incidence of cardiovascular and urinary tract abnormalities or oral clefts in their infants. Figures concerning NTDs were not reported. Recently three women taking valproate during pregnancy have been described who gave birth to children with NTDs despite periconceptional folate intake at a daily dose of 3.5–5 mg (Craig *et al.* 1999; Duncan *et al.* 2001). Clearly, prospective trials with large numbers of epileptic mothers taking AEDs are needed to examine whether the preventative effect of folate in this population is as large as in women at high risk for other reasons.

If AED treatment is unavoidable then it is likely that the risk of NTDs, as for congenital abnormalities in general, can be reduced by the use of a single AED at as low a dose as possible with multiple dosing to reduce peak plasma levels.

AED exposure *in utero* and psychomotor development

Whereas exposure to AED's in the first trimester can cause disturbance in the gross structure of the nervous system, teratogenic effects in the second half of pregnancy may interrupt neuronal migration and synaptic organization and result in some degree of cognitive dysfunction (Barrett and Richens 2003). Data from both retrospective and prospective studies of psychomotor development in children exposed to AEDs *in utero* have been conflicting. Some have reported a high prevalence of developmental delay compared to controls (Hill *et al.* 1982; Gaily *et al.* 1988; Hanson *et al.* 1976; Rovet *et al.* 1995), others have only found transient impairments (Normura *et al.* 1984) or no deficits at all (Nelson and Ellenberg 1982; Shapiro *et al.* 1976).

This lack of agreement is due to generally small sample sizes and methodological differences, such as varying treatment regimens, the wide range of ages when children were tested, and differences in the developmental and cognitive testing material. In addition, other factors that may affect the development of children of epileptic mothers have sometimes not been taken into account. These include the influence of maternal and paternal intelligence, genetic traits associated with epilepsy and psychosocial problems caused by the maternal seizure frequency. Prolonged generalized seizures of the mother may also lead to foetal brain damage complicating the picture. There is no evidence, however, that brief convulsive or non-convulsive seizures would cause cognitive problems in the exposed children (Barrett and Richens 2003). The question of a possible neuro-developmental disadvantage is important and a topic of several ongoing prospective studies (Barrett and Richens 2003).

Because of the uncertainty in this area, the question arises whether a pregnant woman should take AEDs in the second and third trimester. This should be discussed with the woman as well as other treatment options.

Lithium and heart defects

Clinical features

Lithium has been associated with various abnormalities in the development of the large vessels and Ebstein's anomaly. The latter is characterized by a downward displacement of the tricuspid valve into the right ventricle. This can cause tricuspid regurgitation, arrhythmia and congestive heart failure. Ebstein's anomaly is often associated with other cardiac anomalies. Lithium may also increase the risk of non-cardiac malformations.

Incidence

Following earlier case reports of cardiovascular abnormalities in infants born to mothers taking lithium in pregnancy, a lithium baby register was established in 1968 in Denmark. It was later expanded to other Scandinavian countries, the United States and Canada and data collection was completed in 1979. The register included 225 babies exposed to lithium in the first trimester (Weinstein 1980). Twenty-five (11 per cent) children were born with major congenital abnormalities. Of these, 7 cases (3 per cent) had non-cardiac abnormalities (which is consistent with the rate in the general population) and 18 (8 per cent) had cardiac defects. Of these 18 infants 12 had various abnormal developments of the heart and the large vessels but 6 (2.7 per cent) had the otherwise rare Ebstein's anomaly. In the general population the incidence of Ebstein's is estimated to be only about 1:20 000 live births.

Because the lithium baby register was a voluntary reporting system the incidence of anomalies is likely to have been over-estimated. However, further evidence for an association of lithium with Ebstein's anomaly comes from a report by Nora *et al.* (1974). They observed that two mothers who had given birth to children with Ebstein's had taken lithium in the first trimester of pregnancy. Lithium exposure during the two years in which these two cases were ascertained was recorded only in these two instances out of 733 teratogenic histories obtained.

Several studies have since attempted to estimate the magnitude of the risk. Kallen and Tandberg (1983) retrospectively linked the psychiatric and obstetric registers in Sweden and identified 287 women with bipolar affective disorder who had given birth. Of the 228 infants not exposed to lithium 9 (4 per cent) had congenital malformations compared to 7/59 (12 per cent) in the lithium exposed group ($P < 0.03$). Cardiac defects occured significantly more frequently following lithium exposure (6.8 per cent vs 0.9 per cent, $P < 0.02$) but did not include specifically Ebstein's. Interestingly, the incidence of cardiac defects in the unexposed infants was consistent with the general population rate in live newborns of 0.8 per cent (Mitchell *et al.* 1971).

Jacobson *et al.* (1994) summarized the results of a cohort study with subjects from four Teratogen Information Centres in North America; 148 women treated with lithium in the first trimester were compared with age-matched controls exposed to non-teratogenic drugs. In both groups there were three live infants with congenital malformations but in the exposed group one pregnancy was terminated due to a prenatal diagnosis of Ebstein's.

Four case control studies have looked for an association with lithium in children born with Ebstein's (Kallen 1988; Sipek 1989; Edmonds and Oakley 1990; Zalstein *et al.* 1990). Taking all 251 cases together, there were none who were exposed to the drug. In a fifth small case control study Kallen (1991) took a different approach. He compared children who had bipolar mothers and were born with heart defects ($N = 11$) and without heart defects ($N = 16$). There was no difference in lithium exposure (3 vs 4 cases). However, the only case of Ebstein anomaly occurred in an unexposed infant, raising the possibility that this defect may be associated with bipolar disorder itself rather than treatment with lithium.

These studies indicate that the lithium-related incidence of Ebstein's anomaly is likely to be smaller than the 2.7 per cent found in the Lithium Baby Register. Because of the limited sample sizes and the design of the published studies it is at present not known how much smaller the risk is. It has been suggested that lithium may only lead to a tenfold increase above the background rate, i.e. 1:2000 (Cohen *et al.* 1994). Further studies are urgently needed to provide better risk estimates for this serious complication. Of concern is also the threefold increase in the incidence of all congenital abnormalities and the eightfold increase of all cardiac malformations in the well-designed study of bipolar women by Kallen and Tandberg (1983).

Pharmacological mechanism

Lithium freely crosses the placenta in animals and humans and serum concentrations in maternal and fetal blood are similar. The pharmacological mechanism that may link lithium with disturbances in cardiovascular development is not known.

Management

In an infant exposed to lithium in the first trimester gross structural abnormalities of the heart can be detected sonographically with the four chamber view from about the 11th week of gestation. Most major vascular connections are visible from 18 weeks onwards. Fetal lithium exposure is also an indication for fetal echocardiography which allows detailed structural and functional assessments. This may be done from 14 weeks of gestation onwards but in later scans more subtle defects can be visualized (Silverman and Hanley 2001). Referral to a tertiary fetal scanning center may be recommended in lithium exposed pregnancies. If the diagnosis of Ebstein's anomaly is confirmed no fetal interventions are currently recommended (Silverman and Hanley 2001). Neonates with Ebstein's have a high mortality rate and most of the survivors require corrective surgery. As with other major fetal malformations, women require detailed advice and support.

Risk factors and prevention

No risk factors that effect the risk of cardiac malformations occurring with lithium have been identified. The only preventative strategy is to avoid lithium prior to conception and during the first trimester. It is essential that women of childbearing age are provided with advice regarding the teratogenic risk associated with lithium before commencing treatment. The importance of reliable contraception should be discussed. The psychiatrist should emphasize that should the patient wish to conceive at some future date they should discuss this with the psychiatric team first so that appropriate preconception counselling can be arranged.

Pre-conception counselling

Perinatal psychiatrists are increasingly asked for advice on the management of women who have recurrent psychiatric disorders, take prophylactic medication and wish to have a child. Most of these requests relate to women with histories of affective disorders, in particular bipolar affective disorder (Wieck unpublished data). Teratogenicity is only one of many aspects to be considered. One of the questions arising is the effect of childbearing on the course of a woman's illness. A recent study suggests that when women with bipolar disorder are gradually withdrawn from lithium in the beginning of pregnancy the course of the illness does not alter until after childbirth, when they are at high risk of becoming ill again (Viguera et al. 2000). It is therefore important to carefully review whether a woman requires continuation of drug therapy before conception and during pregnancy, taking into account the frequency and severity of past episodes, her response to treatment and the presence of stressful life circumstances. If in the opinion of the clinician psychotropic medication should be continued and the woman is taking a potentially teratogenic mood stabilizer, the most reasonable approach needs to be defined between the clinician, the patient and the partner. Attitudes to taking risks for the child vary not only between women but also the clinicians advising them.

If patient and doctor agree that a mood stabilizer should be discontinued, other treatment options need to be considered. The alternatives most likely to be chosen are the typical antipsychotics chlorpromazine, stelazine and haloperidol, because of their relative safety in pregnancy and their known class effect in acute mania. If a patient has a history of significant side effects in response to these agents, such as prolactin-induced amenorrhoea, parkinsonian or orthostatic symptoms, an atypical antipsychotic may have to be considered. To date little is known about their safety in pregnancy. At present most data are available for olanzapine. Infant outcomes reported for 144 prospectively followed pregnancies exposed to this agent, mostly in the first trimester, have not shown an increased rate of congenital malformations (Data on file, Lilly Research Laboratories). Olanzapine also has the advantage of being licensed for maintenance treatment in bipolar disorder. Other antipsychotics have yet been little tested in the prophylaxis of bipolar recurrences, but this also applies to all mood stabilizers except for lithium.

Summary: Anticonvulsant syndrome

Definition	A constellation of congenital abnormalities following first trimester anticonvulsant exposure.
Incidence	For all AEDs together incidence of congenital malformations is increased about two to threefold irrespective of maternal epilepsy.
	No reliable data for individual drugs.
Drugs causing the syndrome	Carbamazepine, valproate, phenytoin
	Insufficient information on other AEDs.
Key features	Dysmorphic facial features
	Finger and toe dysplasias
	Associated problems include:
	Growth retardation and microcephaly
	Heart defects
Pharmacological mechanism	Unknown. May be due to antifolate action of AEDs
Investigations (prenatal diagnosis)	Screening ultrasound for abnormalities at the end of 1st trimester and targeted ultrasound between 18–23 weeks of pregnancy, fetal echocardiography for suspected heart defects.

Management	Aim for prevention (advice to patient regarding risk and need for contraception; if AED mood stabilizer unavoidable use in monotherapy and in lowest possible dose; avoid doses of valproate >1000 mg; efficacy of dietary folate (5 mg/day) in the three months before and after conception in prevention is unclear)
	Counselling for patient regarding condition, prognosis and management options
	Facial dysmorphisms resolve in time
	If diagnosed prenatally and other abnormalities are severe the patient may consider termination
Further reading	Jones KL, Lacro RV, Johnson KA, *et al.* (1989) Pattern of malformations in the children of women treated with carbamazepine during pregnancy. *The New England Journal of Medicine*, **320**, 1661–6.
	Di Liberti JR, Farndon PA, Dennis NR, *et al.* (1984) The foetal valproate syndrome. *American Journal of Medical Genetics*, **19**, 483–91.

Summary: Neural tube defects

Definition	Congenital CNS abnormalities caused by a failed closure of the neural tube
Incidence	General population incidence: 0.06 % of all live births
	After 1st trimester carbamazepine exposure: 0.5–1.0%
	After 1st trimester valproate exposure: 1–2%
Drugs causing the syndrome	Carbamazepine, valproate
Key features	Mostly anencephaly and spina bifida (meningocele, myelomeningocele, closed defects)
	Associated abnormalities: hydrocephalus. Also in gastrointestinal tract, cardiovascular system, urogenital system, lower extremities
Pharmacological mechanism	Probably antifolate action of AEDs interacting with genetic predisposition
Investigations (prenatal diagnosis)	Screening ultrasound for abnormalities at the end of 1st trimester
	Targeted ultrasound between 18–23 weeks gestation
	Maternal alpha-fetoprotein levels
	Amniocentesis: measurement of amniotic alpha-fetoprotein and acetylcholinesterase levels

Management	Aim for prevention (advice to patient regarding risk and need for contraception; if AED mood stabilizer unavoidable use in monotherapy and in lowest possible dose; avoid doses of valproate >1000 mg; efficacy of dietary folate (5 mg/day) in the three months before and after conception in prevention is unclear)
	Counselling for patient regarding condition, prognosis and management options
	Anencephaly: usually termination
	Fetal surgery for myelomeningocele in development
	Surgery and management of neurological deficits and associated abnormalities ongoing from birth
Further reading	Omtzigt JC, Nau H, and Los FJ (1992). The disposition of valproate and its metabolites in the late first trimester and early second trimester of pregnancy in maternal serum, urine and amniotic fluid: effect of dose, co-medication and the presence of spinal bifida. *European Journal of Clinical Pharmacology*, **43,** 381–8.
	Goldstein RB and Caponigro M (2001). The role of sonography in the evaluation of pregnant women with high maternal serum alpha-fetoprotein. *Applied Radiology*, **30,** 9–18.
	Matalon S, Schechtmann S, Goldzweig G, *et al.* (2002). The teratogenic effect of carbamazepine: a meta-analysis of 1255 exposures. *Reproductive Toxicology*, **16,** 9–17.

Summary: Heart defects associated with lithium

Definition	Abnormalities of intra-uterine cardiovascular development caused by first trimester exposure to lithium
Incidence	All heart defects in the general population: 0.8% of all live births
	All heart defects after 1st trimester lithium exposure: Relative risk increased 7.7 fold
	Ebstein's anomaly in general population: 1:20,000
	Ebstein's anomaly after 1st trimester exposure: no reliable data, estimated as 1:2000
Key features	Ebstein's anomaly: downward displacement of the tricuspid valve into the right ventricle causing tricuspid regurgitation, arrhythmia and congestive heart failure. Usually associated with other cardiovascular defects
Pharmacological mechanism	Unknown

Investigations (prenatal diagnosis)	Sonographic screening for gross abnormalities at the end of 1st trimester
	Targeted ultrasound between 18–23 weeks gestation
	Fetal echocardiography from 14 weeks onwards
Management	Aim for prevention (advice to patient regarding risk and need for contraception; consider switch to alternative treatment prior to conception)
	Counselling of patient regarding condition, prognosis and management options
	Depending on severity of defect patient may decide to terminate pregnancy
	Surgical treatment of cardiac defects
Further reading	Weinstein MR (1980). Lithium treatment of women during pregnancy and the post-delivery period. In Johnson FN, ed. *Handbook of lithium* therapy, pp. 421–9. MTP Press, Lancaster.
	Cohen LS, Friedman JM, Jefferson JW, *et al.* (1994). A re-evaluation of risk of in utero exposure to lithium. *JAMA*, **271**, 146–50.

References

Altshuler LL, Cohen L, Szuba MP, *et al.* (1996). Pharmacologic management of psychiatric illness during pregnancy: dilemmas and guidelines. *Am J Psychiatry*, **153**, 592–606.

Barrett C and Richens A (2003). Epilepsy and pregnancy: report of an epilepsy research foundation workshop. *Epilepsy Res*, **52**, 147–87.

Beller FK and deProsse CA (1992). Confusion of trimester viability. Consequences for abortion laws in the United States. *J Reprod Med*, **37**, 537–40.

Centers for Disease Control (1992). Recommendations for the use of folic acid to reduce the number of cases of spina bifida and other neural tube defects. *MMWR*, **41**, RR-14.

Cohen LS, Friedman JM, Jefferson JW, *et al.* (1994). A reevaluation of risk of in utero exposure to lithium. *JAMA*, **271**, 146–50.

Craig J, Morrison P, Morrow J, *et al.* (1999). Failure of periconceptional folic acid to prevent a neural tube defect in the offspring of a mother taking sodium valproate. *Seizure*, **8**, 253–4.

Department of Health (1992). *Folic Acid and the Prevention of Neural Tube Defects. Report from an Expert Advisory Group.* HMSO: London.

Dicke JM (1978). Teratology: principles and practice. *Med Clin North Am*, **27**, 567–82.

Di Liberti JR, Farndon PA, Dennis NR, *et al.* (1984). The foetal valproate syndrome. *Am J Med Genet*, **19**, 483–91.

Duncan S, Mercho S, Lopes-Cendes, *et al.* (2001). Repeated neural tube defects and valproate monotherapy suggest a pharmacologic abnormality. *Epilepsia*, **52**, 750–3.

Edmonds LD and Oakley GP (1990). Ebstein's anomaly and maternal lithium exposure during pregnancy. *Teratology*, **41**, 551–2.

Ellenbogen RG (2002). Neural tube defects in the neonatal period. *http://emedicine.com/ped/topic2805.htm.*

Finnell RH, Gould A, and Spiegelstein O (2003). Pathobiology and genetics of neural tube defects. *Epilepsia*, **44** (Suppl. 3), 14–23.

Frey L and Hauser WA (2003). Epidemiology of neural tube defects. *Epilepsia*, **44** (Suppl. 3), 4–13.

Gaily E, Kantola-Sorsa E, and Granstroem ML (1988). Intelligence of children of epileptic mothers. *J Pediatr*, **113**, 677–84.

Goldstein RB and Caponigro M (2001). The role of sonography in the evaluation of pregnant women with high maternal serum alpha-fetoprotein. *Appl Radiol*, **30**, 9–18.

Hanson JW and Smith DW (1975). The foetal hydantoin syndrome. *J Pediatri*, **87**, 285–90.

Hanson JW, Myrianthopoulos NC, Harvey MAS, *et al.* (1976). Risks to offspring of women treated with hydantoin anticonvulsants with emphasis on the foetal hydantoin syndrome. *J Paediatr*, **89**, 662–8.

Hansen WF, Peacock AE, and Yankowitz J (2002). Safe prescribing in pregnancy and lactation. *J Midwifery Wom Heal*, **47**, 409–20.

Hernandez-Diaz S, Werler MM, Walker AM, *et al.* (2000). Folic acid antagonists during pregnancy and the risk of birth defects. *New Engl J Med*, **343**, 1608–14.

Hill R, Verniaud W, Rettig G, *et al.* (1982). Relationship between antiepileptic drug exposure of the infant and development potential. In D Janz (ed.), *Epilepsy and the Child*, pp. 409–17. Raven Press: New York.

Holmes LB, Harvey EA, Coull BA, *et al.* (2001). The teratogenicity of anticonvulsant drugs. *New Engl J Med*, **344**, 1132–8.

Jablensky A (2000). Epidemiology of schizophrenia: the global burden of disease and disability. *Eur Arch Psychiatry Clin Neurosci*, **250**, 274–85.

Jacobson SJ, Jones K, Johnson K, *et al.* (1992). Prospective multicentre study of pregnancy outcome after lithium exposure during first trimester. *Lancet*, **339**, 530–3.

Jones KL, Lacro RV, Johnson KA, *et al.* (1989). Pattern of malformations in the children of women treated with carbamazepine during pregnancy. *New Engl J Med*, **320**, 1661–6.

Kallen B (1988). Comments on teratogen update: lithium. *Teratology*, **38**, 597.

Kallen B (1991). Lithium therapy and congenital malformations. In *Lithium in Biology and Medicine: New Applications and Developments*, M Schrauzer and FK Klippel (ed.), pp. 121–30. VCH Verlagsgesellschaft: Weinheim.

Kallen B and Tandberg A (1983). Lithium and pregnancy: a cohort study on manic-depressive women. *Acta Psychiatr Scand*, **68**, 134–9.

Kaneko S, Battino D, Andermann E, *et al.* (1999). Congenital malformations due to antiepileptic drugs. *Epilepsy Res*, **33**, 145–58.

Kennedy DL (2001). Post marketing surveillance in the new millenium. DIA Workshop – Adverse Experience, 9 January 2001. Pregnancy Labeling Task Force, Food and Drug Administration. *http://www.fda.gov/cder/present/dia1–2001/dkennedy/tsld001.htm.*

Koren G, Pastuszak A, and Ito S (1998). Drugs in pregnancy. *New Engl J Med*, **338**, 1128–37.

Lamner EC, Sever LE, and Oakley GP (1987). Teratogen update: valproic acid. *Teratology*, **35**, 465–7.

Lindhout D, and Schmidt D (1986). In-utero exposure to valproate and neural tube defects. *Lancet* **1**, 1392–3.

Lindhout D, Meinardi H, Meijer JW, *et al.* (1992). Antiepileptic drugs and teratogenesis in two consecutive cohorts: changes in prescription policy paralleled by changes in pattern of malformations. *Neurology*, **42** (Suppl. **5**), 94–110.

Lo WY and Friedman JM (2002). Teratogenicity of recently introduced medications in human pregnancy. *Obstet Gynecol*, **100**, 465–73.

Lumley J, Watson L, Watson M, *et al.* (2001). Periconceptional supplementation with folate and/or multivitamins for preventing neural tube defects (Cochrane Review). In *The Cochrane Library*, Issue **3**, 2003. Oxford: Update Software.

Matalon S, Schechtmann S, Goldzweig G, *et al.* (2002). The teratogenic effect of carbamazepine: a meta-analysis of 1255 exposures. *Reprod Toxicol*, **16**, 9–17.

Mitchell SC, Korones SB, and Berendes HW (1971). Congenital heart disease in 56, 109 births. Incidence and natural history. *Circulation*, **43**, 323–32.

MRC Vitamin Study Research Group (1991). Prevention of neural tube defects: results of the Medical Research Council Vitamin Study. *Lancet*, **338**, 131–7.

Nakano KK (1973). Anencephaly: a review. *Devel Med Child Neurol*, **15**, 383–400.

Nakane Y, Okuma T, Takahashi R, *et al.* (1980). Multi-institutional study on the teratogenicity and fetal toxicity of antiepeleptic drugs: a report of a collaborative study group in Japan. *Epilepsia*, **21**, 663–80.

Nelson K and Ellenberg J (1982). Maternal seizure disorder, outcome of pregnancy, and neurodevelopmental abnormalities in the children. *Neurology*, **32**, 1247–54.

Nelson K and Holmes LG (1989). Malformations due to presumed spontaneous mutations in newborn infants. *New Engl J Med*, **320**, 19–23.

Nora JJ, Nora AG, and Toews WH (1974). Lithium, Ebstein's anomaly, and other congenital heart defects. *Lancet* **1**, 594–5.

Normura Y, Takebe Y, Normura Y, *et al.* (1984). The physical and mental development of infants born to mothers treated with antiepileptic drugs. In *Antiepileptic Drugs and Pregnancy*, T Sato and S Shinagawa (ed.), pp. 187–95. Excerpta Medica: Amsterdam.

Nulman I, Rovet J, Stewart DE, *et al.* (1997). Neurodevelopment of children exposed *in utero* to antidepressant drugs. *New Engl J Med*, **336**, 258–62.

Omtzigt JC, Nau H, and Los FJ (1992). The disposition of valproate and its metabolites in the late first trimester and early second trimester of pregnancy in maternal serum, urine and amniotic fluid: effect of dose, co-medication and the presence of spinal bifida. *Eur J Clin Pharmacol*, **43**, 381–8.

Robert E, Reuvers M, and Schaefer C (2001). Antiepileptics. In *Drugs During Pregnancy and Lactation*, C Schaefer (ed.), pp. 46–57. Elsevier: Amsterdam.

Rosa FW (1991). Spina bifida in infants of women treated with carbamazepine during pregnancy. *New Engl J Med*, **324**, 674–7.

Rovet J, Cole S, Nulman I, *et al.* (1995). Effects of maternal epilepsy on children's neuro-development. *Child Neuropsychol*, 1, 150–7.

Royal College of Physicians of London (1997). Adults with poorly controlled epilepsy. Clinical guidelines for treatment and practical tools for aiding epilepsy management.

Samren EB, van Duijn CM, Koch S, *et al.* (1997). Maternal use of antiepileptic drugs and the risk of major congenital malformations: a joint European prospective study of human teratogenesis associated with maternal epilepsy. *Epilepsia*, 38, 957–8.

Samren EB, van Duijn CM, Christiaens GC, *et al.* (1999). Antiepileptic drug regimens and major congenital abnormalities in the offspring. *Ann Neurol*, 46, 739–46.

Shapiro S, Slone K, Hartz SC, *et al.* (1976). Anticonvulsants and parental epilepsy in the development of birth defects. *Lancet* 1, 272–5.

Silverman NH and Hanley FL (2001). The fetus with congenital heart disease. In *The Unborn Patient. The Art and Science of Fetal Therapy*, MR Harrison, MI Evans, NS Adzick and W Holzgreve (ed.), pp. 379–416. WB Saunders: Philadelphia.

Sipek A (1989). Lithium and Ebstein's anomaly. *Cor Vasa*, 31, 149–56.

Smith AL and Weissman MM (1992). Epidemiology. In *Handbook of Affective Disorders*, ES Paykel (ed.), pp. 111–30. Churchill Livingstone: Cambridge.

Tanganelli P and Regesta G (1992). Epilepsy, pregnancy and major birth anomalies. *Neurology*, 42 (Suppl. 5), 89–93.

Viguera A, Nonacs R, Cohen LS, *et al.* (2000). Risk of recurrence of bipolar disorder in pregnant and non-pregnant women after discontinuing lithium maintenance. *Am J Psychiatry*, 157, 179–84.

Weinstein MR (1980). Lithium treatment of women during pregnancy and the post-delivery period. In *Handbook of Lithium Therapy*, FN Johnson (ed.), pp. 421–9. MTP Press: Lancaster.

Wieck A, Haddad P, Denham P, *et al.* (1999). Lithium treated patients: Knowledge and attitude to lithium and the relationship to side-effects. *Eur Neuropsychopharmacol*, 9 (Suppl. 5), S250.

Zalzstein E, Koren G, Einarson T, *et al.* (1990). A case-control study of the association between first trimester exposure of lithium and Ebstein's anomaly. *Am J Cardiol*, 65, 817–18.

Chapter 10

Antidepressant discontinuation syndromes

Peter M Haddad, Ian Anderson, and Jerrold Rosenbaum

Introduction

In November 1957 imipamine was launched in Switzerland: it was the first tricyclic antidepressant to enter clinical practice. Soon after it was noted to be associated with a variety of 'withdrawal' or discontinuation symptoms (Mann and MacPherson 1959; Andersen and Kristiansen 1959). Subsequent reports described discontinuation symptoms with other tricyclic antidepressants (TCAs) (e.g. Dilsaver *et al.* 1983*a,b*) and monoamine reuptake inhibitors (MAOIs) (e.g. Le Gassicke *et al.* 1965). However the area attracted little interest until the mid-1990s, when it was recognized that a discontinuation syndrome could occur with the selective serotonin reuptake inhibitors (SSRIs) (Schatzberg *et al.* 1997). Since then antidepressant discontinuation syndromes have attracted increasing interest, both in the scientific literature and in the lay media. Despite this there is a paucity of systematic research and much of our current knowledge derives from case reports or small case series, a far from ideal situation. Methodologically sound studies are needed to investigate this area and provide a stronger evidence base. To date discontinuation symptoms have been reported with at least 22 different antidepressants (Table 10.1).

Terminology and relation to addiction/dependence

At the outset it is important to address the twin issues of terminology and whether antidepressants are addictive. Some authors refer to antidepressant 'withdrawal' syndromes and others to 'discontinuation' syndromes. Both terms refer to the same phenomenon and they are likely to continue to be used interchangeably; the main issue is to be clear about the meaning. We prefer 'discontinuation syndrome' as it does not imply that antidepressants are addictive

Table 10.1 Antidepressants reported as causing discontinuation symptoms

Tricyclic and related compounds
Amineptine
Amitryptyline
Amoxapine
Clomipramine
Desipramine
Doxepin
Imipramine
Nortriptyline
Protriptyline
Trazodone

Monoamine oxidase inhibitors
Isocarboxazid
Moclobemide
Phenelzine
Tranylcypromine

Selective serotonin reuptake inhibitors
Citalopram
Fluoxetine
Fluvoxamine
Paroxetine
Sertraline

Miscellaneous antidepressants

Mirtazapine (noradrenergic and specific serotonergic antidepressant, NaSSA)
Nefazodone
Venlafaxine (serotonin and noradrenaline reuptake inhibitor, SNRI)

This list is based on the authors' review of the published literature. All the drugs that appear have been reported to cause discontinuation symptoms in either a study or case report.

or cause a dependence syndrome. In contrast the term 'withdrawal syndrome' is synonymous, in many people's minds, with addiction/dependence. This may lead to unwarranted implications about antidepressant use and is inconsistent with current definitions.

Both ICD-10 (World Health Organization 1992) and DSM-IV (American Psychiatric Association 1994) differentiate between a diagnosis of substance dependence and a drug withdrawal state where substance dependence criteria are not met. In both classification systems substance dependence is a syndrome, withdrawal symptoms are neither sufficient nor mandatory for the diagnosis and behavioural features and a compulsive pattern of drug use underlie most of the diagnostic criteria. In DSM-IV these include excessive time being spent using the drug, inability to control drug use, drug use

Table 10.2 Criteria for substance dependence adapted from DSM-IV (American Psychiatric Association 1994)

A maladaptive pattern of substance use, leading to clinically significant impairment or distress as manifested by three or more of the following, occurring at any time in the same 12-month period:

1 Tolerance
2 Occurrence of withdrawal syndrome
3 Substance taken in larger amounts or over longer periods than intended
4 Persistent desire or unsuccessful attempts to cut down or control use
5 Excessive time spent obtaining, using or recovering from effects of substance
6 Substance takes priority over social, occupational or recreational activities
7 Substance use continues despite persistent or recurrent harm.

---

taking priority over other activities and drug use continuing despite persistent harmful consequences (Table 10.2). These features rarely occur in patients taking antidepressants and in terms of these definitions antidepressants in general have no clinically significant potential to cause dependence (Haddad 1999; Haddad and Anderson 1999; Tyrer 1999).

Two exceptions are amineptine and tranylcypromine, rarely prescribed antidepressants with dopaminergic effects (Haddad 1999). Case reports noted the addictive potential of both drugs shortly after they entered clinical practice (e.g. Le Gassicke *et al.* 1965), something that has not happened with other antidepressants despite these being prescribed in far greater amounts. It is worth noting that all addictive drugs cause some immediate gratification or reward after initial consumption e.g. relaxation with alcohol, excess energy with amphetamines, euphoria with opiates etc. Stimulant effects are likely to account for the 'dependence' noted with amineptine and tranylcypromine and, as most antidepressants have no such effects, they appear to be the exceptions that prove the rule.

Antidepressants apart, many drugs cause discontinuation symptoms but are not associated with addiction or a dependence syndrome e.g. anticonvulsants, beta-blockers, nitrates, diuretics, centrally acting antihypertensives, sympathomimetics, heparin (Routledge and Bialas 1997), tamoxifen (Kerr and Myers 1999), dopaminergic agents (Keyser and Rodnitzky 1991) and antipsychotics (Gardos *et al.* 1978; Tranter and Healy 1998). Conversely some highly addictive drugs, including freebase (crack) cocaine and nicotine, cause only relatively minor withdrawal syndromes.

Although most antidepressant discontinuation syndromes are mild and short-lived, some patients experience severe symptoms that make it very difficult for them to stop their antidepressant. Similar prolonged discontinuation reactions occasionally occur with antipsychotics (Tranter and Healy 1998).

How often this occurs and why some patients experience severe problems when most do not remain un-researched. These areas warrant further investigation. However, as these patients do not fulfil criteria for addiction/dependence, we would not regard them as being addicted to their antidepressant, even though their discontinuation syndrome makes it difficult for them to stop antidepressant treatment. Some may regard this differentiation as semantic but we do not agree; there are important practical differences that are meaningful to patients and their families. Such patients do not show the behavioural features that are seen in addiction and once the discontinuation syndrome has resolved they do not crave their antidepressant.

A major problem is that the words 'dependence' and 'addiction' carry individual and varied meanings when used casually by both health professionals and patients, ranging from becoming an 'addict' or 'junkie' to concern about tolerance to the beneficial effects of medication with the need for escalating doses to control the illness. One solution we have suggested (Haddad and Anderson 1999), based on work by Heather (1998), is to avoid the terms 'addiction' and 'dependence' where possible and instead describe component elements i.e. does a drug cause physiological changes (tolerance and/or a withdrawal/discontinuation syndrome), cognitive changes (abnormal desire or craving for the drug) or behavioural changes (i.e. compulsive use, persistent breaking of resolve to stop drug use)? Antidepressants, like many drugs, often cause withdrawal/discontinuation effects but rarely tolerance. Craving and behavioural changes do not occur and in this respect antidepressants differ from alcohol, benzodiazepines, opiates, amphetamines and other 'addictive' drugs.

Core clinical features

Antidepressant discontinuation syndromes share several common features. These include:

1 Characteristic symptoms (see next section).

2 Onset shortly after stopping the antidepressant or, less commonly, reducing the dose.

3 Short duration when untreated.

4 Being distinct from a reappearance of the underlying disorder for which the antidepressant was prescribed.

5 Rapid suppression by restarting the offending antidepressant or a drug with a similar pharmacodynamic profile.

Symptoms usually appear within a few days of stopping an antidepressant. Onset more than 1 week later is unusual. In a naturalistic study of 97 patients stopping SSRIs the mean time of onset of symptoms was 2 days after drug discontinuation (Bogetto *et al.* 2002). In a series of 160 adverse drug reaction (ADR) reports of paroxetine discontinuation reactions the median interval between stopping paroxetine and symptom onset was 2.1 days (Price *et al.* 1996). Symptoms occurred within 4 days in 86 per cent and within 1 week in 93 per cent.

Left untreated, most antidepressant discontinuation reactions are short-lived, resolving between 1 day and three weeks. In the prospective study by Bogetto *et al.* (2002) the mean duration of SSRI discontinuation symptoms was 5 days. In 71 untreated paroxetine discontinuation reactions reported by doctors as ADRs (Price *et al.* 1996), and presumably representing the severer end of the spectrum of reactions, the median duration was 8 days (range 1–52 days). Symptoms usually resolve within 24 hours if the original antidepressant is re-commenced.

Specific syndromes

A diverse range of antidepressant discontinuation symptoms have been described and these vary somewhat between different antidepressant classes. A review of all case reports of SSRI discontinuation reactions published up to October 1996 ($n = 47$) noted over 50 different symptoms (Haddad 1998). The severity of discontinuation reactions occurs on a spectrum in terms of number and degree of symptoms, ranging from an isolated symptom to a cluster and from mild to severely disabling. As with many syndromes, including most psychiatric disorders, this raises the issue of a 'threshold' issue for defining discontinuation syndromes. Provisional operational criteria for an SSRI discontinuation syndrome have been proposed but there is no accepted definition (Haddad 1998; Black *et al.* 2000). The situation is made more complex as different symptom clusters, or discontinuation syndromes, can occur. These are reviewed below.

SSRI discontinuation syndrome

The most common syndrome seen with the SSRIs comprises a mixture of physical and psychological symptoms, the former predominating. We will refer to this as the 'general' SSRI discontinuation syndrome to differentiate it from other SSRI discontinuation syndromes. Six main symptom groups are recognized within this syndrome (Table 10.3). The commonest symptoms are dizziness, nausea, lethargy and headache (Haddad 1998). This syndrome was initially reported in case reports and ADR reports, but its features have been confirmed in several well conducted double-blind studies in which SSRI

Table 10.3 Key symptom groups of the 'general' SSRI discontinuation syndrome

---

1 Sensory symptoms*
Paraesthesia
Numbness
Electric-shock like sensations
Rushing noise 'in head'
Palinopsia (visual trails)

2 Dysequilibrium*
Light headedness/dizziness
Vertigo
Ataxia

3 General somatic symptoms
Lethargy
Headache
Tremor
Sweating
Anorexia

4 Sleep disturbance
Insomnia
Nightmares
Excessive dreaming

5 Gastrointestinal symptoms
Nausea
Vomiting
Diarrhoea

6 Affective symptoms
Irritability
Anxiety/agitation
Low mood
Tearfulness

The table lists common or highly characteristic symptoms, many others have been reported. Groups 3 to 6 make up the 'general' TCA discontinuation syndrome. Patients vary in the number and combination of symptoms that they show.

* Some patients experience sensory symptoms (e.g. electric shock-like sensations) or symptoms of dysequilibrium (e.g. dizziness) in brief bursts when they move their head or eyes. When this occurs it is highly characteristic of the SSRI discontinuation syndrome.

treatment is briefly interrupted with placebo (Rosenbaum *et al.* 1998; Michelson *et al.* 2000; Judge *et al.* 2002). The syndrome can be accompanied by impairment of cognitive function (Hindmarch 2000). A similar discontinuation syndrome occurs with venlafaxine (Fava *et al.* 1997).

TCA discontinuation syndrome

This shares four of the six SSRI symptom groups (Table 10.3). The remaining two SSRI groups, sensory abnormalities and problems with equilibrium, are rare with TCAs and can be regarded as SSRI specific. Whether the 'general' SSRI and TCA discontinuation syndromes would be better regarded as several sub-syndromes is unclear.

MAOI discontinuation syndrome

Discontinuation reactions with MAOIs, particularly tranylcypromine, are often more severe than with other antidepressants. An acute confusional state with disorientation, paranoid delusions and hallucinations may occur (Liskin *et al.* 1984, 1985; Roth 1985; Halle and Dilsaver 1993). Anxiety symptoms and perceptual disturbance (hyperacusis, depersonalization) can occur (Tyrer 1984). A worsening of depressive symptoms, exceeding the severity of the state that originally led to treatment, is also recognized (Halle and Dilsaver 1993).

Uncommon syndromes

Several rare discontinuation syndromes have been reported and are discussed below. The only evidence for these syndromes is case reports, i.e. these syndromes have not been seen in systematic studies.

Hypomania/mania

A sudden onset of mania/hypomania can complicate termination of TCAs (e.g. Mirin *et al.* 1981), SSRIs (e.g. Landry and Roy 1997), MAOIs (e.g. Rothschild 1985) and miscellaneous antidepressants including mirtazepine (Callender and McCall 1999) and venlafaxine (Goldstein *et al.* 1999). The phenomenon has been reported in patients with unipolar depression and bipolar disorder. There have been two case reports with paroxetine (Bloch *et al.* 1995) and one with fluvoxamine (Szabadi 1992) in which hypomanic symptoms formed the first stage of a biphasic discontinuation syndrome, the second stage consisting of aggressive feelings. None of the three patients had a past history of hypomania. Discontinuation-hypomania has been reported to resolve spontaneously without treatment (Mirin *et al.* 1981; Bloch *et al.* 1995). Rapid resolution has also been noted following reinstatement of the original TCA (Lejoyeux *et al.* 1996; Nelson *et al.* 1983).

Extrapyramidal syndromes

Parkinsonian symptoms (bradykinesia, shuffling gait, cogwheel rigidity) have been described after missed doses of desipramine with resolution once the drug was given (Dilsaver *et al.* 1983*b*). Dystonic reactions have occurred on stopping paroxetine (D'Arcy 1993) and fluoxetine (Stoukides and Stoukides 1991). Akathisia has been reported on stoppage of venlafaxine (Wolfe 1997), fluvoxamine (Hirose 2001) and imipramine (Sathananthan and Gershon 1973) and in all three cases it resolved within hours of restarting the antidepressant.

Miscellaneous syndromes

Kasantikul (1995) reported a patient who experienced an episode of delirium on two consecutive occasions that he attempted to stop fluoxetine; both episodes rapidly resolved after fluoxetine was restarted. Delirium has also been reported on abrupt termination of doxepin (Santos and McCurdy 1980). Cardiac arrhythmias have been reported following abrupt termination of amitriptyline (Ceccherini-Nelli *et al.* 1993), imipramine (Boisvert and Chouinard 1981) and clomipramine (Van Sweden 1988) but have not been reported with SSRI stoppage. There is one report of generalized seizures following stoppage of tranylcypromine (Vartzopulos and Krull 1991). Occasional reports of auditory (Louie *et al.* 1996; Parker and Blennerhassett 1998) and visual hallucinations (Agelink *et al.* 1997) complicating venlafaxine termination have appeared. Irregularities in blood pressure have been noted as discontinuation effects with venlafaxine (Agelink *et al.* 1997) and sertraline (Amsden and Georgian 1996). Panic attacks have been attributed to amitriptyline termination (Gawin and Markoff 1981). In all these examples the small number of reports make it difficult to be sure that the relationship with drug termination is causal rather than a spurious association.

Incidence

Discontinuation symptoms are common, at least with certain antidepressants. Older antidepressants associated with a high incidence of one or more discontinuation symptoms include imipramine (100.0 per cent) (Law *et al.* 1981), amitriptyline (80.0 per cent) (Bialos *et al.* 1982), clomipramine (33.3 per cent) (Diamond *et al.* 1989) and phenelzine (32.2 per cent) (Tyrer 1984). Turning to newer antidepressants, Fava *et al.* (1997) reported that during the 3 days following stoppage of venlafaxine and placebo under double-blind conditions, seven (78 per cent) of nine venlafaxine treated subjects and two (22 per cent) of nine placebo-treated patients reported the emergence of adverse events, a statistically significant difference. Among the SSRIs paroxetine is associated with the highest incidence of discontinuation symptoms and fluoxetine the lowest. This is a consistent finding in analyses of spontaneous ADR reports (Price *et al.* 1996; Stahl *et al.* 1997) and retrospective (Coupland *et al.* 1996) and prospective studies (Rosenbaum *et al.* 1998; Michelson *et al.* 2000; Judge *et al.* 2002; Bogetto *et al.* 2002; Tint *et al.* 2002).

Rosenbaum *et al.* (1998) reported on patients, successfully treated for a depressive illness, whose SSRI treatment was interrupted in a double-blind fashion so that they received placebo substitution for 5 to 8 days. Adverse events were monitored using the Discontinuation Emergent Signs and

Symptoms (DESS) checklist and depressive symptoms assessed using the Hamilton Depression Rating Scale (HDRS28) and the Mongomery Asberg Depression Rating Scale (MADRS). Prior to interruption patient groups treated with paroxetine, fluoxetine and sertraline showed no significant difference in the mean scores on these three measures. Following interruption the mean change in the number of DESS events, the HDRS28 score and the MADRS score were significant for patients treated with sertaline ($P < 0.001$) and paroxetine ($P < 0.001$) but not with fluoxetine ($P = 0.578$ to 0.943). Patients were regarded as experiencing a 'discontinuation syndrome' if the number of DESS checklist events increased by 4 or more during the interruption period. The incidence of an SSRI discontinuation syndrome was 14 per cent in the fluoxetine-treated group, 60 per cent in the sertraline-treated group and 66 per cent in the paroxetine-treated group ($P < 0.001$).

It has been suggested that the onset of fluoxetine discontinuation symptoms is delayed due to the drug's long half-life and as such the symptoms go unrecognized i.e. the apparent low propensity of fluoxetine to cause discontinuation symptoms is an artefact. However, a double-blind study found no evidence of a clinically significant discontinuation syndrome emerging within the first 6 weeks after stoppage of fluoxetine (Zajecka *et al.* 1998).

Clinical relevance

Discontinuation symptoms can cause significant morbidity, may be misdiagnosed leading to inappropriate treatment and can adversely effect future antidepressant compliance.

Morbidity

Most discontinuation reactions are mild and do not reach medical attention. However a minority are severe and cause considerable morbidity. In the SSRI discontinuation syndrome ataxia can cause falls (Einbinder 1995) and electric shock-like sensations can impair activities such as walking and driving (Frost and Lal 1995). Symptoms may lead to urgent consultations and attendance at A&E departments (Pacheco *et al.* 1996; Haddad *et al.* 2001). Occasionally inpatient admission is required, though nearly all such reports relate to MAOI discontinuation syndromes (e.g. Liskin *et al.* 1985; Roth 1985). Less marked symptoms can still cause impaired functioning. In 2 double-blind studies (Michelson *et al.* 2000; Judge *et al.* 2002) placebo-interruption of SSRI treatment for 3 to 5 days led to the appearance of characteristic discontinuation symptoms accompanied by a deterioration in social and occupational functioning. Most discontinuation symptoms are short-lived but there are occasional reports of symptoms lasting several months (Frost and Lal 1995; Haddad *et al.* 2001).

Misdiagnosis

A discontinuation syndrome may be misdiagnosed leading to inappropriate management. Examples include:

- ◆ Discontinuation symptoms that follow antidepressant switching may be incorrectly attributed to side effects of the new antidepressant (Haddad and Qureshi 2000) which is stopped on the assumption that the patient cannot tolerate it. This is more likely to occur when switching occurs across antidepressant classes.

- ◆ Discontinuation symptoms that follow recovery from depression and termination of antidepressant treatment may be misdiagnosed as a recurrence i.e. a further depressive episode. This may lead to unnecessary reinstatement of the antidepressant and a more negative prognosis with significant social implications.

- ◆ Discontinuation symptoms due to covert non-compliance with acute antidepressant treatment may be mistaken as worsening depressive symptoms and lead the doctor to incorrectly conclude that treatment is ineffective. As a result the antidepressant dose may be increased, an augmentation strategy adopted or an unnecessary switch made to another antidepressant.

- ◆ Most discontinuation symptoms are physical, not psychological (Table 10.2). Failure to recognize the syndrome may lead to unnecessary referrals and investigations in an attempt to identify a 'physical' problem. Examples of this situation have been reported with fluoxetine (Einbinder 1995), venlafaxine (Haddad *et al.* 2000) and sertraline (Rosenstock 1996).

Misdiagnosis means that the discontinuation symptoms go untreated and the patient could be managed inappropriately with potentially harmful results. It is unknown how often misdiagnosis occurs. In the authors' experience the correct diagnosis is rarely difficult to make and misdiagnosis results from clinicians' unfamiliarity with antidepressant discontinuation syndromes so that it is not considered as a differential diagnosis.

Effect on compliance

Patients often miss consecutive antidepressant doses for several days. Demyttenaere *et al.* (2001) found that, over a 9-week period, 31 per cent of patients had at least one 3-day 'drug holiday' from their antidepressant. Such breaks may precipitate discontinuation symptoms. It has been reported that some patients find this beneficial as it reminds them to take their medication. However the experience may lead other patients to stop their medication, particularly if they worry that the symptoms indicate that they are becoming addicts. Thus discontinuation symptoms can result from, and also cause, poor compliance.

Pharmacological basis

Long-term administration of a psychotropic drug will result in compensatory adjustments within the central nervous system (CNS). When the drug is rapidly withdrawn the adapted systems have to establish a new homeostasis and this manifests as discontinuation symptoms. Adaptation is most likely in the neurotransmitter systems that the drug acts directly on but there may also be far removed 'down-stream' effects on other systems. It is reasonable to postulate that these secondary effects will vary greatly between individuals, reflecting differences in genetic make-up and life experiences. This may explain why individuals vary markedly in the nature, severity and duration of discontinuation effects that they show on drug stoppage. In summary, both pharmacological properties of a drug and constitutional factors in the individual are relevant to the pathogenesis of discontinuation syndromes. Personality and cognitive factors will also influence how individuals interpret and act upon their symptoms.

Some SSRI discontinuation symptoms may reflect a sudden serotonin deficiency at down-regulated serotonin receptors. Dizziness and paraesthesia may relate to the apparent role of serotonin in coordinating autonomic and sensory function with gross control of skeletal and facial muscles (Jacobs and Fornal 1993). Serotonin pathways modulate dopamine neurotransmission and altered activity in these pathways may explain why extrapyramidal syndromes can appear on SSRI stoppage (Lane 1998).

Changes in regional cerebrovascular blood flow in the left prefrontal cortex and left caudate nucleus have been shown to correlate with the emergence of discontinuation symptoms and increased depressive symptoms following brief interruption of paroxetine treatment in patients with remitted depression (Henry *et al.* 2003). These are brain areas implicated in depression and known to have extensive serotonergic innervation.

The TCAs have a significant antimuscarinic action that leads to post-synaptic supersensitivity. Withdrawal of these drugs can lead to excess cholinergic activity (cholinergic rebound) and this may account for the prominent abdominal cramping and nausea that often forms part of the general TCA discontinuation syndrome. Monoaminergic excess, secondary to cholinergic overdrive, has been proposed as the explanation for TCA discontinuation mania (Dilsaver and Greden 1984). Mania occurring with MAOI termination has been suggested as reflecting hyperdopaminergic function (Rothschild 1985).

Pharmacokinetic differences may partly explain the variation in the incidence of the discontinuation syndrome between different SSRIs (Haddad 1998). Fluoxetine, associated with a low incidence of discontinuation symptoms, has the longest half-life of the SSRIs and an active metabolite with an even longer half-life. In contrast paroxetine, associated with a high incidence of discontinuation symptoms, has the shortest half-life of the SSRIs and no active metabolite, resulting in a rapid drop in plasma concentration on abrupt discontinuation.

Differential diagnosis

The diagnosis of an antidepressant discontinuation syndrome is usually straightforward; the key features are (i) the abrupt onset of (ii) characteristic symptoms within (iii) a few days of the antidepressant being stopped or reduced in dose. Antidepressant non-compliance is common and often covert unless inquired about. Consequently a discontinuation syndrome should also be considered when unexpected physical or psychological symptoms arise in a patient currently prescribed an antidepressant. Clinical judgement will determine when a physical examination and investigations, particularly blood tests, are needed to exclude physical disorders.

A discontinuation syndrome that occurs when an antidepressant is stopped following recovery from a depressive illness must be distinguished from a recurrence i.e. a new episode of depression. If there are doubts over diagnosis, and symptoms are not severe, then the clinician and patient can monitor the course of the symptoms and reserve a definitive diagnosis to a later date. If adopting this approach the clinician should give a full explanation to the patient.

When a patient with unipolar depression stops an antidepressant and mania occurs as a discontinuation syndrome then bipolar illness is a differential diagnosis. The rapid onset of symptoms within days of antidepressant stoppage is the main indicator. However as the symptoms are identical, differentiation is not as clear as with the general SSRI or TCA syndrome. If the treatment adopted for the presumed discontinuation-mania is antidepressant reinstatement then it is advisable to monitor the patient closely, ideally as an inpatient, because if the diagnosis is incorrect and the patient actually has a bipolar disorder then the antidepressant may exacerbate the manic symptoms. The situation is even more difficult in a bipolar patient with mania/hypomania on antidepressant discontinuation. Whether or not to restart the antidepressant in this situation depends on careful balancing of probability as to whether it was the antidepressant or its discontinuation that triggered the elevated mood. Management of the mania/hypomania with anticonvulsants and/or antipsychotics is probably the best first step, but awareness of the phenomenon suggests consideration should be given to reinstating the antidepressant in cases of non-response or severe continuing mood instability.

Management

The treatment of a discontinuation syndrome depends on (i) whether or not further antidepressant medication is warranted and (ii) the severity of the symptoms. If an antidepressant is needed (i.e. the patient is still depressed or at high risk of relapse/recurrence) then the treatment of choice is to restart the antidepressant; this scenario usually follows non-compliance with medication. If further antidepressant treatment is not clinically indicated, management depends on the severity of the discontinuation syndrome. A mild syndrome, the majority, only requires that the patient is reassured about its benign nature. With moderate cases, symptoms can be treated symptomatically. For example insomnia may be treated with a short course of a benzodiazepine. Antimuscarinic agents can help treat gastrointestinal symptoms following TCA discontinuation (Dilsaver *et al.* 1983a, 1983b) which is consistent with these symptoms being due to cholinergic rebound. If symptoms are severe then the antidepressant can be reinstated and withdrawn more cautiously. Symptoms usually resolve within 24 hours of restarting the offending antidepressant. Treatment should always include an appropriate explanation of the symptoms to the patient.

These principals of treatment apply not only to the 'general' TCA and SSRI discontinuation syndromes, but also to rare discontinuation syndromes, though the evidence is only from case reports. For example discontinuation-hypomania due to TCAs and SSRIs has been reported to resolve spontaneously after a short duration without treatment (Mirin *et al.* 1981; Bloch *et al.* 1995). Extrapyramidal symptoms associated with venlafaxine (Wolfe 1997), fluvoxamine (Hirose 2001), imipramine (Sathananthan and Gershon 1973) and desipramine (Dilsaver *et al.* 1983*b*) have resolved when the responsible antidepressant has been restarted. Similarly hypomanic symptoms have been reported to resolve following reintroduction of clomipramine (Lejoyeux *et al.* 1996) and desipramine (Nelson *et al.* 1983). Antipsychotics can be used to treat a discontinuation-mania (Mirin *et al.* 1981).

Discontinuation effects of MAOIs include confusion and psychotic symptoms. Treatment options include restarting the MAOI or symptomatic treatment with an antipsychotic.

Risk factors

There is no reliable data to allow one to predict which patient is more likely to develop a discontinuation syndrome should antidepressant treatment be stopped. Discontinuation symptoms can occur whenever antidepressants are prescribed irrespective of the underlying disorder. Personality status is an important predictor of the severity of benzodiazepine discontinuation symptoms, with symptoms being more marked in those with personality disorders, particularly dependent ones (Murphy and Tyrer 1991). No one, to our knowledge, has investigated this possibility with antidepressant discontinuation syndromes. A small open study in patients with dysthymia suggested that an earlier age of onset of illness was associated with an increased risk of a subsequent SSRI discontinuation syndrome (Bogetto *et al.* 2002).

Prevention

Tapering at the end of treatment

Several case reports describe discontinuation symptoms being suppressed by re-introduction of the antidepressant, with subsequent tapering preventing their re-emergence (e.g. Dominguez and Goodnick 1995; Benazzi 1996). Tapering antidepressants at the end of treatment, as opposed to abrupt stoppage, is recommended as standard practice by several authorities (*British National Formulary* 2003; *Drug and Therapeutics Bulletin* 1999, *British Association of Psychopharmacology* (Anderson *et al.* 2000) and in the Summary of Product Characteristics of many antidepressants. Recommendations on taper length vary. For example the *British National Formulary* (2003) recommends that antidepressants administered for 8 weeks or more should, wherever possible, be reduced over a 4-week period. Other authorities recommend more cautious tapers. In reality there is no controlled data to recommend the effectiveness of tapering, the length of time over which it should occur or the minimum dose that one should taper to. Furthermore individual patients vary in their requirements.

A open randomized study reported by Tint *et al.* (2002) showed no benefit in tapering venlafaxine and SSRIs over 14 days as opposed to 3 days in preventing discontinuation symptoms. This implies that if tapering is beneficial, and intuitively one would expect it to be, then it needs to be in excess of 14 days.

Several factors will influence the rate of taper including:

- the antidepressant,
- the duration of treatment,
- whether the patient has a previous history of discontinuation symptoms,
- and the degree of urgency associated with stoppage.

Discontinuation symptoms are relatively uncommon with fluoxetine and it has been suggested that, in contrast to other antidepressants, routine tapering is not required (Rosenbaum and Zajecka 1997). Venlafaxine and paroxetine are associated with particularly high rates of discontinuation symptoms.

Discontinuation symptoms are more likely with longer periods of treatment (e.g. Kramer *et al.* 1961). Routine tapering appears unnecessary when antidepressants have been prescribed for less than 5 weeks. Discontinuation symptoms are probably more common following termination of higher doses though this has not been formally examined.

Some individuals require very gradual tapers (Louie *et al.* 1996; Amsden and Georgian 1996; Koopowitz and Berk 1995). The rate of reduction may need to be reduced towards the end of the taper period. If discontinuation symptoms appear during or at the end of the taper, one should consider increasing the dose back to the lowest dose that was preventing their reappearance before commencing a slower taper. Liquid formulations, if available, can allow very gradual tapers. When managing SSRI and venlafaxine discontinuation symptoms another strategy to consider is switching to fluoxetine. Anecdotal data indicates that fluoxetine can suppress discontinuation symptoms associated with other SSRIs (Keuthen *et al.* 1994; Rosenblatt and Rosenblatt 1996) and venlafaxine (Giakas and Davis 1997; Haddad *et al.* 2001) though this is not always the case (Phillips 1995). If the switch is successful, fluoxetine can usually be stopped after several weeks of treatment without symptoms reappearing. Presumably the effectiveness of this strategy reflects the long half-life of fluoxetine and its active metabolite norfluoxetine as discussed previously.

Tapering in other situations

Employing a long taper after successful treatment of an affective disorder is straightforward. However when switching antidepressants due to lack of efficacy, the risks of discontinuation symptoms secondary to rapid stoppage need to be balanced against the benefits of starting a new antidepressant quickly. If the patient and clinician are aware that discontinuation symptoms may occur, a rapid taper, or even an abrupt switch, is acceptable; many of the problems of discontinuation symptoms arise when they are unexpected or misdiagnosed. The potential for drug interactions and the need for washout periods also need to be considered when switching antidepressants.

Discontinuation symptoms are less likely when switching between antidepressants with similar pharmacodynamic profiles, but can still occur. The authors practice is not to taper when switching between SSRIs unless problems have been noted in previous attempts. Abrupt antidepressant stoppage is justified if a patient has developed serious side effects, there is a medical emergency warranting stoppage or the antidepressant has induced mania.

Education

In a survey of UK general practitioners conducted in 1998 (Haddad *et al.* 1999) 30 per cent of respondents rated themselves as poorly aware of antidepressant discontinuation symptoms and, from other questions, it was apparent that many of the remainder had over-rated their knowledge. Other surveys have demonstrated that a substantial proportion of psychiatrists (Young and Currie 1997) and pharmacists (Donoghue and Haddad 1999) are unfamiliar with this area. Increased awareness is essential to allow clinicians to adopt preventative strategies and facilitate diagnosis and treatment when symptoms do arise.

Patients should be informed that antidepressant treatment should not be stopped or interrupted abruptly as this can lead to discontinuation symptoms. They should be aware that it is standard practice to taper antidepressants at the end of treatment to prevent or minimize such symptoms. It should also be explained to patients that although antidepressants can cause discontinuation or withdrawal symptoms they do not cause craving, tolerance and behavioural problems and it for this reason that antidepressants are not regarded as addictive in the way that alcohol and illicit drugs such as heroin are. This advice is likely to reduce patient distress and prevent problems associated with misdiagnosis should a discontinuation syndrome occur. Although discontinuation symptoms are unlikely when antidepressants have been used for less than 5 weeks (Haddad 1998) it is rare to plan to prescribe antidepressants for such a short period and it is difficult to know in advance whether the period may be extended. Consequently the best plan is to warn all patients about discontinuation symptoms when starting on antidepressants and also when discontinuation is being contemplated.

Drug holidays have been suggested as a way of managing the sexual side effects associated with SSRIs (Rothchild 1995) but risk precipitating discontinuation symptoms. The clinician and patient must consider the relative risks and benefits before adopting this technique.

There have been reports of possible discontinuation symptoms in babies born to mothers who took antidepressants, both SSRIs and TCAs, up to the time of birth (e.g. Cowe *et al.* 1982; Nordeng *et al.* 2001). Symptoms have included irritability, constant crying, shivering, increased tonus, eating and sleeping difficulties and convulsions. However, as is often the case with anecdotal reports, the diagnosis is debatable. The symptoms may be unrelated to medication. If they are the result of antidepressant medication they may represent a toxicity syndrome, in particular serotonin toxicity, rather than a withdrawal syndrome. The two mechanisms (i.e. withdrawal and toxicity) may occur for symptoms in different cases. The possibility of discontinuation symptoms arising in breast-fed infants whose mothers suddenly stop taking an antidepressant has been raised (Kent and Laidlaw 1995). Despite the uncertainties we recommend that the possibility of neonatal symptoms, due to maternal antidepressant use, should be discussed, where possible, with pregnant or breastfeeding mothers who are contemplating antidepressant treatment. The possible risks need to be balanced against the benefits associated with antidepressant treatment and breastfeeding and decisions should be made on an individual basis.

Choice of antidepressant

If a patient has previously experienced a severe discontinuation syndrome or is known to comply poorly with medication then one should consider prescribing an antidepressant with a low propensity to cause discontinuation symptoms, e.g. fluoxetine. However many other factors need to be considered when selecting an antidepressant including past efficacy, tolerability, the potential for drug interactions and any cautions or contraindications to prescribing.

Conclusions

Antidepressant discontinuation syndromes have been recognized for over 40 years and occur with all antidepressant classes. A common core discontinuation syndrome occurs with SSRIs and, with some differences, TCAs. This is readily recognizable and clinicians should be aware of it and strategies for its minimization and management. In addition they need to be aware that rarer discontinuation syndromes must be considered in differential diagnosis, especially of extrapyramidal syndromes (akathisia, dystonia and parkinsonian symptoms), mania/hypomania and delirium and psychotic symptoms.

Preventative strategies include ensuring that patients take antidepressants consistently and tapering antidepressants at the end of treatment (though the effectiveness of tapering has not been sufficiently tested). When syndromes do occur, prompt diagnosis and reassurance are often all that is required. More severe symptoms should be treated symptomatically or the antidepressant re-started in which case symptoms usually resolve within 24 hours. A more cautious taper can then follow.

Summary: Antidepressant discontinuation syndrome

Definition	Characteristic symptoms that commence shortly after stopping or reducing the dose of an antidepressant and are unrelated to the underlying psychiatric disorder. Untreated the duration is usually short. Remission occurs within 24 hours on restarting causal antidepressant.

Incidence	Variable depending on definition, antidepressant, length of treatment, rate of taper prior to stoppage and possibly dose. Abrupt stoppage of many antidepressants leads to >33% of patients spontaneously reporting one or more discontinuation symptoms. In one study incidence of discontinuation syndrome (4 or more new or worsened symptoms) was approx 66% with paroxetine and sertraline (Rosenbaum et al. 1998).
Drugs causing syndrome	Occurs with all antidepressant classes i.e. TCAs, MAOIs, SSRIs, SNRIs. Particularly high incidence with paroxetine and venlafaxine.
Key symptoms	Very variable. Several syndromes can occur. Commonest syndrome with TCAs and SSRIs (the 'general' syndrome) involves physical and psychological symptoms, the former predominate. Commonest SSRI symptoms are dizziness, nausea, lethargy and headache while paraesthesia is highly characteristic.
Pharmacological mechanism	Sudden disruption of CNS systems that had adapted to antidepressant treatment. Pharmacodynamic, pharmacokinetic and constitutional factors influence presentation.
Investigations to confirm diagnosis	Accurate history, particularly close temporal relationship of symptom onset versus decrease in dose or termination of antidepressant. Symptoms rarely start more than one week after dose reduction or termination of treatment.
Management	Four options: 1 Education/support and allow symptoms to spontaneously resolve 2 Symptomatic treatment 3 Re-start antidepressant and taper more slowly 4 With intractable 'general' SSRI discontinuation syndromes switch to fluoxetine which can usually be stopped without major problems.
Further reading	Haddad P (1998). The SSRI discontinuation syndrome. *Journal of Psychopharmacology*, **12**, 305–13. Rosenbaum JF, Fava, M, Hoog SL, et al. (1998). Selective serotonin reuptake inhibitor discontinuation syndrome: a randomized clinical trial. *Biological Psychiatry*, **44**, 77–87. Stahl NMS, Lindquist M, Petterson M, et al. (1997). Withdrawal reactions with selective serotonin reuptake inhibitors as reported to the WHO system. *Eur J Clin Pharmacol* **53**, 163–9.

References

Agelink MW, Zitselsberger A, and Kleiser E (1997). Withdrawal symptoms after discontinuation of venlafaxine (letter). *Am J Psychiatry*, **154**, 1473–74.

American Psychiatric Association. *Diagnostic and Statistical Manual of Mental Disorders*, 4th edn. Washington, DC: American Psychiatric Association.

Amsden GW and Georgian F (1996). Orthostatic hypotension induced by sertraline withdrawal. *Pharmacotherapy*, **16**, 684–86.

Andersen H and Kristiansen ES (1959). Tofranil treatment of endogenous depressions. *Acta Psychiatr Scand*, **34**, 387–97.

Anderson IM, Nutt DJ, and Deakin JF (2000). Evidence-based guidelines for treating depressive disorders with antidepressants: a revision of the 1993 British Association for Psychopharmacology guidelines. British Association for Psychopharmacology. *J Psychopharmacol*, **14**, 3–20.

Benazzi F (1996). Venlafaxine withdrawal symptoms. *Can J Psychiatry*, **41**, 487.

Bialos D, Giller E, Jatlow P, *et al.* (1982). Recurrence of depression after discontinuation of amitriptyline. *Am J Psychiatry*, **139**, 325–29.

Black DW, Wesner R, and Gabel J (1993). The abrupt discontinuation of fluvoxamine in patients with panic disorder. *J Clin Psychiatry*, **54**, 146–9.

Black K, Shea C, Dursun S, *et al.* (2000). Selective serotonin reuptake inhibitor discontinuation syndrome: proposed diagnostic criteria. *J Psychiatry Neurosci*, **25**, 255–61.

Bloch M, Stager SV, Braun AR, *et al.* (1995). Severe psychiatric symptoms associated with paroxetine withdrawal. *Lancet*, **346**, 57.

Bogetto F, Bellino S, Revello RB, *et al.* (2002). Discontinuation syndrome in dysthymic patients treated with selective serotonin reuptake inhibitors: a clinical investigation. *CNS Drugs*, **16**, 273–83.

Boisvert D and Chouinard G (1981). Rebound cardiac arrhythmia after withdrawal from imipramine: a case report. *Am J Psychiatry*, **138**, 985–86.

British National Formulary (2000). British Medical Association and Royal Pharmaceutical Society of Great Britain. Section 4.3 '*Antidepressant Drugs: withdrawal*'. London: The Pharmaceutical Press.

Callender J and MacCall C (1999). Mirtzapine withdrawal causing hypomania. *Br J Psychiatry*, **175**, 390.

Ceccherini-Nelli A, Bardellini L, Guazzalli M, *et al.* (1993). Antidepressant withdrawal phenomena: prospective findings. *Am J Psychiatry*, **150**, 165.

Coupland NJ, Bell CJ, and Potokar JP (1996). Serotonin reuptake inhibitor withdrawal. *J Clin Psychopharmacol*, **16**, 356–62.

Cowe L, Lloyd DJ, and Dawling S (1982). Neonatal convulsions caused by withdrawal from maternal clomipramine. *BMJ (Clin Res Ed)* **284**, 1837–38.

D'Arcy PF (1993). Dystonia and withdrawal symptoms with paroxetine (letter*). Int Pharm J* **7**, 140.

Demyttenaere K, Mesters P, Boulanger B, *et al.* (2001). Adherence to treatment regimen in depressed patients treated with amitriptyline or fluoxetine. *J Affect Disorders*, **65**, 243–52.

Diamond BI, Borison RL, Katz R, *et al.* (1989). Rebound reactions due to clomipramine. *Psychopharmacol Bull*, **255**, 209–12.

Dilsaver SC and Greden JF (1984). Antidepressant withdrawal-induced activation (hypomania and mania): mechanisms and theoretical significance. *Brain Res*, **319**, 29–48.

Dilsaver SC, Feinberg M, and Greden JF (1983*a*). Antidepressant withdrawal symptoms treated with anticholinergic agents. *Am J Psychiatry*, **140**, 249–51.

Dilsaver SC, Kronfol Z, Greden JF, *et al.* (1983*b*). Antidepressant withdrawal syndromes: evidences supporting the cholinergic overdrive hypothesis. *J Clin Psychopharm*, **3**, 157–64.

Dominguez RA and Goodnick PJ (1995). Adverse events after the abrupt discontinuation of paroxetine. *Pharmacotherapy*, **15**, 778–80.

Donoghue J and Haddad P (1999). Pharmacists lack knowledge of antidepressant discontinuation symptoms. *J Clin Psychiatry*, **60**, 124–5.

Drug and Therapeutics Bulletin (1999). Withdrawing patients from antidepressants. *Drug and Therapeutics Bulletin*, **37**, 49–52.

Einbinder E (1995). Fluoxetine withdrawal? *Am J Psychiatry*, **152**, 1253.

Fava M, Mulroy R, Alpert J, *et al.* (1997). Emergence of adverse effects following discontinuation of treatment with extended-release venlafaxine. *Am J Psychiatry*, **154**, 1760–2.

Frost L and Lal S (1995). Shock-like sensations after discontinuation of selective serotonin reuptake inhibitors. *Am J Psychiatry*, **152**, 810.

Gardos G, Cole JO, and Tarsy D (1978). Withdrawal syndromes associated with antipsychotic drugs. *Am J Psychiatry*, **135**, 1321–4.

Giakas WJ and Davis SM (1997). Intractable withdrawal from venlafaxine treated with fluoxetine. *Psychiat Ann*, **27**, 85–6.

Goldstein TR, Frye MA, Denicoff KD, *et al.* (1999). Antidepressant discontinuation-related mania: critical prospective observation and theoretical implications in bipolar disorder. *J Clin Psychiatry*, **60**, 563–7.

Haddad P (1998). The SSRI discontinuation syndrome. *J Psychopharmacol*, **12**, 305–13.

Haddad P (1999). Do antidepressants have any potential to cause addition? *J Pychopharmacol*, **13**, 300–7.

Haddad P and Anderson I (1999). Antidepressants aren't addictive: clinicians have depended on them for years. *J Psychopharmacol*, **13**, 291–2.

Haddad PM and Qureshi M (2000). Misdiagnosis of antidepressant discontinuation symptoms. *Acta Psychiatr Scand*, **102**, 466–8.

Haddad PM, Devarajan S, and Dursun SM (2001). Antidepressant discontinuation symptoms presenting as 'stroke'. *J Psychopharmacol*, **15**, 139–41.

Haddad P, Tylee A, and Young A (1999). General Practitioners' knowledge of antidepressant discontinuation reactions (abstract). *J Psychopharmacol*, **13**, 3 (Suppl. A), A44 P137.

Halle MT and Dilsaver SC (1993). Tranylcypromine withdrawal phenomena. *J Psychiat Neurosci*, **18**, 49–50.

Heather N (1998). A conceptual framework for explaining drug addiction. *J Psychopharmacol*, **12**, 3–7.

Henry ME, Kaufman MJ, Hennen J, *et al.* (2003). Cerebral blood volume and clinical change on the third day of placebo substitution for SSRI treatment. *Biol Psychiatry*, **53**, 100–5.

Hindmarch I, Kimber S, and Cockle SM (2000). Abrupt and brief discontinuation of anti-depressant treatment: effects on cognitive function and psychomotor performance. *Int Clin Psychopharmacol*, **15**, 305–18.

Hirose S (2001). Restlessness related to SSRI withdrawal. *Psychiatry Clin Neurosci*, **55**, 79–80.

Gawin FH and Markoff RA (1981). Panic anxiety after abrupt discontinuation of amitriptyline. *Am J Psychiatry*, **138**, 117–18.

Jacobs BL and Fornal CA (1993). 5-HT and motor control: a hypothesis. *Trends Neurosci*, **16**, 346–52.

Judge R, Parry MG, Quail D, *et al.* (2002). Discontinuation symptoms: comparison of brief interruption in fluoxetine and paroxetine treatment. *Int Clin Psychopharmacol*, **17**, 217–25.

Kasantikul D (1995). Reversible delirium after discontinuation of fluoxetine. *J Med Assoc Thailand*, **78**, 53–4.

Kent LSW and Laidlaw JDD (1995). Suspected congenital sertraline dependence. *Br J Psychiatry*, **167**, 412–13.

Kerr B and Myers P (1999). Withdrawal syndrome following long-term administration of tamoxifen. *J Psychopharmacol*, **13**, 419.

Keuthen NJ, Cyr P, Ricciardi JA, *et al.* (1994). Medication withdrawal symptoms in obsessive-compulsive disorder patients treated with paroxetine. *J Clin Psychopharm*, **14**, 206–7.

Keyser DL and Rodnitzky RL (1991). Neuroleptic malignant syndrome in Parkinon's disease after withdrawal or alteration of dopaminergic therapy. *Arch Intern Med*, **151**, 794–6.

Koopowitz LF and Berk M (1995). Paroxetine induced withdrawal effects. *Hum Psychopharmacol*, **10**, 147–8.

Kramer JC, Klein DF, and Fink M (1961). Withdrawal symptoms following discontinuation of imipramine therapy. *Am J Psychiatry*, **118**, 549–50.

Landry P and Roy L (1997). Withdrawal hypomania associated with paroxetine. *J Clin Pychopharm*, **17**, 60–1.

Lane RM (1998). SSRI-induced extrapyramidal side-effects and akathisia: implications for treatment. *J Psychopharmacol*, **12**, 192–214.

Law W, Petti TA, and Kazdin A (1981). Withdrawal symptoms after gradual cessation of imipramine in children. *Am J Psychiatry*, **118**, 647–50.

Le Gassicke J, Ashcroft GW, Eccleston D, *et al.* (1965). The clinical state, sleep and amine metabolism of a tranylcypromine (Parnate) addict. *Br J Psychiatry*, **3**, 357–64.

Lejoyeux M, Ades J, Mourad I, *et al.* (1996). Antidepressant withdrawal syndrome: recognition, prevention and management. *CNS Drugs*, **5**, 278–92.

Liskin B, Roose SP, Walsh BT, *et al.* (1985). Acute psychosis following phenelzine discontinuation. *J Clin Psychopharm*, **5**, 46–7.

Louie AK, Lannon RA, Kirsch MA, *et al.* (1996). Venlafaxine withdrawal reactions. *Am J Psychiatry*, **153**, 1652.

Mann AM and MacPherson A (1959). Clinical experience with imipramine (G22355) in the treatment of depression. *Can Psychiatr Assoc J*, **4**, 38–47.

Michelson D, Fava M, Amsterdam J, *et al*. (2000). Interruption of selective serotonin reuptake inhibitor treatment. Double-blind, placebo-controlled trial. *Br J Psychiatry* **176**, 363–8.

Mirin SM, Schatzberg AF, and Creasey DE (1981). Hypomania and mania after withdrawal of tricyclic antidepressants. *Am J Psychiatry*, **138**, 87–9.

Murphy SM and Tyrer P (1991). A double-blind comparison of the effects of gradual withdrawal of lorazepam, diazepam, and bromazepam in benzodiazepine dependence. *Br J Psychiatry*, **158**, 511–16.

Nelson JC, Schottenfeld RS, and Conrad ED (1983). Hypomania after desipramine withdrawal. *Am J Psychiatry*, **140**, 624–5.

Nordeng H, Lindemann R, Perminov KV, *et al*. (2001). Neonatal withdrawal syndrome after in utero exposure to selective serotonin reuptake inhibitors. *Acta Paediatr*, **90**, 288–91.

Pacheco L, Malo P, Aragues E, *et al*. (1996). More cases of paroxetine withdrawal syndrome. *Br J Psychiatry*, **169**, 384.

Parker G and Blennerhassett J (1998). Withdrawal reactions associated with venlafaxine. *Aust NZ J Psychiatry*, **32**, 292–4.

Philips SD (1995). A possible paroxetine withdrawal syndrome. *Am J Psychiatry*, **152**, 645–6.

Price JS, Waller PC, Wood SM, *et al*. (1996). A comparison of the post-marketing safety of four selective serotonin re-uptake inhibitors, including the investigation of symptoms occurring on withdrawal. *Br J Clin Pharmacol*, **42**, 757–63.

Rosenbaum JF and Zajecka J (1997). Clinical management of antidepressant discontinuation. *J Clin Psychiatry*, **58** (Suppl. 7), 37–40.

Rosenbaum JF, Fava M, Hoog SL, *et al*. (1998). Selective serotonin reuptake inhibitor discontinuation syndrome: a randomised clinical trial. *Biol Psychiatry*, **44**, 77–87.

Rosenblatt JE and Rosenblatt NC (1996). Paroxetine withdrawal after slow dosage taper. *Curr Affect Illness*, **15**, 8–9.

Rosenstock HA (1996). Sertraline withdrawal in two brothers: a case report. *Int Clin Psychopharmacology*, **11**, 58–9.

Roth SD (1985). More on psychosis following phenelzine discontinuation. *J Clin Psychopharmacol*, **5**, 360–1.

Rothchild AJ (1995). Selective serotonin reuptake inhibitor-induced sexual dysfunction: efficacy of a drug holiday. *Am J Psychiatry*, **152**, 1514–16.

Rothschild AJ (1985). Mania after withdrawal of isocarboxazid. *J Clin Psychopharm* **5**, 340–2.

Routledge PA and Bialas MC (1997). Adverse reactions to drug withdrawal. *Adverse Drug Reaction Bulletin*, **187**, 711–14.

Santos AB Jr and McCurdy L (1980). Delirium after abrupt withdrawal from doxepin: case report. *Am J Psychiatry*, **137**, 239–40.

Sathananthan GL and Gershon S (1973). Imipramine withdrawal: an akathisia-like syndrome. *Am J Psychiatry*, **130**, 1286–7.

Schatzberg AF, Haddad P, Kaplan EM, *et al.* (1997). Serotonin reuptake inhibitor discontinuation syndrome: a hypothetical definition. *J Clin Psychiatry*, **58** (Suppl. 7), 5–10.

Stahl NMS, Lindquist M, Petterson M, *et al.* (1997). Withdrawal reactions with selective serotonin re-uptake inhibitors as reported to the WHO system. *Eur J Clin Pharmacol*, **53**, 163–9.

Stoukides JA and Stoukides CA (1991). Extrapyramidal symptoms upon discontinuation of fluoxetine. *Am J Psychiatry*, **148**, 1263.

Szabadi E (1992). Fluvoxamine withdrawal syndrome. *Br J Psychiatry*, **160**, 283–4.

Tint AK, Haddad PM, Anderson IM, *et al.* (2002). SSRI/venlafaxine discontinuation symptoms during antidepressant switching: an interim analysis. *J Psychopharmacol*, **16**, 3, (Suppl.) A44.

Tranter R and Healy D (1998). Neuroleptic discontinuation syndromes. *J Psychopharmacol*, **12**, 401–6.

Tyrer P (1984). Clinical effects of abrupt withdrawal from tricyclic antidepressants and monoamine oxidase inhibitors after long term treatment. *J Affect Disorders*, **6**, 1–7.

Tyrer P (1999). Stress diathesis and pharmacological dependence. *J Psychopharmacol*, **13**, 294–5.

Van Sweden B (1988). Rebound antidepressant cardiac arrhythmia. *Biol Psychiatry*, **24**, 363–4.

Vartzopulos D and Krull F (1991). Dependence on monoamine oxidase inhibitors in high dose. *Br J Psychiatry*, **158**, 856–7.

Wolfe RM (1997). Antidepressant withdrawal reactions. *Am Fam Physician*, **56** (2), 452–62.

World Health Organization (1992). *The ICD-10 Classification of Mental and Behavioural Disorders*. Geneva: World Health Organization.

Young AH and Currie A (1997). Physicians' knowledge of antidepressant withdrawal effects: a survey. *J Clin Psychiatry*, **58**, (Suppl. 7), 28–30.

Zajecka J, Fawcett J, Amsterdam J, *et al.* (1998). Safety of abrupt discontinuation of fluoxetine: a randomized, placebo-controlled study. *J Clin Psychopharmacol*, **18**, 193–7.

Chapter 11

Antipsychotic discontinuation syndromes

Salman Karim and Shôn Lewis

Much of the evidence for the existence of antipsychotic discontinuation syndromes comes from studies done in the 1960s (Brooks 1959; Greenberg and Roth 1964). For instance, in the late 1950s chlorpromazine was thought to have anti-tuberculous properties and was used in patients suffering from tuberculosis. Hollister *et al.* (1960) reported that following 6 months treatment with 300 mg of chlorpromazine in a placebo controlled double-blind protocol, the treatment was discontinued due to no beneficial effect on illness. This led to a withdrawal syndrome in 5 of the 17 subjects and was characterized by nausea, vomiting, restlessness and sleeplessness that could be mitigated by restarting chlorpromazine.

In the early literature, these symptoms were labeled as 'withdrawal syndromes' as the symptoms occurred within a brief time of stopping the drug and abated if the medication was restarted. Later on, the term 'withdrawal syndrome' became associated with drugs, particularly drugs of abuse, that were associated with craving and tolerance as well as withdrawal symptoms. Recently there has been a resurgence of interest, although little new data, in the symptoms associated with discontinuation of antipsychotics and the term 'discontinuation syndrome' is popularly used to describe them.

Clinical features

Antipsychotics other than clozapine

Dilsaver and Alessi (1988) reviewed the literature on symptoms that develop within the first seven days of discontinuation of an antipsychotic, in order to differentiate them from the symptoms of psychotic relapse. They quoted early studies mostly involving conventional antipsychotics (Whittaker and Hay 1964; Rothstein 1960; Morton 1968) which appeared to show discontinuation symptoms, given that the probability of a psychotic relapse is minimal in a stable patient within the first two weeks of stopping antipsychotics. The most common symptoms were nausea, vomiting and anorexia. Diaphoresis, headache, insomnia, restlessness, anxiety and agitation were also common. Less frequently noted symptoms were vertigo, alternating feelings of warmth and cold, myalgia, parasthesia and hyperalgesia. These symptoms began within one to four days of stopping of medication and subsided spontaneously within one to two weeks.

Most of the early studies did not take into account the possibility of a base rate of symptoms that could lead to an over-estimation of withdrawal symptoms. Reidenberg and Lowenthal (1968) measured 25 common symptoms in 175 drug-free normal subjects and found that only 18 per cent of subjects did not report any symptom. Lacoursiere *et al.* (1976) addressed this issue by measuring the withdrawal symptoms before and after the withdrawal of antipsychotic medication. The results showed that 11 per cent of subjects had reported withdrawal-like symptoms before the discontinuation and a significantly higher 38 per cent reported symptoms after the discontinuation.

In one of the better studies, Battegay (1967) studied a population of 88 patients from whom antipsychotics were withdrawn in a placebo-controlled double-blind fashion. The emergent symptoms were recorded and 55 (68 per cent) out of 88 developed withdrawal symptoms. Out of the 55 symptomatic subjects 11 developed dyskinesias, 2 developed dystonic syndromes and 39 had a combination of sweating, vertigo, alternating feelings of warmth and cold, tachycardia and tendency to collapse. Eight had headaches, 26 had nausea and vomiting and 16 had insomnia. The duration of the symptoms was difficult to judge as the symptoms in 46 of the 55 cases were so severe that drug treatment had to be restarted within a week.

Viguera *et al.* (1997) divided antipsychotic discontinuation symptoms into acute and chronic motor and non-motor symptoms. The motor symptoms include the acute dystonias, dyskinesias and akathisia and the subsequent establishment of chronic tardive dyskinesia or akathisia. Variants of dyskinesias such as 'rabbit syndrome', twitching of perioral muscles, have been described on discontinuation with risperidone (Nishimura *et al.* 2001).

Further evidence of the existence of antipsychotic discontinuation symptoms comes from case reports of the use of dopamine blocking drugs in non-psychiatric patients. Grimes (1981) reported seven cases of orobuccolingual dyskinesias following withdrawal of metoclopramide, an antiemetic, and Patel (1986) reported a case of tardive dyskinesia on metoclopramide withdrawal.

Tardive motor syndromes have not been classically described as discontinuation syndromes. They usually occur during treatment and can occur with drug naive subjects. However they are exacerbated by dose reduction of an antipsychotic and often become obvious when medication is discontinued. The risk of developing tardive dyskinesia increases with age, female gender, mood disorder, organic brain dysfunction, type II diabetes mellitus and occurrence of extrapyramidal side effects with antipsychotics (Jeste and Caligiuri 1993; Marsalek 2000). An association has been claimed between intermittent treatment and an increased risk of tardive dyskinesia and higher rates of psychotic and dysphoric symptoms (Jeste and Caligiuri 1993). The association of tardive syndromes with the dose reduction and discontinuation of antipsychotics makes a strong case for the view that these are a variant of antipsychotic discontinuation syndrome (Tranter and Healy 1998).

Clozapine discontinuation syndromes

Clozapine is an atypical antipsychotic with unique properties of minimal extrapyramidal side effects, less likelihood of causing tardive dyskinesia, effectiveness in treatment resistance schizophrenias and (possibly) improving negative symptoms (Goudie 2000). Clozapine has an unusal side effect profile, which includes sedation, weight gain, tachycardia, seizures, hypertension, fever, nausea and hyper-salivation. Its best-known side effect is agranulocytosis which in early series occurred in about 0.5 per cent of cases. Routine hematological monitoring effectively precludes this side effect having fatal consequences, though if significant neutropaenia appears then clozapine must be discontinued.

Clozapine has the best-described discontinuation syndrome of all antipsychotic drugs. Data on the effects of rapid withdrawal of clozapine suggest that symptoms often start within two to three days, usually within two weeks. Anxiety, insomnia, motor restlessness or mute withdrawal, altered consciousness, confusion, nausea and diaphoresis have been reported since the early days of its use (Simpson and Vraga 1974, Borison *et al.* 1998, Eklund 1987). Clozapine discontinuation can also induce movement disorders, although most cases of withdrawal dystonias and dyskinesias on sudden stopping of clozapine have been described in the patients with prior history of tardive dyskinesia before commencing clozapine (Ahmed *et al.* 1998). Withdrawal tics and a Tourettes'-like picture have also been described (Poyurovsky *et al.* 1998).

The clozapine discontinuation symptoms as described above can also resemble the 'serotonin syndrome', which is seen with SSRIs and can complicate the clinical picture if the patient is on an SSRI along with clozapine (Zerjav-Lacombe and Dewan 2001).

The notion of a clozapine-specific rebound psychosis remains prevalent but unproven. Clinicians and several authors have been impressed by the apparently high rate of swift and difficult to treat relapse after clozapine discontinuation

(Baldessarini *et al.* 1995; Meltzer *et al.* 1996). This has been labeled as 'rebound' or 'super sensitivity psychosis'. Meltzer *et al.* (1997) reported a 79 per cent relapse rate in neuroleptic responsive patients and 39.1 per cent in neuroleptic nonresponsive patients after stopping clozapine therapy. Tollefson *et al.* (1999) reported a relapse rate of 25 per cent after clozapine discontinuation in a double-blind clinical trial. However, the status of rebound psychosis remains unclear: whether it is a true phenomenon with some specificity to clozapine; whether it is simply the re-emergence of psychosis following antipsychotic cessation; or whether in part is actually a cholinergic rebound, remains unproven.

Pharmacological basis

Pharmacology of antipsychotics

According to the dopamine hypothesis, antipsychotic drugs exert at least part of their therapeutic effects through post-synaptic dopamine D_2 receptor blockade in the mesolimbic system. Several lines of evidence support the role of D_2 receptors in mediating this antipsychotic action. *In vitro* binding studies have revealed a direct correlation between antipsychotic potency and the drug's affinity for D_2 receptors (Peroutka and Synder 1980). Such a direct relationship has not been found for any other receptor system. Johnstone *et al.* (1978) showed that the steroeisomer of flupenthixol which was active at D_2 receptors was clinically effective in treating acutely relapsed patients, whereas the chemically identical but D_2 inactive isomer was similar to placebo. The early PET studies revealed high blockade of striatal D_2 receptors by 12 distinct classes of antipsychotic drugs (Farde *et al.* 1989). In a double-blind PET study of schizophrenic patients the likelihood of a good clinical response to the antipsychotic drug raclopride increased with the increasing levels of D_2 receptor blockade (Nordstorm *et al.* 1993). However, since then several *in vivo* studies have complicated the picture. Patients failing to respond to classical antipsychotics have been shown to have the same levels of D_2 blockade as patients who are responders (Wolkin *et al.* 1989; Pilowsky *et al.* 1993).

The atypical antipsychotic clozapine has been shown to have modest D_2 occupancy *in vivo* despite having produced excellent clinical responses in patients resistant to classical antipsychotics (Pilowsky *et al.* 1992; Farde *et al.* 1992). Recent studies on atypical antipsychotics have revealed their higher occupancy of 5-HT_2 receptors and in some cases higher occupancy of other dopamine receptors including D_3 and D_4 (Kapur *et al.* 1999, 2000; Meltzer *et al.* 1999). Furthermore, some atypical antipsychotic drugs appear to show preferential occupancy of limbic cortical D_2 receptors. There is good reason to suppose that cortical dopamine D_2 receptors may be the common site of action for all antipsychotic drugs (Pilowsky 2001). Abi-Dargham *et al.* (1998; 2000) used alpha-methyl-para-tyrosine to deplete synaptic dopamine and showed that the resulting increase in D_2 receptor availability was larger in untreated schizophrenic patients than in controls and that it predicted treatment response in patients. Although antipsychotic drugs may exert their therapeutic effect chiefly at the postsynaptic dopamine receptor, current evidence is that the core dopamine abnormalities in schizophrenia are pre-synaptic, for example in terms of markedly increased release of dopamine secondary to experimental amphetamine administration (Laruelle *et al.* 1996).

Antipsychotic drugs are not selective. The blockade of dopamine receptors in non-target pathways causes the well-described extrapyramidal syndromes such as acute dystonia, akathisia, parkinsonism and tardive dyskinesia (see Chapter 1) and endocrine problems such as hyperprolactinaemia (see Chapter 5). Along with blockade of various dopamine receptors the antipsychotics variously block serotonin ($5HT_2$), alpha-adrenergic, muscarinic and histamine receptors. Their affinity for these different types of receptors varies from one compound to another. For example the atypical antipsychotics risperidone, olanzapine, clozapine and quetiapine have high affinity to serotonin $5HT_2A$ receptors (Nyberg *et al.* 1993; Travis *et al.* 1998; Jones *et al.* 2000).

Mechanisms for discontinuation syndromes

Considering the wide range of effects on different receptors by antipsychotics, and the secondary up-regulation of corresponding receptors especially during chronic administration, one should expect a variety of symptoms to appear on their discontinuation. Discontinuation symptoms seem most likely to reflect the affinity of antipsychotics to muscarinic, alpha-adrenergic and dopamine receptors (Miller and Hilly 1974; Peroutka and Synder 1980).

A study of the role of super sensitivity of cholinergic receptors by Luchins *et al.* (1980) suggested that the antipsychotic drugs with greater anti-muscarinic (M1) effects were more apt to produce withdrawal symptoms. Phenothiazines of the aliphatic and piperidine groups and chlorprothixenes are known to be more anti-muscarinic as compared to piprazine phenothiazines and butyrophenones (Dilsaver and Alessi 1988). However this issue is complicated by the concomitant use of anticholinergic drugs, commonly used to control the extrapyramidal symptoms caused by antipsychotics. The anticholinergics can produce cholinergic rebound discontinuation symptoms of their own and are often stopped at the same time as the antipsychotic drug. Cholinergic rebound symptoms can produce a flu-like syndrome though the symptoms can be more varied. They include myalgia, diaphoresis, malaise, rhinitis, parasthesia, gastrointestinal distress, headaches, anxiety, insomnia, dysphoria, nightmares and fatigue. Simpson *et al.* (1965) and Melnytt *et al.* (1965) showed that patients who had antipsychotic and anticholinergic drugs discontinued together showed a higher number of symptoms compared to those who were withdrawn from antipsychotics alone.

Clozapine is also strongly anticholinergic. Some of the symptoms of the acute clozapine discontinuation syndrome, in particular nausea, abdominal cramps, insomnia and anxiety, may reflect 'cholinergic overdrive' (Verghese *et al.* 1996). These discontinuation symptoms resemble those that can occur on stopping tricyclic antidepressants that are also known to have strong anticholinergic properties (Dilsaver and Greden 1984).

Clozapine induced alterations in D_2 receptors (Waldenberg and Seeman 1999) and super sensitivity of GABA receptors (Coward *et al.* 1989) have been suggested as possible mechanisms for causing motor symptoms on clozapine discontinuation.

A number of mechanisms for clozapine 'rebound' psychosis have been suggested. Seeman and Tallerico (1999) have argued that because clozapine has a relatively weak association with D_2 receptors, it is readily displaced by endogenous dopamine at the D_2 receptors and this may cause a rapid relapse of psychotic symptoms. They have further argued that the swift dissociation time of clozapine at the D_2 receptors may be disguising a higher D_2 receptor occupancy than that estimated with receptor imaging studies and this may predispose to rapid psychotic relapse after withdrawal. Alternatively Baldessarini *et al.* (1995) have suggested the mechanism of dopamine super sensitivity involving up-regulated D_4 receptors for which clozapine has a high sensitivity. Meltzer (1997) has suggested that the 'rebound' psychosis may reflect serotonergic receptor alterations that occur during clozapine treatment with a hyper-serotonergic state occurring after clozapine withdrawal.

Differential diagnosis

Anxiety, restlessness, agitation, insomnia and confusion can occur as antipsychotic discontinuation symptoms and also as symptoms of schizophrenia and other psychotic illnesses. In the case of these discontinuation symptoms the most important differential diagnosis is early relapse of psychosis (Dilsaver and Alessi 1988). An important guide to differentiation can be the time of symptom onset. Antipsychotic discontinuation symptoms usually occur within the first week of stopping medication. In contrast the recurrence of psychotic symptoms is rare in the first week of discontinuation. A clinically stable patient, recently withdrawn from antipsychotics, who becomes agitated, restless, anxious and experiences insomnia is more likely to be suffering from a discontinuation syndrome (Dilsaver and Alessi 1988). Another useful guide is the presence of physical symptoms such as nausea, headaches and abdominal cramps. These often form part of an antipsychotic discontinuation syndrome but are not characteristic of psychotic relapse. The simultaneous appearance of these physical symptoms makes it more likely that psychological symptoms commencing within a few days of stopping an antipsychotic represent a discontinuation syndrome.

When new symptoms arise within a few days of switching antipsychotic it is important that the clinician considers whether the symptoms are side effects of the new drug or discontinuation symptoms from the antipsychotic that was stopped. Of course another possibility is that the symptoms are not drug-related.

Management

Patients who are stopping an antipsychotic or switching between antipsychotics should be warned about the potential for discontinuation symptoms to occur. Strategies for prevention should be considered (see next section). Many discontinuation symptoms are relatively mild and short lived and no specific treatment may be necessary. Some symptoms are amenable to symptomatic treatment, for example the cholinergic rebound symptoms as described above can be controlled by the use of anticholinergic drugs. Reassurance to the patient that the symptoms might not be a sign of relapse and short term use of hypnotics for sleep disturbance may also be helpful. If symptoms are severe and persistent then it may be necessary to reinstate the antipsychotic and then withdraw it more gradually.

Risk factors and prevention

Considering the present evidence, it is difficult to state whether certain patients are more at risk of developing antipsychotic discontinuation symptoms. Most of the conventional and atypical antipsychotics have been reported to show discontinuation symptoms on occasions, and so all patients stopping these drugs should be considered at risk.

Studies conducted on animals have shown differences in the propensity of antipsychotics to trigger withdrawal effects (Antkiewicz-Michaluk et al. 1995). In general, low potency drugs are more likely to give non-motor symptoms and high potency more likely to give motor effects on withdrawal (Luchins et al. 1980).

To our knowledge no systematic studies or guidelines have been published on withdrawal and switching strategies of antipsychotics. It is not clear whether gradual withdrawal of an antipsychotic minimizes the risk and severity of discontinuation symptoms but one would expect that it would and a gradual withdrawal strategy seems more logical. As typical and atypical antipsychotics differ in their receptor profiles, it might be important for the clinician to keep them in mind while planning the future course of action. Typical antipsychotics have overlapping receptor profiles and exact receptor profiles may not be important while switching from one typical antipsychotic to another as long as the dose is adequate. The atypicals have a wider variation in receptor profiles and clinicians need to aware of the withdrawal effects of a particular drug when discontinuing it and whether the new agent being introduced shares a similar receptor profile to cover the withdrawal effects (Verghese *et al.* 1996). In one study a randomized comparison of four switching methods from a conventional antipsychotic to olanzapine was conducted. The results showed that gradual discontinuation combined at the start with an initial full (rather than incremental) dose of the new drug had the best combination of efficacy and tolerability (Kinon *et al.* 2000).

Simultaneously stopping anticholinergic agents with an antipsychotic drug adds to the risk of discontinuation symptoms occurring (Simpson *et al.* 1965; Melnytt *et al.* 1965). Consequently, as a general rule, if it has been decided to stop both an antipsychotic and an anticholinergic it is best to do this in sequence, first withdrawing the antipsychotic and then the anticholingic agent. This minimizes the likelihood of the patient developing extrapyramidal symptoms due to a period of 'untreated' antipsychotic treatment.

Clozapine warrants special consideration due to the severity of the discontinuation syndrome that can occur including the possibility of discontinuation psychosis. The British National Formulary recommends that clozapine be withdrawn over 1 to 2 weeks to minimize the risk of rebound psychosis but based on our experience and anecdotal reports we would recommend a slower taper. Szafranski and Gmurkowski (1999) have suggested that clozapine discontinuation should be done by 50 mg per week. It has also been recommended that to prevent relapse, a new antipsychotic be started overlapping with the clozapine withdrawal. There has been debate over which is the most appropriate antipsychotic to switch to.

Baldessarini *et al.* (1995) suggested the use of thioridazine because it has anticholinergic properties, has the ability to block D_4 receptors and is administered in doses similar to clozapine. However following concerns about a relationship with sudden deaths the 'Summary of Product Characteristics' for thioridazine has been altered and its use is restricted. Consequently it can no longer be recommended as the first option for switching to when clozapine is stopped. Amongst the newer antipsychotics olanzapine, in a double-blind clinical trial, has been reported to have significantly lowered the relapse rates after clozapine withdrawal as compared to placebo (Tollefson *et al.* 1999). Risperidone, because of its equal potency for D_2 and D_4 receptors has also been suggested and Baldessarini *et al.* (1995) have reported successful transfer of patients from clozapine to risperidone if clozapine is removed gradually and risperidone is increased slowly. In cases of sudden withdrawal of clozapine, anticholinergics should be used to prevent cholinergic rebound.

Summary: Antipsychotic discontinuation syndromes

Definition	Characteristic symptoms that commence shortly after stopping or reducing the dose of an antipsychotic and are unrelated to the underlying psychiatric disorder.
Incidence	Variable. Depends on definition. Also likely to vary depending on antipsychotic, length of treatment, rate of taper prior to stoppage and dose. In some studies over half of patients develop discontinuation symptoms on stopping antipsychotic treatment.
Drugs causing syndrome	Occurs with all antipsychotics.
Key symptoms	Very variable. With conventional antipsychotics and clozapine common symptoms include gastrointestinal symptoms (nausea, vomiting, anorexia), general somatic distress (sweating, headache, insomnia), insomnia and anxiety and agitation. Clozapine termination has also been associated with muteness and confusion. Psychosis often appears soon after stopping clozapine; it is unclear whether this is a relapse of underlying illness or a discontinuaion effect. Extrapyramidal syndromes (akathisia, dystonia, tardive dyskinesia) can occur on stopping conventional antipsychotics and less commonly atypicals.
Pharmacological mechanism	Sudden disruption of CNS systems that had adapted to antipsychotic treatment. Anticholinergic rebound may explain gastrointestinal symptoms, insmonis and agitation.
Investigations to confirm diagnosis	Accurate history, particularly close temporal relationship of symptom onset versus decrease in dose or termination of antipsychotic.
Management	Three options: 1 Education/support and allow symptoms to spontaneously resolve 2 Symptomatic treatment 3 Re-start antipsychotic and taper more slowly
Further reading	Borison RL, Diamond BI, Sinha D, *et al.* (1998). Clozapine withdrawal rebound psychosis. *Psychopharmacology Bull*, **24,** 260–3.

Dilsaver SC and Alessi NE (1988). Antipsychotic withdrawal symptoms: Phenomenology and pathophysiology. *Acta Psychiatr Scand*, **77**, 241–6.

Tollefson GD, Dellva MA, Mattler CA, *et al.* (1999). Controlled, double-blind investigation of the clozapine discontinuation symptoms with conversion to either olanzapine or placebo. The Collaborative Crossover Study Group. *J Clin Psychopharmacol*, **19**, 435–43.

References

Abi-Dargham A, Gil R, Krystal J, *et al.* (1998). Increased striatal dopamine transmission in schizophrenia: confirmation in a second cohort. *Am J Psychiatry*, **155**, 761–7.

Abi-Dargham A, Rodenhiser J, Printz D, *et al.* (2000). Increased baseline occupancy of D_2 receptors by dopamine in schizophrenia. *Proc Natl Acad Sci USA*, **97**, 8104–9.

Ahmed S, Chengappa KN, Naidu VR, *et al.* (1998). Clozapine withdrawal-emergent dystonias and dyskinesias: a case series. *J Clin Psychiatry*, **59**, 472–7.

Antkiewicz-Michaluk L, Karolewicz B, Michaluk J, *et al.* (1995). Differences between haloperidol and Pimozide-induced withdrawal syndrome: a role for Ca channels. *Eur J Pharmac*, **294**, 459–67.

Baldessarini RJ, Gardner DM, and Garver DL (1995). Conversion from clozapine to other antipsychotic drugs. *Arch Gen Psychiatry*, **52**,1071–2.

Battegay R (1967). Drug dependence as a criterion for differentiation of psychotropic drugs. In *Neuropsychopharmacology*, H Brill, JO Cole, P Deniker, H Hippius, PB Bradley (ed.), pp. 244–52. Excerpta Medica: Amsterdam.

Borison RL, Diamond BI, Sinha D, *et al.* (1998). Clozapine withdrawal rebound psychosis. *Psychopharmacol Bull*, **24**, 260–3.

Brooks GW (1959). Withrawal from neuroleptic drugs. *Am J Psychiatry*, **16**, 931–2.

Coward DM, Imperato A, Urwyler S, *et al.* (1989). Biochemical and behavioural properties of clozapine. *Psychopharmacology*, **99**, S6–12.

Dilsaver SC and Alessi NE (1988). Antipsychotic withdrawal symptoms: Phenomenology and pathophysiology. *Acta Psychiatr Scand*, **77**, 241–6.

Dilsaver SC and Greden JF (1984). Antidepressant withdrawal phenomena. *Biol Psychiatry*, **19**, 237–56.

Eklund K (1987). Supersensitivity and clozapine withdrawal. *Psychopharmacology*, **91**, 135.

Farde L, Nordstorm AL, Weisel A, *et al.* (1992). Positron emission tomography analysis of central d1 and D2 dopamine receeotor occupancy in patients treated with classical neuroleptics and clozapine: relation to extrapyramidal side-effects. *Arch Gen Psychiatry*, **49**, 538–43.

Farde L, Weisel F-A, Nordstrom A-L, *et al.* (1989). D_1 and D_2 dopamine receptor occupancy during treatment with conventional and atypical neuroleptics. *Psychopharmacology*, **99**, S28–31.

Goudie AJ (2000). What is the clinical significance of the discontinuation syndrome seen with clozapine? *J Psychopharmacol*, **14**, 188–92.

Greenberg LM and Roth S (1964). Differential effects of abrupt versus gradual withdrawal of chlorpromazine in hospitalised chronic schizophrenic patients. *Am J Psychiatry*, **121**, 491–3.

Grimes JD (1981). Parkinsonism and tardive dyskinesia associated with longterm metoclopramide therapy. *New Engl J Med*, **305**, 1417.

Hollister LE, Eikenberry DT, and Raffel S (1960). Chlorpromazine in nonpsychotic patients with pulmonary tuberculosis. *Am Rev Resp Dis*, **81**, 562–3.

Jeste DV and Caligiuri MP (1993). Tardive dyskinesia. *Schizophr Bull*, **19**, 303–15.

Johnstone EC, Crow TJ, Frith CD, *et al.* (1978). Mechanism of the antipsychotic effect in the treatment of acute schizophrenia. *Lancet*, **1** (8069), 848–51.

Jones HM, Travis MJ, Mullighan R, *et al.* (2000). *In vivo* serotonin 5-HT2A receptor occupancy and quetiapine. *Am J Psychiatry*, **157**, 148.

Kapur S, Zipursky R, Jones C, *et al.* (2000). A positron emission tomography study of quetiapine in schizophrenia. *Arch Gen Psychiatry*, **57**, 553–9.

Kapur S, Zipursky RB, and Remington G (1999). Clinical and theoretical implications of 5-HT$_2$ and D$_2$ receptor occupancy of clozapine, risperidone, and olanzapine in schizophrenia. *Am J Psychiatry*, **156**, 286–93.

Kinon BJ, Basson BR, Gilmore JA, *et al.* (2000). Strategies for switching from conventional antipsychotic drugs or risperidone to olanzapine. *J Clin Psychiatry*, **61**, 833–40.

Lacoursiere RB, Spohn HE, and Thompson K (1976). Medical effects of abrupt neuroleptic withdrawal. *Compr Psychiatry*, **17**, 285–94.

Laruelle M, Abi-Dargham A, Van-Dyck H, *et al.* (1996). Single photon emission computerised tomography imaging of amphetamine induced dopamine release in drug free schizophrenic subjects. *Proc Natl Acad Sci USA*, **93**, 9235–40.

Luchins DJ, Freed MH, and Wyatt RJ (1980). The role of cholinergic supersensitivity in the medical symptoms associated with withdrawal of antipsychotic drugs. *Am J Psychiatry*, **137**, 1395–8.

Marsalek M (2000). Tardive drug-induced extrapyramidal syndromes. *Pharmacopsychiatry*, **33** (Suppl. 1), 14–33.

Melnytt WT, Worthington AG, and Laverty (1965). Abrupt withdrawal of chlorpromazine and thioridazine from schizophrenic patients. *Can Psychiatr Assoc*, **6**, 347–51.

Meltzer HY (1997). Clozapine withdrawal: serotonergic or dopaminergic mechanisms? *Arch Gen Psychiatry*, **54**, 760–1.

Meltzer HY, Lee MA, Ranjan R, *et al.* (1996). Relapse following clozapine withdrawal: effect of cyproheptadine plus neuroleptic. *Psychopharmacology*, **124**, 176–87.

Meltzer HY, Park S, and Kessler R (1999). Cognition, schizophrenia and the typical antipsychotic drugs. *Proc Natl Acad Sci USA*, **96**, 13591–3.

Miller RJ and Hilly CR (1974). Antimuscarinic properties of neuroleptics and drug induced Parkinsonism. *Nature*, **248**, 596–7.

Morton MR (1968). A study of withdrawal of chlorpromazine in chronic schizophrenia. *Am J Psychiatry*, **124**, 1585–8.

Nishimura K, Tsuka M, and Horikawa N (2001). Withdrawal-emergent rabbit syndrome during dose reduction of risperidone. *Eur Neuropsychopharmacol*, **11**, 323–4.

Nordstorm AL, Fared L, Weisel FA, *et al.* (1993). Central D$_2$ dopamine receptor occupancy in relation to antipsychotic drug effects: a double blind PET study of schizophrenic patients. *Biol Psychiatry*, **33**, 227–35.

Nyberg S, Farde L, Eriksson L, *et al.* (1993). 5-HT$_2$ and D$_2$ dopamine receptor occupancy by risperidone in the living human brain. *Psychopharmacology*, **110**, 265–72.

Patel M (1986). Long term neurologic complications of metoclopramide. *N Y State J Med*, **86**, 210.

Peroutka SJ and Synder SH (1980). Relationship of neuroleptic drug effects at brain dopamine, serotonin, alpha-adrenergic and histaminergic receptors to clinical potency. *Am J Psychiatry*, **137**, 1518–22.

Pilowsky LS (2001). Probing targets for antipsychotic drug action with PET and SPET receptor imaging. *Nuc Med Commun*, **22**, 829–33.

Pilowsky LS, Costa DC, Ell PJ, *et al.* (1992). Clozapine, single photon emission tomography and the D2 dopamine receptor blockade hypothesis of schizophrenia. *Lancet*, **340**, 199–202.

Pilowsky LS, Costa DC, Ell PJ, *et al.* (1993). Antipsychotic medication, D2 dopamine receptor blockade and clinical response-a 123I IBZM SPET (single photon emission tomography) study. *Psychol Med*, **23**, 791–9.

Poyurovsky M, Bergman Y, Shoshani D, *et al.* (1998). Emergence of obsessive – compulsive symptoms and tics during clozapine withdrawal. *Clin Neuropharmacol*, **21**, 97–100.

Reidenberg MM and Lowenthal DT (1968). Adverse non-drug reactions. *New Engl J Med*, **279**, 678–9.

Rothstein C (1960). An evaluation of the effects of discontinuation of chlorpromazine. *New Engl J Med*, **262**, 67–9.

Seeman P and Tallerico T (1999). Rapid release of antipsychotic drugs from dopamine D$_2$ receptors: an explanation for low receptor occupancy and early clinical relapse upon withdrawal of clozapine or quetiapine. *Am J Psychiatry*, **156**, 876–84.

Simpson GM, Amin M, and Konz E (1965). Withdrawal effects of phenothiazines. *Compr Psychiatry*, **6**, 347–51.

Simpson GM and Varga E (1974). Clozapine – a new antipsychotic agent. *Curr Ther Res*, **16**, 679–86.

Szafranski T and Gmurkowski K (1999). Clozapine withdrawal. A review. *Psychiatr Pol*, Jan-Feb, **33**, 51–67.

Tollefson GD, Dellva MA, Mattler CA, *et al.* (1999). Controlled, double-blind investigation of the clozapine discontinuation symptoms with conversion to either olanzapine or placebo. The Collaborative Crossover Study Group. *J Clin Psychopharmacol*, **19**, 435–43.

Tranter R and Healy D (1998). Neuroleptic discontinuation syndromes. *J Psychopharmacol*, **12**, 401–6.

Travis MJ, Busatto GF, Pilowsky LS, *et al.* (1998). 5-HT$_2$A receptor blockade in patients with schizophrenia treated with risperidone or clozapine. A SPET study using the novel 5-HT$_2$A ligand. *Br J Psychiatry*, **173**, 236–41.

Verghese C, DeLeon J, Nair C, *et al.* (1996). Clozapine withdrawal effects and receptor profiles of typical and atypical neuroleptics. *Biol Psychiatry*, **39**, 135–8.

Viguera AC, Baldessarini RJ, Hegarty JD, *et al.* (1997). Clinical risk following abrupt and gradual withdrawal of maintenance neuroleptic treatment. *Arch Gen Psychiatry*, **54**, 49–55.

Waldenberg M-L and Seeman P (1999). Clozapine pre-treatment enhances raclopride catalepsy. *Eur J Pharmacol*, **377**, R1-R2.

Whittaker CB and Hay RM (1964). Withdrawal of perphenazine in chronic schizophrenia. *Br J Psychiatry*, **109**, 422–7.

Wolkin A, Barouche F, Wolf AP, *et al.* (1989). Dopamine blockade and clinical response: evidence for two biological subgroups of schizophrenia. *Am J Psychiatry*, **146**, 905–8.

Zerjav-Lacombe S and Derwan V (2001). Possible serotonin syndrome associated with clomipramine after withdrawal of clozapine. *Ann Pharmacother*, **35**, 180–2.

Chapter 12

Blood dyscrasias

Hyun-Sang Cho, John H Krystal, and
Deepak Cyril D'Souza

Most adverse effects of psychotropic drugs are related to the primary pharmacological mechanism of a drug. For example, antipsychotic drugs cause extrapyramidal side effects which are related to their primary mechanism of action, dopamine D_2 receptor antagonism. However, some adverse effects are unrelated to the mode of primary pharmacological activity; these are often called idiosyncratic reactions and include blood dyscrasias. These hematologic side effects are generally infrequent but may be severe and even fatal. This section will review the blood dyscrasias associated with psychotropic medications.

The hematopoietic system

Hematopoiesis, the production of blood cells, is a regulated system sensitively and rapidly responsive to various functional demands, such as infection and inflammation, allergic or immune challenges, hemorrhage, hypoxic changes etc. The various blood cell types are produced by hematopoietic stem cells in the bone marrow. These have characteristically high proliferation and differentiation capacity. These cells proliferate and differentiate into a wide variety of mature cell types under the influence of specific colony-stimulating factors (CSF).

Peripheral blood cell types include red blood cells (RBC, erythrocytes), white blood cells (leucocytes), and platelets. Erythrocytes, the most numerous of blood cell types, transport oxygen to various tissues. Leucocytes are involved in inflammatory and immune responses and comprise neutrophils (45–74 per cent), basophils (0–4 per cent), eosinophils (0–7 per cent), lymphocytes (16–45 per cent) and monocytes (4–10 per cent) (Braunwald *et al.* 2001). The so-called granulocytes include neutrophils, basophils and eosinophils. Neutrophils are important to defensive functions against bacterial infection. Eosinophils are thought to play a role in allergic reactions and helminthic infestation. Lymphocytes produce antibodies and monocytes play a role in phagocyting and antigen processing. Platelets participate in coagulation at bleeding sites.

Peripheral white blood cell (WBC) count is maintained between 5,000 and 10,000 per mm^3. The platelet count is normally maintained between 150,000–450,000 cells per mm^3.

Definitions and clinical features

Psychotropic drugs have been reported to be associated with various blood dyscrasias. Some of these blood dyscrasias are well recognized and have established rates of occurrence whereas others are rare with sporadic cases reported in the literature. The frequently reported psychotropics-induced blood dyscrasias include neutropenia, leucopenia, agranulocytosis, eosinophilia, thrombocytopenia, and aplastic anemia. Other rare events include leucocytosis, thrombocytosis, and hemolytic anemia.

- *Leucocytosis* is defined as an increased count beyond normal limits (>10,000 cells/ mm^3) and is accompanied by increased neutrophil counts (neutrophilia).

- *Leucopenia* is defined as a reduction in white blood cells less than 3,000 white blood cells/mm^3. The term leucopenia is generally used when a differential white blood cell count is not available.

- *Neutropenia* is defined as a neutrophil count less than 1,500 cells/mm^3. When the neutrophil count falls below 1,000 cells/mm^3, the vulnerability to various infectious diseases significantly increases.

- *Agranulocytosis* is a severe state of neutropenia, when the absolute neutrophil count falls below 500 cells/mm^3. When this occurs, there is a risk that the body may lose control over the normal bacterial flora. Clinical signs and symptoms include headache, fever, sore throat, stomatitis (or oral ulceration), diarrhea, malaise, chills, myalgia, arthralgia, urinary frequency and bleeding gums (Oyesanmi *et al.* 1999; Andres *et al.* 2002). Sometimes there are no symptoms, so that the abnormal findings in a full blood cell count (FBC) (i.e. complete blood count – CBC in the United States) may be the only clue (Chengappa *et al.* 1996). However, in some instances because of its rapid onset, monitoring FBC may not be useful. Early pretreatment with antibiotics may attenuate the signs of agranulocytosis. If unchecked, agranulocytosis may be fatal as a result of a massive overwhelming infection.

- *Eosinophilia* is defined as an eosinophil count greater than 300 or 500 cells/mm^3 (Pisciotta 1992; Holland and Gallin 2001). It is a common manifestation of allergy to many drugs and tends to be more prevalent in individuals with a history of allergies. The affected organs may include the heart, lungs, skin, joints, gut and central nervous system. Eosinophils infiltrate the involved tissues and are thought to cause tissue damage. Thus, the signs and symptoms vary according to the involved organ system.

- *Thrombocytopenia* is defined as a platelet count less than 100,000 cells/mm^3. The most common site to observe bleeding is in the skin and mucous membranes. Thrombocytopenia may manifest as petechiae, ecchymoses (common bruises), oral hemorrhagic bullae and hematomas. Prodromal signs may include fever, chills, nausea, vomiting and fatigue. Platelet counts of 50,000 – 100,000 cells per mm^3 prolong the bleeding time mildly, and bleeding occurs only in severe trauma. When the platelet count is less than 50,000 cells per mm^3, easy bruising after minor trauma can occur, and when the platelet count is less than 20,000 cells per mm^3 spontaneous bleeding may occur sometimes manifesting as intracranial hemorrhage (Handin 2001).

- *Thrombocytosis* is generally asymptomatic but may cause thrombosis, especially in elderly persons (Williams 1995).

- *Aplastic anemia* or *pancytopenia* is the state when hematopoiesis fails, counts of *all* blood cell types are extremely low, and biopsy of the bone marrow shows a marked reduction in the number of cells with a normal appearance of the scanty remaining cells. This is generally diagnosed with the combination of a peripheral blood count and a bone marrow biopsy. It is defined by the presence of two of three criteria: a neutrophil count less than 500 cells/mm^3, a platelet count less than 20,000 cells/mm^3, and a reticulocyte (slightly immature RBC) count less than 1 per cent. The pathophysiology of aplastic anemia is now believed to be immune-mediated, with active destruction of blood-forming cells by lymphocytes. Aplastic anemia manifests with fatigue, dyspnea, and cardiac symptoms related to reduced oxygenation due to a paucity of RBCs; increased susceptibility to infection related to neutropenia; and easy bruising and mucosal bleeding related to thrombocytopenia (reviewed in Young 2002).

Pharmacological basis

While the precise nature of the pathophysiology of blood dyscrasias associated with psychotropics is yet to be determined in most instances, there are some general principles that may be applicable. Two main types of drug-induced blood dyscrasias are suggested based on pathophysiology. The first type is a dose-related toxicity and is often nonspecific. It is elicited by interference of the drug, its metabolites, and free radicals with protein synthesis and cell replication in highly proliferative cells, for example bone marrow progenitor cells. The second type may not be dose related and is believed to have an allergic or immunological basis. The offending drug sensitizes cells e.g., neutrophils or their precursors to immune-mediated peripheral destruction. However, drug-induced thrombocytopenia is induced mostly by an immune response with complement activation.

Dyscrasias and psychiatric drugs

Antipsychotics

Clozapine

The psychotropic-induced blood dyscrasia best characterized is clozapine-induced agranulocytosis. After the occurrence of several cases of fatal agranu-locytosis occurred in clozapine-treated patients in Europe, clozapine was withdrawn from the market but was later reintroduced for use in treatment refractory schizophrenia. Clozapine is associated with agranulocytosis in about 0.8 per cent of patients (Alvir et al. 1993; Atkin et al. 1996) and neu-tropenia in 2.9 per cent of patients (Atkin et al. 1996). The incidence of agra-nulocytosis is about 10 times that of phenothiazine drugs. This incidence was reduced to 0.38 per cent with weekly WBC count monitoring in the United Sates (Honigfeld et al., 1998). More than 84 per cent of cases of agranulocyto-sis occur within 3 months of initiation treatment and over 90 per cent within the first 6 months (Alvir et al. 1993). However the problem may occur at any point during treatment, hence the importance of regular blood monitoring for as long as clozapine is prescribed. About 3 per cent of cases with agranulo-cytosis will result in death. With regular WBC count monitoring, mortality rates have dropped from 1 per cent to 0.01 per cent.

There has been debate about whether the mechanism underlying clozapine-induced agranulocytosis is an immune or toxic reaction. The association with human leukocyte antigens (HLA) haplotypes (HLA-B38, DR4, DRB1, DQB1, and DQA1 in Jewish subjects and DR2 in non-Jewish Caucasian patients) (Yunis et al. 1995; Amar et al. 1998; Dettling et al. 2001) and the major histo-compatibility complex (MHC) regions marked by heat shock protein 70, vari-ants and tumor necrosis factor loci (Corzo et al. 1995; Turbay et al. 1997) suggests the involvement of genetic and immune mechanisms. However, N-desmethylclozapine, the major metabolite of clozapine, is believed to be toxic to haematopoietic precursors resulting in cytotoxicity of granulocytes (Gerson et al. 1994). Clozapine also undergoes bioactivation to a toxic nitreni-um ion by P450 and peroxidase enzymes. This direct toxic mechanism effect is believed to be more consistent with clinical and laboratory findings than an immune mechanism (Gerson and Meltzer 1992; Williams *et al.* 2000). Bone marrow shows a normal compartment of the hematopoietic stem cells committed to granulocyte production, but not of the intermediate mature forms, and normal quantities of erythroid and megakaryocyte precursor cells (Gerson 1993).

Clozapine is also associated with eosinophilia, leucopenia, leucocytosis, thrombocytopenia and thrombocytosis (Deliliers 2000). It is suggested that eosinophilia or thrombocytosis may be predictors of impending agranulocytosis or neutropenia (Galletly *et al.* 1996; Lucht and Rietschel 1998; Hampson 2000). Eosinophilia appears to be a significant risk in women and usually occurs early in therapy, spontaneously resolves (Banov *et al.* 1993). This event can result in acute myocarditis, cardiomyopathy, colitis, pancreatitis and pleural effusion (Chatterton 1997).

Other atypical antipsychotics

While there are case reports about agranulocytosis, neutropenia and thrombocytopenia (Assion *et al.* 1996; Dernovsek and Tavcar 1997; Finkel *et al.* 1998*a*) associated with risperidone, it is not significantly associated with hematotoxicity (Umbricht and Kane 1996). A recent review of case reports suggested the possibility that olanzapine may be associated with agranulocytosis, and neutropenia or leucopenia (Tolosa-Vilella *et al.* 2002). Also, according to case reports, olanzapine may prolong granulocyte depression during recovery from clozapine-induced granulocytopenia (Flynn *et al.* 1997; Konakanchi *et al.* 2000). However, the rate of agranulocytosis associated with olanzapine is extremely low and hence does not warrant monitoring. Further, patients who develop agranulocytosis after treatment with typical and atypical antipsychotics have been successfully treated with olanzapine without recurrence of agranulocytosis (Finkel *et al.* 1998*b*; Swartz *et al.* 1999; Oyewumi and Al-Semaan 2000). Other rare dyscrasias reported to be associated with olanzapine include eosinophilia and possibly thrombocytopenia (Bogunovic and Viswanathan 2000; Mathias *et al.* 2002). There are case reports of agranulocytosis and neutropenia associated with quetiapine (Ruhe *et al.* 2001). Finally, there are no published case reports of blood dyscrasias associated with ziprasidone, amisulpride and aripiprazole.

Typical antipsychotics

The risk of agranulocytosis associated with these drugs is estimated at 0.01–0.14 per cent. The highest risks of blood dyscrasias appear to be associated with the aliphatic phenothiazine derivatives chlorpromazine. Chloropromazine directly damages the bone marrow microenvironment or myeloid precursor cells by the parent drug or a drug metabolite (Pisciotta 1992).

Mood stabilizers

Lithum

Lithium salts have been demonstrated to cause leucocytosis. Lithium has been reported to enhance the proliferation of hematopoietic cells (Gallicchio and Chen 1982; Ballin *et al.* 1998), and this increase is mediated by enhancement of CSF (Harker *et al.* 1977; Gallicchio and Chen 1982). Lithium is also reported to be associated with thrombocytosis. These effects are not considered a clinically significant problem in the use of lithium as a mood stabilizer. In fact lithum's capacity to enhance hemoproliferation has been used to manage various hematologic problems and disorders (malignancies). For example, lithium can produce a reversal of carbamazepine-induced leucopenia and increasing leukocyte (predominantly neutrophil) counts (Kramlinger and Post 1990). However, lithium does not have a protective effect on clozapine-induced agranulocytosis (Gerson 1994). Although very rare, there are also reports of aplastic and megaloblastic anemia associated with lithium.

Carbamazepine

Uncommon but serious hematologic side effects with carbamazepine include agranulocytosis, aplastic anemia and thrombocytopenia, which usually appear within first 3 weeks of intiating treatment (Sobotka *et al.* 1990; Tohen *et al.* 1995). Due to the rapid onset of these blood dyscrasias, frequent laboratory tests and informing patients to watch for early signs and symptoms are necessary. Leucopenia develops more slowly, occurring in 2–14 per cent (Ballenger 1988; Post 1990; Tohen *et al.* 1995) and approximately 12 per cent of children and 7 per cent of adults (Sobotka *et al.* 1990). Mild asymptomatic leucopenia is not related to serious idiopathic dyscrasias, so that it usually resolves spontaneously even with continued treatment or dose reduction (American Psychiatric Association 2002). Thrombocytopenia is less frequent than leucopenia.

Valproate

The most common hematologic effect of valproate is subclinical thrombocytopenia. Thrombocytopenia has been reported in 6–33 per cent of adult patients with epilepsy on valproate (Neophytides *et al.* 1979; Covanis *et al.* 1982) and about 12 per cent in general psychiatric patients (Conley *et al.* 2001). The decrease in platelet count and prolongation of bleeding time is reported to be correlated to valproate dose and its plasma concentration

(Gidal *et al.* 1994; Kaufman and Gerner 1998). In a recent report, more than half of elderly patients show thrombocytopenia, and hence the need for routine monitoring is suggested (Trannel *et al.* 2001). As with carbamazepine, cases of mild asymptomatic thrombocytopenia or leucopenia are usually reversible upon dose reduction or discontinuation (American Psychiatric Association 2002).

Other anti-epileptic drugs

Agranulocytosis, leucopenia, and thrombocytopenia have been described as possible hematological side effects of lamotrigine in a few cases (Mackay *et al.* 1997; Damiani and Christensen 2000; Solvason 2000). There are no published case reports of blood dyscrasias associated with topiramate and gabapentin. One case report shows a possibility of thrombocytopenia secondary to tiagabine (Willert *et al.* 1999).

Antidepressants

Tricyclic antidepressants (TCAs)

The occurrence of leucopenia was reported to be 0.3 per cent with TCAs, lower than carbamazepine and similar to valproate (Tohen *et al.* 1995). TCA-induced agranulocytosis is rare but there are case reports for clomipramine, desipramine, amitriptyline and imipramine. Nomifensin is reported to induce hemolytic anemia and mianserin is believed to be associated with granulocytopenic disorders. As a result nomifensin was withdrawn in Britain. Mianserin remains available in Britain, but FBC monitoring is advised during the first few months of treatment and patients should be warned to report signs that may indicate neutropenia at any time during treatment (*British National Formulary* 2003).

Selective serotonin reuptake inhibitors (SSRIs)

SSRIs have been reported to be associated with bleeding (Skop and Brown 1996) in particular upper gatrointestinal bleeding (De Abajo *et al.* 1999). The elderly appear to be at highest risk for bleeding (van Walraven *et al.* 2001). In childhood and adolescence these drugs have been associated with bruising or epistaxis (Lake *et al.* 2000). De Abajo *et al.* (1999) showed a threefold increase in the relative risk (1 case per 8,000 prescriptions) of bleeding episodes similar to low dose ibuprofen in clomipramine or the SSRIs. Peripheral serotonin, released from platelets, promotes thrombogenesis by enhancing platelet aggregation and vasocostriction. During treatment with SSRIs, the intraplatelet serotonin content is reduced as a result of inhibition of the serotonin reuptake mechanism and thereby reduces platelet plug formation

(Hergovich *et al.* 2000). However, during treatment with SSRIs there is no evidence supporting an increased risk of either intracerebral hemorrhage or a decreased risk of ischemic stroke (Bak *et al.* 2002). In general the risk of bleeding is not clinically significant. However, with higher doses of SSRIs, pre-existing platelet abnormalities and combination with other serotonergic drugs (Skop and Brown 1996), the potential for clinically significant bleeding abnormalities increases. Further, if bleeding time is increased, it is recommended that fluoxetine and other SSRIs should be discontinued temporarily in the event of elective surgery (Beliles and Stoudemire 1998). Neutropenia associated with SSRIs is rare.

Mirtazapine

Agranulocytosis caused by mirtazapine, a tetracyclic antidepressant, occurred in approximately 1/1,000 during premarketing trials. But this incidence is no higher than the incidence of agranulocytosis with other antidepressants. Hence, routine FBC monitoring is not recommended but may be obtained as on and as needed basis (Hartmann 1999).

Miscellaneous antidepressants

There are case reports of eosinophilia associated with venlafaxine and bupropion (Malesker *et al.* 1995; Fleisch *et al.* 2000).

Other psychotropic drugs

Agranulocytosis associated with benzodiazepines is relatively rare. There have been case reports of thrombocytopenia with clonazepam and diazepam (Balon and Berchou 1986), and decreased platelet aggregation with chlordiazepoxide and diazepam (Oyesanmi *et al.* 1999). Reports of blood dyscrasias associated with cholinesterase inhibitors are rare. Naltrexone and acamprosate, drugs used in the treatment of alcoholism, have not been associated with blood dyscrasias. Finally, newborn infants born to mothers using methadone may have been reported to present with thrombocytosis (Hanssler and Roll 1994).

Differential diagnosis

A definite diagnosis of drug-induced blood dyscrasia is often difficult and is generally one of exclusion. Further, because psychotropics are often combined with each other and with other nonpsychotropic medications that have been associated with blood dyscrasias, it is often challenging to identify the offending agent conclusively.

Since most blood dyscrasias resolve spontaneously, identifying the offending agent can often be facilitated by drug discontinuation. However, this becomes difficult with polypharmacy. The reintroduction of the questioned drug may be helpful in clarifying causality but generally is not recommended. In fact when agranulocytosis or neutropenia develops with clozapine treatment, reinitiation of clozapine is contraindicated because of the risk of recurrence.

Neutrophil counts may be decreased in acute viral infections (infectious mononucleosis and infectious hepatitis), acute bacterial sepsis, acute leukemia and aplastic anemia. A drug-related etiology is more probable when (1) there appears a temporal relation between onset of neutropenia and initiation of treatment with a drug (2) there is known association between a drug and neutropenia (e.g., clozapine) (3) the dyscrasia resolves upon drug discontinuation, and (4) when specific bone marrow findings exist (Solal-Céligny 1994). Important differential diagnoses of isolated drug-associated thrombocytopenia include idiopathic thrombocytopenic purpura, aplastic anemia, liver disease, alcoholism and infection including AIDS. Finally, with eosinophilia one should consider parasitic (helminthic) infestation, pruritic skin illnesses including atopic dermatitis and respiratory allergies in the differential diagnosis.

Management

Most psychotropic-induced blood dyscrasias spontaneously resolve within several days or weeks following discontinuation of the offending drug. Treatment includes observation for the consequences of the specific dyscrasia, monitoring of blood counts, prevention of risks and general support.

For clozapine-induced neutropenia, the drug should be discontinued and neutrophil counts should be monitored on a daily basis until the count returns to normal levels. Patients should be instructed to avoid situations that might expose them to infection and immediately report any symptoms suggestive of infection including fever, malaise, sore throat, etc.

Similarly for clozapine-induced agranulocytosis, the drug should be immediately discontinued and neutrophil counts should be monitored on a daily basis until the count returns to normal levels. Consultation with a hematologist and infectious disease specialist should be sought. Prophylactic antibiotics, inverse isolation, and the institution of broad-spectrum antibiotics when febrile neutropenia develops are important (Gerson 1994). It is still unclear whether granulocyte colony-stimulating factor (G-CSF) shortens the period of clozapine-associated agranulocytosis, though some reports suggest that administration of G-CSF reduces recovery time to 1 week. Even without G-CSF treatment, agranulocytosis is reported to last 3–11 days (Chengappa *et al.* 1996). After recovery, re-administration of clozapine is contraindicated.

For drug-induced thrombocytopenia, discontinuation of the offending drug usually suffices, as recovery is spontaneous. A normal platelet count is usually restored within one week and subsequent mild thrombocytosis may be seen. Immunoglobulin and plasmapheresis may be helpful in severe cases of thrombocytopenia. In valproate-induced mild thrombocytopenia lowering the dose may restore the platelet count (American Psychiatric Association 2002).

The occurrence of aplastic anemia is rare but potentially fatal, and makes consultation with a hematologist and infectious disease specialist critical. The probable offending drug should be immediately discontinued. Typical measures include erythrocyte and platelet transfusions, isolation, antibiotics and CSF. Sometimes immunosuppression and bone marrow transplantation may be necessary (Young 2002).

The treatment of eosinophilia is withdrawal of the offending drug and glucocorticoids in severe cases. The reduction of eosinophil may not normalize in atopic persons.

Risk factors and prevention

Generally, patients with a history of hematologic adverse events to any drug and the elderly may be at higher risk. In the elderly, this higher risk is probably due to changes in pharmacokinetics and pharmacodynamics associated with ageing, multiple drug use, frequent comorbid condition and severe illness status (Nolan and O'Malley 1989).

The risk of clozapine-induced agranulocytosis increases with age and is higher in women (Alvir et al. 1993). There is a tendency for white blood cell count to spike upward before declining to levels of agranulocytosis (Alvir and Lieberman 1994). Clozapine treatment should not be initiated in persons with <3,500/mm^3 and those with a history of myeloproliferative disorder or clozapine-induced neutropenia. A history of other psychotropic-induced hematologic side effects may increase vulnerability (Idanpaan-Heikkila et al. 1977) to clozapine-induced agranulocytosis, but this is not an absolute contraindication.

Clozapine should not be prescribed concurrently with other drugs that have a substantial potential for causing agranulocytosis such as carbamazepine, chloramphenicol, co-trimoxazole, sulphonamides, pyrazolone analgesics (e.g. azapropazone), penicilllamine or cytotoxics. Long-acting depot antipsychotics should also be avoided due to their myelosupressive potential.

Patients prescribed clozapine, and their families, have to be educated to report immediately any early sign of infection including flu-like symptoms. In Britain leucocyte and differential blood counts must be monitored weekly for the first 18 weeks then at least fortnightly. After 1 year of treatment, if blood counts have been stable, monitoring can be reduced to every 4 weeks

Table 12.1 Monitoring for blood dyscrasias

Drugs	Recommended monitoring	Monitoring if abnormal blood cell counts	
Clozapine	WBC and differential blood counts prior to starting clozapine, weekly for the first 18 weeks of treatment, every 2 weeks between weeks 18 and 52, and every 4 weeks thereafter. Continue monitoring for 4 weeks after stopping treatment or until haematological recovery has occurred.	If WBC 3000–3500/mm^3 or absolute neutrophil count (ANC) 1500–2000/mm3	Continue clozapine, sample blood twice weekly until WBC and differential counts stabilize or increase
		If WBC <3000/mm^3 or ANC <1500/mm^3	Immediately stop clozapine, sample blood daily until haematological abnormality is resolved, monitor for symptoms suggestive of infection. If WBC <2000/mm^3 or ANC <1000/mm^3 management should be guided by a haematologist. Consider protective isolation, culture and antibiotics depending on clinical state and blood results. Re-starting clozapine is contraindicated.
Other antipsychotics	Not needed		
Lithium	Not needed		
Carbamazepine	WBC count very 2 weeks for the first 2 months, thereafter, at least every 3–6 months	If WBC or platelet counts decreased, close monitoring is needed; If WBC count >3000/mm^3 and ANC <1500/mm^3, and mild asymptomatic thrombocytopenia, dose reduction or discontinuation	
Valproic acid	Platelet counts at least every 6 months; close monitoring is needed in elderly	If platelet count between 50-100,000/mm^3 monitor more closely and check bleeding time. If platelet count falls below 50,000/mm^3, discontinue valproate and monitor	
Mianserin	FBC is recommended every 4 weeks during the first 3 months of treatment with subsequent clinical monitoring for symptoms that may indicate neutropenia		
Other tricyclic antidepressants	Not needed		
SSRIs and clomipramine	Not needed; in a cardiovascular-diseased patient who is anticoagulated, checking prothrombin time and bleeding time before any surgical procedure is recommended.		

Table 12.1 (continued) Monitoring for blood dyscrasias (continued)

Drugs	Recommended monitoring	Monitoring if abnormal blood cell counts
Mirtazapine	Routine FBC monitoring not recommended but patients should be advised to report fever, sore throat, stomatitis or other signs of infection at which point FBC should be obtained	
Benzodiazepines	Not needed	

(*British National Formulary* 2003). Similar, though more frequent monitoring is required in the United States. Currently, monitoring is required for as long as the patient is treated with clozapine. Monitoring should be continued for 1 month after discontinuation.

Decreasing the dose may be helpful when valproate-associate blood dyscrasia, especially thrombocyopenia (Conley *et al.* 2001) or prolonged bleeding time in patients with SSRIs occurs. Platelet count estimation every 6 months is recommended in patients taking valproate.

In order to prevent drug-induced blood dyscrasia, careful evaluation before starting drugs, close monitoring of laboratory tests, and encouragement of patients and their families to report any sign of blood dyscrasia are very important. Recommended FBC monitoring for early detection and prevention of progression of blood dyscrasias is summarized in Table 12.1.

Summary: Blood dyscrasia

Definition	Neutropenia: neutrophil count <1500 cells/mm^3
	Agranulocytosis: neutrophil count <500 cells/mm^3
	Eosinophilia: eosinophil count >500 cells/mm^3
	Thrombocytopenia: platelet count <100,000 cells/mm^3
Incidence	Clozapine-induced agranolocytosis and neutropenia, 0.8% and 2.9%, respectively; carbamazepine-induced leucopenia, 2–14%; valproate-induced thrombocytopenia, 12%
Drugs causing syndrome	Clozapine, chlorpromazine, carbamazepine, valproic acid. Blood dyscrasias can occur with many non-psychiatric drugs e.g. chloramphenicol and aplastic anaemia.
Key symptoms	Depends on nature of dyscrasia. Neutropenia and agranulocytosis manifest with increased susceptibility to

infection. Thrombocytopenia manifests with bleeding, petechiae and purpura. If RBC count is low, for example in aplastic anaemia, there will be symptoms of anaemia such as tiredness and dyspnoea. Presentation of eosinophilia varies according to organs involved.

Pharmacological mechanism	Direct cytotoxicity or immune-mediated mechanism, by the drug itself or its metabolites.
Investigations to confirm diagnosis	FBC with differential count, platelet count, bleeding time, and bone marrow examination if necessary.
Management	Stop causal drugs and consult hematologist. With agranulocytosis and aplastic anaemia considered isolation, antibiotics, colony stimulating factor (agranulocytosis and aplastic anaemia) and transfusion.
Further reading	Oyesanmi O, Kunkel EJ, Monti DA, *et al.* (1999) Hematologic side effects of psychotropics, *Psychosomatics*, **40**, 414–21.
	Skop BP and Brown TM (1996) Potential vascular and bleeding complications of treatment with selective serotonin reuptake inhibitors, *Psychosomatics*, **37**, 12–16.
	Tohen M, Castillo J, Baldessarini RJ, *et al.* (1995) Blood dyscrasias with carbamazepine and valproate: a pharmacoepidemiological study of 2,228 patients at risk, *Am J Psychiatry*, **152**, 413–18.

References

Alvir JM and Lieberman JA (1994). Agranulocytosis: incidence and risk factors. *J Clin Psychiatry*, **55** (Suppl. B), 137–8.

Alvir JM, Lieberman JA, Safferman AZ, *et al.* (1993). Clozapine-induced agranulocytosis. Incidence and risk factors in the United States. *New Engl J Med*, **329**, 162–7.

Amar A, Segman RH, Shtrussberg S, *et al.* (1998). An association between clozapine-induced agranulocytosis in schizophrenics and HLA-DQB1*0201. *Int J Neuropsychopharmcology*, **1**, 41–4.

American Psychiatric Association (2002). Practice guideline for the treatment of patients with bipolar disorder (revision). *Am J Psychiatry*, **159** (Suppl. 4), 1–50.

Andres E, Kurtz JE, and Maloisel F (2002). Nonchemotherapy drug-induced agranulocytosis: experience of the Strasbourg teaching hospital (1985–2000). and review of the literature. *Clin Lab Haematol*, **24**, 99–106.

Assion HJ, Kolbinger HM, Rao ML, *et al.* (1996). Lymphocytopenia and thrombocytopenia during treatment with risperidone or clozapine. *Pharmacopsychiatry*, **29**, 227–8.

Atkin K, Kendall F, Gould D, *et al.* (1996). Neutropenia and agranulocytosis in patients receiving clozapine in the UK and Ireland. *Br J Psychiatry*, **169**, 483–8.

Bak S, Tsiropoulos I, Kjaersgaard JO, *et al.* (2002). Selective serotonin reuptake inhibitors and the risk of stroke: a population-based case-control study. *Stroke*, **33**, 1465–73.

Ballenger JC (1988). The clinical use of carbamazepine in affective disorders. *J Clin Psychiatry*, **49** (Suppl.), 13–21.

Ballin A, Lehman D, Sirota P, *et al.* (1998). Increased number of peripheral blood CD34+ cells in lithium-treated patients. *Br J Haematol*, **100**, 219–21.

Balon R and Berchou R (1986). Hematologic side effects of psychotropic drugs. *Psychosomatics*, **27**, 119–27.

Banov MD, Tohen M, and Friedberg J (1993). High risk of eosinophilia in women treated with clozapine. *J Clin Psychiatry*, **54**, 466–9.

Beliles K and Stoudemire A (1998). Psychopharmacologic treatment of depression in the medically ill. *Psychosomatics*, **39**, S2–19.

Bogunovic O and Viswanathan R (2000). Thrombocytopenia possibly associated with olanzapine and subsequently with benztropine mesylate. *Psychosomatics*, **41**, 277–8.

Braunwald E, Fauci AS, Hauser SL, *et al.* (2001). *Harrison's Principles of Internal Medicine*, 15th edn. McGraw-Hill: New York. Appendix A.

British National Formulary (2003). British Medical Association and Royal Pharmaceutical Society of Great Britain. Pharmaceutical Press: London.

Chatterton R (1997). Eosinophilia after commencement of clozapine treatment. *Aust N Z J Psychiatry*, **31**, 874–6.

Chengappa KN, Gopalani A, Haught MK, *et al.* (1996). The treatment of clozapine-associated agranulocytosis with granulocyte colony-stimulating factor (G-CSF). *Psychopharmacol Bull*, **32**, 111–21.

Conley EL, Coley KC, Pollock BG, *et al.* (2001). Prevalence and risk of thrombocytopenia with valproic acid: experience at a psychiatric teaching hospital. *Pharmacotherapy*, **21**, 1325–30.

Corzo D, Yunis JJ, Salazar M, *et al.* (1995). The major histocampatibility complex region marked by HSP70–1 and HSP70–2 variants is associated with clozapine-induced agranulocytosis in two different ethnic groups. *Blood*, **86**, 3835–40.

Covanis A, Gupta AK, and Jeavons PM (1982). Sodium valproate: monotherapy and polytherapy. *Epilepsia*, **23**, 693–720.

Damiani JT and Christensen RC (2000). Lamotrigine-associated neutropenia in a geriatric patient. *Am J Geriatr Psychiatry*, **8**, 346.

De Abajo FJ, García Rodríguez LA, and Montero D (1999). Association between selective serotonin reuptake inhibitors and upper gastrointestinal bleeding: population based case-control study. *BMJ*, **319**, 1106–9.

Deliliers GL (2000). Blood dyscrasia in clozapine-treated patients in Italy. *Hematologica*, **85**, 233–7.

Dernovsek Z and Tavcar R (1997). Risperidone-induced leucopenia and neutropenia. *Br J Psychiatry*, **171**, 393–4.

Dettling M, Cascorbi I, Roots I, *et al.* (2001). Genetic determinants of clozapine-induced agranulocytosis: recent results of HLA subtyping in a non-Jewish Caucasian sample. *Arch Gen Psychiatry*, **58**, 93–4.

Finkel B, Lerner A, Oyffe I, *et al.* (1998*a*). Olanzapine treatment in patients with typical and atypical neuroleptic-associated agranulocytosis. *Int Clin Psychopharmacol*, **13**, 133–5.

Finkel B, Lerner AG, Oyffe I, *et al.* (1998*b*). Risperidone-associated agranulocytosis. *Am J Psychiatry*, **155**, 855–6.

Fleisch MC, Blauer F, Gubler JG, *et al.* (2000). Eosinophilic pneumonia and respiratory failure associated with venlafaxine treatment. *Eur Respir, J* **15**, 205–8.

Flynn SW, Altman S, MacEwan GW, *et al.* (1997). Prolongation of clozapine-induced granulocytopenia associated with olanzapine. *J Clin Psychopharmacol*, **17**, 494–5.

Galletly C, Wilson D, and McEwen S (1996). Eosinophilia associated with decreasing neutrophil count in a clozapine-treated patient (letter). *J Clin Psychiatry*, **57**, 40–1.

Gallicchio VS and Chen MG (1982). Cell kinetics of lithium-induced granulopoiesis. *Cell Tissue Kinet*, **15**, 179–86.

Gerson SL (1993). Clozapine – deciphering risks (editorial). *New Engl J Med*, **329**, 204–5.

Gerson SL (1994). G-CSF and the management of clozapine-induced agranulocytosis. *J Clin Psychiatry*, **55** (Suppl. B), 139–42.

Gerson SL, Arce C, and Meltzer HY (1994). N-desmethylclozapine: a clozapine metabolite that suppresses haemopoiesis. *Br J Haematol*, **86**, 555–61.

Gerson SL and Meltzer HY (1992). Mechanisms of clozapine-induced agranulocytosis. *Drug Saf*, **7** (Suppl. 1), **17**–25.

Gidal B, Spencer N, Maly M, *et al.* (1994). Valproate-mediated disturbances of hemostasis: relations to dose and plasma concentration. *Neurology*, **44**, 1418–22.

Hampson ME (2000). Clozapine-induced thrombocytosis (letter). *Br J Psychiatry*, **176**, 400.

Handin RI (2001). Bleeding and thrombosis. In *Harrison's Principles of Internal Medicine*, 15th edn, E Braunwald, AS Fauci, SL Hauser, DL Longo and JL Jameson (ed.), pp. 354–60. McGraw-Hill: New York.

Hanssler L and Roll C (1994). Increased thrombocyte count in newborn infants of drug-dependent mothers. *Klin Padiatr*, **206**, 55–8.

Harker WG, Rothstein G, Clarkson D, *et al.* (1977). Enhancement of colony-stimulating activity production by lithium. *Blood*, **49**, 263–7.

Hartmann PM (1999). Mirtazapine: a newer antidepressant. *Am Fam Physician*, **59**, 159–61.

Hergovich N, Aigner M, Eichler HG, *et al.* (2000). Paroxetine decreases platelet serotonin storage and platelet function in human beings. *Clin Pharmacol Ther*, **68**, 435–42.

Holland SM and Gallin JI (2001). Disorders of granulocytes and monocytes. In *Harrison's Principles of Internal Medicine*, E Braunwald, AS Fauci, SL Hauser, *et al.* (ed.), 15th edn, pp. 366–74. McGraw-Hill: New York.

Honigfeld G, Arellano F, Sethi J, *et al.* (1998). Reducing clozapine-related morbidity and mortality: 5 years of experience with the Clozaril National Registry. *J Clin Psychiatry*, **59** (Suppl. 3), 3–7.

Idanpaan-Heikkila J, Alhava E, Olkinuora M, *et al.* (1977). Agranulocytosis during treatment with chlozapine. *Eur J Clin Pharmacol*, **11**, 193–8.

Kaufman KR and Gerner R (1998). Dose-dependent valproic acid thrombocytopenia in bipolar disorder. *Ann Clin Psychiatry*, **10**, 35–7.

Konakanchi R, Grace JJ, Szarowicz R, *et al.* (2000). Olanzapine prolongation of granulocytopenia after clozapine discontinuation. *J Clin Psychopharmacol*, **20**, 703–4.

Kramlinger KG and Post RM (1990). Addition of lithium carbonate to carbamazepine: hematological and thyroid effects. *Am J Psychiatry*, **147**, 615–20.

Lake MB, Birmaher B, Wassick S, *et al.* (2000). Bleeding and selective serotonin reuptake inhibitors in childhood and adolescence. *J Child Adolesc Psychopharmacol*, **10**, 35–8.

Lucht MJ and Rietschel M (1998). Clozapine-induced eosinophilia: subsequent neutrope-nia and corresponding allergic mechanisms. *J Clin Psychiatry*, **59**, 195–7.

Mackay FJ, Wilton LV, Pearce GL, *et al.* (1997). Safety of long-term lamotrigine in epilepsy. *Epilepsia*, **38**, 881–6.

Malesker MA, Soori GS, Malone PM, *et al.* (1995). Eosinophilia associated with bupropion. *Ann Pharmacother*, **29**, 867–9.

Mathias S, Schaaf LW, and Sonntag A (2002). Eosinophilia associated with olanzapine. *J Clin Psychiatry*, **63**, 246–7.

Neophytides AN, Nutt JG, and Lodish JR (1979). Thrombocytopenia associated with sodi-um valproate treatment. *Ann Neurol*, **5**, 389–90.

Nolan L and O'Malley K (1989). Adverse drug reactions in the elderly. *Br J Hosp Med*, **41**, 446, 448, 452–7.

Oyesanmi O, Kunkel EJ, Monti DA, *et al.* (1999). Hematologic side effects of psychotropics. *Psychosomatics*, **40**, 414–21.

Oyewumi LK and Al-Semaan Y (2000). Olanzapine: safe during clozapine-induced agranulocytosis. *J Clin Psychopharmacol*, **20**, 279–81.

Pisciotta AV (1992). Hematologic reactions associated with psychotropic drugs. In *The Adverse Effects of Psychotropic Drugs*, JH Kane and JA Lieberman (ed.), pp. 376–94. The Guilford Press: New York.

Post RM (1990). Non-lithium treatment for bipolar disorder. *J Clin Psychiatry*, **518** (Suppl.), 9–16.

Ruhe HG, Becker HE, Jessurun P, *et al.* (2001). Agranulocytosis and granulocytopenia associated with quetiapine. *Acta Psychiatr Scand*, **104**, 311–13.

Skop BP and Brown TM (1996). Potential vascular and bleeding complications of treat-ment with selective serotonin reuptake inhibitors. *Psychosomatics*, **37**, 12–16.

Sobotka JL, Alexander B, and Cook BL (1990). A review of carbamazepine's hematologic reactions and monitoring recommendations. *DICP*, **24**, 1214–19.

Solal-Céligny P (1994). Abnormal hematologic values. In *Adverse Drug Reactions: A Practical Guide to Diagnosis and Management*, C Bénichou (ed.), pp. 13–30. John Wiley & Sons: Chichester, England.

Solvason HB (2000). Agranulocytosis associated with lamotrigine. *Am J Psychiatry*, **157**, 1704.

Swartz JR, Ananth J, Smith MW, *et al.* (1999). Olanzapine treatment after clozapine-induced granulocytopenia in three patients. *J Clin Psychiatry*, **60**, 119–21.

Tohen M, Castillo J, Baldessarini RJ, *et al.* (1995). Blood dyscrasias with carbamazepine and valproate: a pharmacoepidemiological study of 2,228 patients at risk. *Am J Psychiatry*, **152**, 413–18.

Tolosa-Vilella C, Ruiz-Ripoll A, *et al.* (2002). Olanzapine-induced agranulocytosis: a case report and review of the literature. *Prog Neuropsychopharmacol Biol Psychiatry*, **26**, 411–14.

Trannel TJ, Ahmed I, and Goebert D (2001). Occurrence of thrombocytopenia in psychi-atric patients taking valproate. *Am J Psychiatry*, **158**, 128–30.

Turbay D, Lieberman JA, Alper CA, *et al.* (1997). Tumor necrosis factor constellation poly-morphism and clozapine-induced agranulocytosis in two different ethnic groups. *Blood*, **89**, 4167–74.

Umbricht D and Kane JM (1996). Medical complications of new antipsychotic drugs. *Schizophr Bull*, **22**, 475–83.

van Walraven C, Mamdani MM, Wells PS, *et al.* (2001). Inhibition of serotonin reuptake by antidepressants and upper gastrointestinal bleeding in elderly patients: retrospective cohort study. *BMJ*, **323**, 655–8.

Willert C, Englisch S, Schlesinger S, *et al.* (1999). Possible drug-induced thrombocytopenia secondary to tiagabine. *Neurology*, **52**, 889.

Williams WJ (1995). Secondary thrombocytosis. In *Williams Hematology*, E Beutler, MA Lichtman, BS Coller, *et al.* (ed.), pp. 1361–3. McGraw-Hill: New York.

Williams DP, Pirmohamed M, Naisbitt DJ, *et al.* (2000). Induction of metabolism-dependent and -independent neutrophil apoptosis by clozapine. *Mol Pharmacol*, **58**, 207–16.

Young NS (2002). Acquired aplastic anaemia. *Ann Intern Med*, **136**, 534–46.

Yunis JJ, Corzo D, Salazar M, *et al.* (1995). HLA associations in clozapine-induced agranulocytosis. *Blood*, **86**, 1177–83.

Chapter 13

Benzodiazepine dependence

Heather Ashton

Recognition

Seldom has a single group of drugs held such therapeutic promise as the benzodiazepines. Their wide range of actions – hypnotic, anxiolytic, anticonvulsant, and muscle relaxant – combined with their low toxicity and alleged lack of dependence potential seemed to make them the ideal 'wonder drugs' for many common conditions affecting millions of people worldwide. These apparent characteristics conferred on benzodiazepines major advantages over their predecessors, mainly barbiturates, which were often lethal in overdose, highly addictive and frequently abused. Thus the benzodiazepines soon replaced barbiturates, as well as their immediate successors (meprobamate, glutethamide, methaqualone and others). Diazepam, just one of the eleven available benzodiazepines at that time, became in the 1970s 'the most widely prescribed of all drugs ever' (Lader 1988).

How the dependence potential of benzodiazepines was overlooked when it was clear that they could replace barbiturates and similarly acting drugs is a matter for amazement and casts shame on the medical profession which claims to be scientifically based. Cross-tolerance between different drugs, for instance between barbiturates and alcohol, was well understood at the time and clearly implied that if one drug could replace another it must have common characteristics and usually a common mode of action. This similarity between benzodiazepines and barbiturates was ignored and doctors were urged in a campaign by the UK medical profession in the 1970s to prescribe benzodiazepines instead of barbiturates (Lader 1993). They complied with such zeal that benzodiazepines, believed to be harmless, were prescribed long term, often for many years, for anxiety, depression, insomnia and ordinary life stresses. By 1979 benzodiazepine prescriptions reached nearly 31 million a year in the UK (usually for a month's supply) for a population of 55 million people (Wells 1993). Expectations by patients and advertisements by drug companies (Medawar 1997) no doubt contributed to the high level of prescriptions.

Then came the backlash. In the early 1980s long-term prescribed benzodiazepine-users themselves realized that over time the drugs lost their efficacy and were associated with adverse effects. In particular, patients found it difficult to stop taking benzodiazepines because of withdrawal effects (Ashton 1984, 1987) and the patients themselves complained that they had become 'addicted'. Controlled clinical trials of such patients (Hallstrom and Lader 1981; Petursson and Lader 1981, 1984; Tyrer *et al.* 1981) demonstrated beyond doubt that withdrawal symptoms from regular 'therapeutic' doses of benzodiazepines were real and that they indicated dependence on the drugs rather than a re-emergence of a pre-existing psychiatric state.

Clinical features

Changing definitions of drug dependence

That benzodiazepines could cause physical and psychological dependence was accepted by the medical profession on the grounds that a withdrawal syndrome occurred on cessation of regular use of high or therapeutic doses, and doctors were advised to reserve them for short-term use in minimal dosage (CSM 1988; Royal College of Psychiatrists 1988). However, definitions of drug dependence have shifted. Until fairly recently, dependence was defined in terms of a drug being associated with tolerance and withdrawal symptoms. However in current classification systems, both ICD-10 and DSM-IV, these two features are no longer regarded as mandatory for a diagnosis of dependence and instead the diagnostic criteria rely heavily on behavioural features associated with drug use. For this reason it is claimed that antidepressants are not addictive, despite the fact that they cause withdrawal reactions (Young and Haddad 2000; Medawar 1997) and the euphemism 'discontinuation reaction' is suggested instead (Haddad *et al.* 1998). Thus the presence of a withdrawal reaction alone is no longer considered sufficient for a diagnosis of drug dependence.

Present criteria for substance dependence (American Psychiatric Association 1994) are shown in Table 13.1. Benzodiazepines meet all these criteria including tolerance, escalation of dosage, continued use despite efforts to stop and knowledge of adverse effects and a withdrawal syndrome. Indeed, it is claimed that 'many long-term benzodiazepine users develop a classic drug-dependence syndrome' (Griffiths and Weerts 1997).

Tolerance

Pharmacodynamic tolerance to benzodiazepines develops at different rates and to different degrees for the various actions. Tolerance to the hypnotic

Table 13.1 Criteria for substance dependence*

A maladaptive pattern of substance use, leading to clinically significant impairment or distress, as manifested by three or more of the following, occurring at any time in the same 12-month period.

Tolerance, as defined by either:
- a need for markedly increased amounts of the substance to achieve the clinical effect.
- markedly diminished effect with continued use of the same amount of the substance.

Withdrawal as manifested by either:
- the characteristic withdrawal syndrome for the substance.
- the same or similar substance is taken to avoid withdrawal symptoms.

The substance is taken in larger amounts or over a longer period than was intended.
There is a persistent desire or unsuccessful attempts to cut down or control substance use.
Time is spent is activities necessary to obtain the substance (e.g. visiting multiple doctors).
Important activities are given up or reduced because of substance use.
The substance use is continued despite knowledge of having a problem caused or exacerbated by the substance.

* Abridged from American Psychiatric Association (1994) *Diagnostic and Statistical Manual of Mental Disorders*, 4th edn, DSM-IV. Washington, DC: APA.

effects develops rapidly, within a few days or weeks of regular use, during which sleep profiles tend to return to pretreatment levels (Petursson and Lader 1984; Kales *et al.* 1978, 1988). Although many poor sleepers report continued efficacy of benzodiazepine hypnotics (Oswald *et al.* 1982), possibly because they prevent rebound insomnia, clinical experience shows that a considerable proportion of hypnotic users increase their dosage, sometimes to above recommended doses.

Tolerance to the anxiolytic effect of benzodiazepines develops more slowly. Such tolerance has been clearly shown in rats after 21 days, but not 5 days, of treatment with chlordiazepoxide (File and Baldwin 1989). In man there is little evidence that benzodiazepines retain their anxiolytic efficacy after four months of regular treatment (Tyrer 1987) and clinical observations show that long-term benzodiazepine use does little to control, and may even aggravate, anxiety (Ashton 1987). There is also evidence of dosage escalation in anxiolytic benzodiazepine users (Ashton 1984): in one clinical study over 25 per cent of the patients were taking two benzodiazepines, the second having been added to the prescription when the first ceased to be effective (Ashton 1987). Although some authors consider long-term use of benzodiazepine anxiolytics appropriate for certain patients (Hollister *et al.* 1993; Schweizer *et al.* 1993), it is likely that the drugs are preventing rebound anxiety or withdrawal symptoms, rather than reducing anxiety (Griffiths and Weerts 1997).

Tolerance to the anticonvulsant effects of benzodiazepines occurs within a few weeks of regular use in a high proportion of patients (Brodie 1990) and also to the muscle relaxant effects when used in spastic disorders (Ashton 1994). Tolerance to electroencephalographic effects and to benzodiazepine suppression of growth hormone response has also been demonstrated in man (Murphy and Tyrer 1988).

However, complete tolerance to the amnesic effects and other cognitive impairments caused by benzodiazepines does not appear to develop, even after years of chronic use. Many studies of long-term benzodiazepine users have shown deficits in learning, memory, attention and visuospatial ability (Golombok et al. 1988; Lucki and Rickels 1988; Curran 1991, 1992; Tata et al. 1994; Gorenstein et al. 1995; Tonne et al. 1995). These effects are most marked in the elderly in whom they may suggest dementia (Lader 1992). Improvement occurs when benzodiazepines are stopped (Salzman et al. 1992) although it may be slow and perhaps incomplete (Tata et al. 1994).

Withdrawal syndrome

The existence of a benzodiazepine withdrawal syndrome has been abundantly demonstrated and described (Busto et al. 1986; Murphy et al. 1984; Owen and Tyrer 1983; Petursson and Lader 1981, 1984; Tyrer et al. 1981, 1983; Hallstrom and Lader 1981; Ashton 1991, 1994). Symptoms include many that are common to anxiety states in general and some more characteristic of benzodiazepine withdrawal (Table 13.2). The syndrome can be mild and short-lived or severe and sometimes protracted (Ashton 1991, 1995a,b; Tyrer 1991). Severity is often associated with prolonged or high dose use, potent benzodiazepines, and certain personality types (Tyrer et al. 1983; Murphy and Tyrer 1991; Ashton and Golding 1989). The reported incidence varies between 30–100 per cent in different reports but many long-term users decline to participate in, or drop out from, withdrawal studies (Ashton 1991). Withdrawal symptoms prolong benzodiazepine use, which often continues for years after the initial reason for taking benzodiazepines has passed. Many long-term users, aware that the drugs are no longer effective or are causing adverse effects, have tried to stop or reduce dosage but have been unsuccessful because of the emergence of withdrawal symptoms (Ashton 1987; Maletzky and Klotter 1976).

Benzodiazepine-dependent populations

In the world population of benzodiazepine users three overlapping types of dependence can be observed:

1 **Therapeutic dose dependence** This population is the largest at present and is composed of long-term users who have inadvertently become dependent

Table 13.2 Some common benzodiazepine withdrawal symptoms

Symptoms common to all anxiety states	Symptoms less common in anxiety states; relatively specific to benzodiazepine withdrawal*
Anxiety, panic attacks, agoraphobia	Perceptual disturbances, sense of movement Depersonalization, derealization
Insomnia, nightmares	Hallucinations (visual, auditory)
Depression, dysphoria	Distortion of body image
Excitability, restlessness	Tingling, numbness, altered sensation
Poor memory and concentration	Formication
Dizziness, light headedness	Sensory hypersensitivity (light, sound, taste, smell)
Weakness 'jelly legs'	Muscle twitches, jerks, fasiculation
Tremor	Tinnitus
Muscle pain, stiffness	Psychotic symptoms**
Sweating, night sweats	Confusion, delirium**
Palpitations	Convulsions**
Blurred or double vision	

* References: Busto *et al*. (1986); Murphy *et al*. (1984); Petursson and Lader (1981); Tyrer *et al*. (1981, 1983, 1990); Ashton (1991, 1995*b*).

** Usually only on rapid or abrupt withdrawal from high doses of benzodiazepines.

on benzodiazepines prescribed by their doctors over months or years. The number of these patients who are dependent is unknown but estimates suggest that there are about one million long-term benzodiazepine users in the UK (Ashton and Golding 1989; Taylor 1987) and recent surveys indicate that there are over 180 patients in every UK general practice who have taken benzodiazepines for 6 months or more (Heather *et al*. 2004), while in the US around 4 million people (2 per cent of the adult population) appear to have been prescribed benzodiazepines regularly for 5–10 years or more (Woods *et al*. 1992). It is likely that at least 50 per cent of these users are dependent. A considerable proportion of such patients are elderly females taking benzodiazepine hypnotics (Heather *et al*. 2004; Taylor 1987) and it is noteworthy that prescriptions for benzodiazepine hypnotics have not declined despite a reduction in prescriptions for benzodiazepine anxiolytics (Chaplin 1988). Other long-term users include patients with physical and psychiatric problems (Ashton and Golding 1989; Taylor 1987; Heather *et al*. 2004).

2 **Prescribed high dose dependence** A minority of patients who start on prescribed benzodiazepines often unintentionally begin to 'require' higher

and higher doses. At first they may persuade their doctors to escalate the pre-scription doses, but on reaching the prescriber's limits, may contact several doctors or hospital departments to obtain further supplies which they then self-prescribe. Sometimes this group combines benzodiazepine misuse with excessive alcohol consumption. Patients in this group tend to be highly anx-ious, depressed and may have psychiatric or personality disorders (Woods *et al.* 1998). They may have a history of other sedative or alcohol misuse. They do not typically use illicit drugs but may resort to 'street' benzodiazepines if other sources fail (Ashton 1997).

3 **Recreational benzodiazepine abuse** Recreational abuse of benzodi-azepines is a growing problem (*Drug and Therapeutics Bulletin* 1997; Griffiths and Weerts 1997). The true prevalence is not known but benzodiazepines commonly form part of a polysubstance abuse pattern. They are taken by at least half of opiate, amphetamine and cocaine users worldwide (Shaw *et al.* 1994; Strang *et al.* 1993, 1994) and are said to be the single most misused category of drug in Scotland (Robertson and Ronald 1992; Ruben and Morrison 1992). Benzodiazepine abuse is also common in alcoholics (Borg *et al.* 1993) and some people use benzodiazepines as their primary recreational drug, bingeing intermittently on high doses or injecting intravenously (Strang *et al.* 1993). Reasons given for taking benzodiazepines in this context are that they enhance the 'high' obtained from illicit drugs, alleviate withdrawal effects from illicit drugs and alcohol, and also produce a 'kick' when taken alone in high doses (especially when injected intravenously) or with alcohol. Many illicit users of benzodiazepines become dependent and show typical withdrawal symptoms which can be severe (Seivewright and Dougal 1993; Seivewright 1998; Stark *et al.* 1987; Scott 1990; Busto and Sellers 1991).

Pharmacological basis

Reinforcement

There is no doubt that benzodiazepines, like other drugs of dependence, can have rewarding or reinforcing effects. Griffiths and Weerts (1997) argue that reinforcement is the major mechanism underlying both chronic long-term use and recreational abuse of benzodiazepines. Reinforcement may be posi-tive, e.g. 'to make one feel good' or negative e.g. 'to reduce tension'. These authors review 26 studies showing reinforcing effects of benzodiazepines in man. In such investigations, the general method is to allow free access to ben-zodiazepines or placebo under various conditions, sometimes requiring some action by the subject, such as riding an exercize bicycle, to obtain the drug.

Reinforcing effects are judged by the likelihood of choice of active drug over placebo or, in some studies, by 'liking scores' of drug compared to placebo or other drugs (Warburton 1988). Reinforcing effects of various benzodiazepines (diazepam, lorazepam, triazolam, alprazolam, flurazepam) were clearly apparent in subjects with histories of drug or alcohol abuse, moderate social alcohol drinkers without alcohol problems, anxious subjects, insomniac subjects and patients undergoing abrupt benzodiazepine withdrawal (Griffiths and Weerts 1997; Warburton 1988; Ashton 1997). In general 'normal' subjects did not prefer benzodiazepines, in keeping with previous observations that certain personality types are most vulnerable (Tyrer 1987; Ashton 1989). On the whole, recreational abusers prefer high doses while therapeutic dose users and anxious subjects prefer low doses of benzodiazepines.

A wealth of laboratory data reviewed by Griffiths and Weerts (1997) shows that benzodiazepines are also reinforcing in rodents and non-human primates and that these animals will, under certain conditions, self-administer the drugs by intravenous, intragastric or oral routes.

Nearly all reinforcing drugs (cocaine, amphetamine, nicotine, alcohol, opioids, cannabis, ecstasy and others) induce dopamine release in the limbic system (nucleus accumbens and/or prefrontal cortex) (Nutt 1996) and it has been argued that dopaminergic activation in these rewarding areas is the final common pathway for all addictive drugs (Di Chiara and Imperato 1988; Wise and Bozarth 1987), although other transmitters are probably also involved (Koob 1992). Benzodiazepines appear to be an exception since in low to moderate doses they do not stimulate dopamine release (Nutt 1996) and GABA-ergic activation actually decreases dopamine release (Haefely *et al.* 1981). However, it seems likely that high doses of benzodiazepines, sufficient to produce a 'kick', do in fact act like other rewarding drugs, producing positive reinforcement (Strang *et al.* 1993). It is noteworthy that recreational benzodiazepine abusers take doses many times greater than therapeutic users, in the range 100–500 mg diazepam or equivalent, often by intravenous injection (Robertson and Ronald 1992; Cole and Chiarello 1990; Ruben and Morrison 1992; Farrell and Strang 1988). In contrast, low doses of benzodiazepines provide negative reinforcement and act essentially as 'depunishing' drugs (Ashton 1989) presumably by decreasing cholinergic and monoaminergic activity in brain 'punishment systems' (Ashton 1992, 2002).

Tolerance and withdrawal effects

The mechanisms underlying tolerance and withdrawal are still not understood. The basic mode of action of benzodiazepines is to enhance central GABA activity by interaction with specific receptor sites on the $GABA_A$ receptor complex. However, the discovery of multiple subtypes of the $GABA_A$ receptor has added considerable complexity to attempts to unravel the possible changes caused by chronic benzodiazepine administration. For example, $GABA_A$ receptors may contain different combinations of at least 18 subunits (including $\alpha 1$–6, $\beta 1$–3, $\gamma 1$–3 and others) (Rudolph *et al.* 2001). Different receptor assemblies have different brain distributions and different affinities for agents that act on them (Bateson 2002). At present it appears from gene 'knockout' experiments in mice, that α_2-containing subtypes mediate anxiolytic effects of benzodiazepines; α_1-containing subtypes mediate sedative and amnesic effects, and α_1-containing, as well as other subtypes, mediate anticonvulsant effects (Rudolph *et al.* 2001).

Early suggestions that benzodiazepine tolerance is due to decreased density (down-regulation) of GABA/benzodiazepine receptors, as measured by diazepam binding studies (e.g. Chiu and Rosenberg 1978; Rosenberg and Chiu 1979), have not been supported by later work (e.g. Preziosa and Neale 1983; Nutt 1986).

Recent research on the subject is reviewed by Bateson (2002) who examines three proposed mechanisms: uncoupling of the linkage between $GABA_A$ and benzodiazepine sites, changes in receptor subtype turnover, and changes in receptor gene expression. Uncoupling and turnover changes have been demonstrated in animals both in *in vitro* and *in vivo* but occur too rapidly (within hours of a single dose) to be the direct cause of the slow development and resolution of tolerance. Changes in gene expression have also been shown to occur after chronic benzodiazepine administration in rodents and provide a longer-lasting response. Bateson (2002) proposes that chronic benzodiazepine administration sets in train a chain of events in which uncoupling leads to preferential degradation of certain $GABA_A$ receptor subunits which become internalized and in turn provide a signal for changes in gene transcription, resulting in a long-term response. The pathway could operate on different time scales depending on the receptor subtype and/or brain region involved and thus give rise to differing rates of development of tolerance to various benzodiazepine actions.

On this model, withdrawal of the benzodiazepine once tolerance has developed would expose the recipient to all the drug-induced alterations in GABA receptors, now no longer opposed by the presence of the drug. The result would be underactivity in the many domains of central function normally modulated by GABA-ergic mechanisms. Since GABA is a universal inhibitor of neural activity and decreases the release of many excitatory neurotransmitters (acetylcholine, noradrenaline, dopamine, serotonin, glutamate) (Haefely *et al.* 1981), there would be a surge in excitatory nervous activity. Increased release of dopamine, noradrenaline and serotonin has been demonstrated in certain areas of rat brain during benzodiazepine withdrawal (Rastogi *et al.* 1976; Hitchcott *et al.* 1990). Such increases, coupled perhaps with adaptive 'downstream' increases in sensitivity of excitatory receptors, may account for many benzodiazepine withdrawal symptoms shown in Table 13.2. The various changes in GABA receptors occurring during tolerance may be slow to reverse after drug withdrawal and may do so at different rates, possibly accounting for the variable time of emergence and duration of individual withdrawal symptoms and the prolonged, and sometimes protracted nature of benzodiazepine withdrawal (Ashton 1991, 1995*a*).

Management

Whatever the mechanisms, the treatment of benzodiazepine dependence remains a clinical problem and is often mismanaged. Long-term benzodiazepine use can give rise not only to dependence but also to many adverse effects including cognitive impairment, depression, increased risk of falls, fractures, traffic and other accidents especially in the elderly, drug interactions and the insidious development of increasing psychological and physical symptoms (Griffiths and Weerts 1997; Ashton 1987, 1995*a,b*). For this reason withdrawal is a desirable option for many long-term users. The management of withdrawal has been reviewed by many authors (Lader and Higgitt 1986; *The Lancet* 1987; Edwards *et al.* 1990; Livingston 1991; Lader 1991; Ashton 1994 and others). All agree that the cornerstones of a successful withdrawal strategy are gradual dosage reduction and psychological support.

Dosage reduction

Benzodiazepine dosage should be tapered gradually since abrupt withdrawal, especially from high doses, can precipitate convulsions, acute psychotic or confusional states, and panic attacks (Breier *et al.* 1984; Levy 1984; Noyes *et al.* 1986; Fyer *et al.* 1987). Even with slow dosage reduction, withdrawal symptoms may appear, and for this reason the rate of tapering should be individually adjusted according to the patient's needs, taking into account factors such as dosage and type of benzodiazepine, duration of use, reasons for prescription, lifestyle, personality, environmental stresses and amount of available support. Various authors suggest optimal times of between 6–8 weeks to a few months for the duration of withdrawal, but some patients may take a year or more (*British National Formulary* 2002; Ashton 1994), controlling their own reduction rate at whatever pace is tolerable. For most patients on therapeutic doses withdrawal is best carried out as an outpatient, allowing time for pharmacological and psychological adjustments to a benzodiazepine-free lifestyle within the patient's own environment.

There are advantages to conducting the actual withdrawal from diazepam because of its long elimination half-life, allowing a gradual fall in blood concentrations, and its availability in low dosage forms, permitting small dosage reductions (Table 13.3). There is clinical evidence that withdrawal is often more difficult from short-acting potent benzodiazepines, such as lorazepam and alprazolam (Murphy and Tyrer 1991; Ashton 1994). Conversion from other benzodiazepines to diazepam can be conducted in stages, allowing for equivalent potencies between different benzodiazepines (Table 13.3). Once converted to diazepam, the size of each reduction depends on the starting dose. *The British National Formulary* (2002) recommends withdrawal in steps of about one eighth (range one tenth to one quarter) of the daily dose every fortnight. In practice, reductions of 1 mg every 1–2 weeks are generally well tolerated from diazepam 20 mg, but when 5 mg is reached decrements of 0.5 mg at a time may be preferred. Further details of conversion and dosage reduction are discussed by Ashton (1994).

Table 13.3 Benzodiazepines: approximate equivalent doses and elimination half-lives

Benzodiazepine	Approximately equivalent dosage (mg)*	Elimination half-life(hrs) (active metabolite)	Available dosage forms in UK (caps/tablets)
Alprazolam	0.5	6–12	0.25, 0.5 mg
Chlordiazepoxide	25	5–30 (36–200)	5, 10, 25 mg
Clonazepam	0.5	18–50	0.5, 2 mg
Diazepam	10	20–100 (36–200)	2, 5, 10 mg (2.5, 5 mg/5 ml liquid)
Flunitrazepam	1	18–26 (36–200)	1 mg
Flurazepam	15–30	(40–250)	15, 30 mg
Loprazolam	1	6–12	1 mg
Lorazepam	1	10–20	1, 2.5 mg
Lormetazepam	1	10–12	0.5, 1 mg
Nitrazepam	10	15–38	5 mg (2.5 mg/5 ml liquid)
Oxazepam	20	4–15	10, 20, 30 mg
Temazepam	20	8–22	10, 15, 20, 30 mg (10 mg/5 ml liquid)

* Clinical potency for hypnotic or anxiolytic effects may vary between individuals; equivalent doses are approximate.

Adjuvant drugs

Various drugs have been tested for their ability to alleviate withdrawal symptoms. Since depression is common both during long-term benzodiazepine use and in withdrawal (Olajide and Lader 1984; Ashton 1987), antidepressant drugs seemed promising. However, both the tricyclic antidepressant dothiepin (Tyrer *et al.* 1996) and the SSRI paroxetine (Zitman and Couvee 2001) were found to be of limited value in placebo controlled trials and did not affect the outcome. Antidepressants may cause an initial exacerbation of anxiety and, if used, should be initiated in low doses (Ashton 1994).

Beta-blockers such as propranolol attenuate some benzodiazepine withdrawal symptoms such as palpitation and tremor but do not reduce subjective anxiety or improve the outcome of withdrawal (Tyrer *et al.* 1981; Abernethy *et al.* 1981; Cantopher *et al.* 1990). The α_2-adrenergic antagonist clonidine was reported to decrease symptom severity in two patients withdrawn from high benzodiazepine doses (Vinogradov *et al.* 1986; Keshaven and Crammer 1985) but not in three other patients withdrawn from more moderate doses (Goodman *et al.* 1986). Podhorna (2002) notes that blockade of noradrenergic neurotransmission with either β-antagonists or α_2 agonists appears to have little effect on anxiety as the predominant symptom of benzodiazepine withdrawal. It is worth noting that antidepressants, propranolol and clonidine are all themselves associated with withdrawal reactions when stopped, especially in anxious patients.

The anxiolytic drug buspirone proved ineffective in several studies of benzodiazepine withdrawal (Schweizer and Rickels 1986; Olajide and Lader 1987; Ashton *et al.* 1990). However, some anticonvulsant drugs with sedative effects may be beneficial in certain cases. In two small open case studies carbamazepine appeared to decrease the severity of, or even prevent withdrawal symptoms in patients on high doses of benzodiazepines, mainly alprazolam (1.5–10 mg daily), who were withdrawn rapidly (over about two weeks) (Ries *et al.* 1989; Klein *et al.* 1986). However, in a double-blind placebo-controlled study in which carbamazepine (200–800 mg daily) was administered for 2–4 weeks before benzodiazepine tapering to 40 patients on moderate therapeutic doses of benzodiazepines which were reduced gradually over five weeks, there were no significant differences from placebo in severity of withdrawal symptoms or outcome at 12 weeks post-withdrawal (Schweizer *et al.* 1991). Patients taking more than 20 mg diazepam equivalent appeared to derive benefit and it was suggested that carbamazepine may have some utility in patients withdrawing from high-dose benzodiazepines. It may also provide anticonvulsant cover for those with a history of epilepsy. Some authors still recommend barbiturate substitution for high dose benzodiazepine users or those with mixed benzodiazepine/alcohol dependence (American Task Force 1990; DuPont and Saylor 1991). The management of polydrug abusers taking benzodiazepines is discussed by Seivewright and Dougal (1993) and Seivewright et al. (1993). A relative newcomer in this field is the anticonvulsant gabapentin which has anxiolytic effects (Pande et al. 1999) and was reported to be effective in controlling anxiety in a patient withdrawing from high doses of alprazolam (12–15 mg/day) (Crockford et al. 2001).

Flumazenil, a competitive antagonist at certain GABA/benzodiazepine receptors (Bateson 2002), presents intriguing possibilities. This drug can precipitate withdrawal reactions when administered acutely to benzodiazepine-dependent animals or humans (Griffiths et al. 1993; Malizia and Nutt 1995; Bernik et al. 1998; Mintzer et al. 1999; Podhorna 2002). However, when administered during chronic benzodiazepine treatment to laboratory animals, it can prevent the development of tolerance. Acute treatment with flumazenil can also reverse some withdrawal effects in rats treated chronically with benzodiazepines (Malizia and Nutt 1995; Podhorna 2002; Baldwin et al. 1990; Gallager et al. 1986) and a few reports suggest that flumazenil can reduce some symptoms during withdrawal of benzodiazepines in benzodiazepine-tolerant patients (Gerra et al. 1996, 2002; Savic et al. 1991). Possible mechanisms for these actions, such as 'resetting' of benzodiazepine receptors by flumazenil, are discussed by Nutt (1990). Two small clinical studies have indicated that flumazenil can reverse or attenuate symptoms persisting after withdrawal in benzodiazepine-dependent patients (Saxon et al. 1997; Lader and Morton 1992). However, the utility of flumazenil in this context is limited by its short duration of action and the need to administer it intravenously. Other drugs acting as agonists at benzodiazepine receptors, such as zopiclone, zolpidem, zaleplon and alpidem, relieve benzodiazepine withdrawal effects but are not realistic treatments since they have many of the same disadvantages as benzodiazepines including tolerance, dependence, abuse and withdrawal effects. Other drugs tested in animal studies are reviewed by Podhorna (2002), but at present there is no ideal drug treatment for benzodiazepine withdrawal in man.

Psychological support

The degree of psychological support required during benzodiazepine withdrawal is variable. For many patients the need is minimal: a single letter from the general practitioner suggesting dosage reduction can be effective in many long-term benzodiazepine users (Heather et al. 2004). For others, the provision of a withdrawal schedule combined with simple encouragement is sufficient. For many patients, withdrawal symptoms, whether 'true' or 'pseudo' (Tyrer et al. 1983), are manifestations of anxiety and for some of these formal cognitive, behavioural or other therapies directed towards anxiety management are indicated. Support should be available not only during dosage reduction but for a prolonged period afterwards since patients remain vulnerable to stress and require time to develop drug-free stress-coping strategies (Tyrer 1991; Ashton 1991, 1994). Patients also require information about withdrawal symptoms and referral to support organizations is often helpful.

Outcome of benzodiazepine withdrawal

With carefully managed withdrawal in motivated patients the success rate for stopping benzodiazepines is high (80–90 per cent) and the relapse rate after 1–5 years is low, perhaps 20 per cent (Ashton 1994). Successful withdrawal is not affected by duration of use, type or dosage of benzodiazepine, severity of symptoms, psychiatric history or the presence of personality disorder or difficulty (Golombok et al. 1987; Ashton 1987; Ashton et al. 1990; Murphy and Tyrer 1991). Mental and physical health improves after withdrawal in most long-term prescribed benzodiazepine users (Ashton 1987; Heather et al. 2004) and there is no evidence of increased alcohol use or psychiatric morbidity.

Risk factors and prevention

The use of higher doses of benzodiazepines and longer courses are both more likely to lead to tolerance and dependence occurring. Patients with personality disorders within the anxious–fearful group (dependent, avoidant, anankastic) tend to develop more severe withdrawal symptoms on benzodiazepine discontinuation than those of normal personality or other personality disorders (Murphy and Tyrer 1991).

Clearly, prevention of benzodiazepine dependence would save a great deal of patient suffering, physicians' and medical workers' time and costs to the national drug bill. Prevention can be achieved by adherence to the advice of the Committee on Safety of Medicines (1988) and Royal College of Psychiatrists (1988) to limit benzodiazepine prescriptions to short-term use (2–4 weeks maximum) or as intermittent brief courses or occasional doses (Ashton 1994). When used short-term, benzodiazepines can have great therapeutic value and dependence is not a problem. Particular care is needed in prescribing benzodiazepines to vulnerable patients such as those with a history of alcohol or drug abuse or 'dependent' personalities (Tyrer 1989a). Stahl (2002) points out that benzodiazepines are still the leading treatments for anxiety and mood disorders and they are often initially helpful, but long-term treatment is more appropriate with antidepressants and/or psychological interventions (Tyrer 1989b). When prescribing benzodiazepines in other psychiatric conditions, such as schizophrenia and bipolar affective disorder, the clinician should examine the benefit–risk ratio early in treatment, so that the risks of dependence can be balanced against the therapeutic benefits (Royal College of Psychiatrists 2002). Finally, doctors should resist the temptation to substitute non-benzodiazepine hypnotics and anxiolytics such as zopiclone, zolpidem or zaleplon as long-term medication for benzodiazepine-dependent patients, since these drugs can also lead to dependence and abuse.

Summary: Benzodiazepine dependence

Definition	Fulfils criteria for DSM IV substance dependence
Incidence	Over 50% of long-term regular prescribed benzodiazepine users; unknown number of recreational benzodiazepine users.
Drugs causing syndrome	All benzodiazepines and other drugs acting similarly on benzodiazepine receptors including zopiclone, zolpidem and zaleplon
Key symptoms	Withdrawal reaction on decreasing dosage or stopping drug including anxiety, insomnia, perceptual disturbance, sensory hypersensitivity, distortion of body image, muscle twitches and others; convulsions on abrupt withdrawal from high doses
Pharmacological mechanism	Benzodiazepine-induced changes in $GABA_A$ receptor subtypes with internalization and alterations in gene transcription
Investigations to confirm diagnosis	History of long-term regular benzodiazepine use; enquire about alcohol or other drug dependence
Management	Gradual dosage reduction combined with psychological support
Further reading	Petursson H and Lader MH (1981) Withdrawal from long-term benzodiazepine treatment. *British Medical Journal* **283**, 643–5.
	Owen RT and Tyrer P (1983) Benzodiazepine dependence: a review of the evidence. *Drugs* **25**, 385–98.
	Bateson AN (2002) Basic pharmacologic mechanisms involved in Benzodiazepine tolerance and withdrawal. *Current Pharmaceutical, Design* **8**, 5–21.

References

Abernethy DR, Greenblatt DJ, and Shader RI (1981). Treatment of diazepam withdrawal syndrome with propranolol. *Ann Intern Med*, **94**, 354–5.

American Psychiatric Association (1994). *Diagnostic and Statistical Manual of Mental Disorders*, (DSM-IV). APA:Washington, DC.

American Task Force (1990). Treatment of benzodiazepine discontinuance symptoms. In *Benzodiazepine Dependence, Toxicity and Abuse, A Task Force Report of the American Psychiatric Association*, pp. 35–8. American Psychiatric Association: Washington, DC.

Ashton H (1984). Benzodiazepine withdrawal: an unfinished story. *BMJ*, **288**, 1135–40.

Ashton H (1987). Benzodiazepine withdrawal: outcome in 50 patients. *Br J Addict*, **82**, 665–71.

Ashton H (1989). Risks of dependence on benzodiazepine drugs: a major problem of long-term treatment. *BMJ*, **198**, 103–4.

Ashton H (1991). Protracted withdrawal syndromes from benzodiazepines. *J Subst Abuse Treat*, **8**, 19–28.

Ashton H (1992). *Brain Function and Psychotropic Drugs*. Oxford University Press: Oxford.

Ashton H (1994). The treatment of benzodiazepine dependence. *Addiction*, **89**, 1535–41.

Ashton H (1995*a*). Protracted withdrawal from benzodiazepines: the post-withdrawal syndrome. *Psychiatr Ann*, **25**, 174–9.

Ashton H (1995*b*). Toxicity and adverse consequences of benzodiazepine use. *Psychiatr Ann*, **25**, 158–65.

Ashton H (1997). Benzodiazepine dependency. In *Cambridge Handbook of Psychology, Health and Medicine*, A Baum, S Newman, J Weinmam, *et al.* (ed.), pp. 376–80. Cambridge University Press: Cambridge.

Ashton CH (2002). Motivation: reward and punishment systems. In *Neurochemistry of Consciousness*, E Perry, H Ashton, and A Young (ed.), pp. 83–104. John Benjamins Publishing Co.: Amsterdam.

Ashton H and Golding JF (1989). Tranquillisers: prevalence, predictors and possible consequences. Data from a large United Kingdom survey. *Br J Addict*, **84**, 541–6.

Ashton CH, Rawlins MD, and Tyrer SP (1990). A double-blind placebo-controlled study of buspirone in diazepam withdrawal in chronic benzodiazepine users. *Br J Psychiatry* **157**, 232–8.

Baldwin HA, Hitchott PK, and File S (1990). The use of flumazenil in prevention of diazepam dependence in the rat. *Hum Psychopharm*, **5**, 57–61.

Bateson AN (2002). Basic pharmacologic mechanisms involved in benzodiazepine tolerance and withdrawal. *Curr Pharm Design*, **8**, 5–21.

Bernik MA, Gorenstein C, and Vieira Filho HG (1998). Stressful reactions and panic attacks induced by flumazenil in chronic benzodiazepine users. *J Psychopharmacol*, **12**, 146–50.

Borg S, Carlsson S, and Lafolie P (1993). Benzodiazepine/alcohol dependence and abuse. In *Benzodiazepine Dependence*, C Hallstrom (ed.), pp. 119–27. Oxford University Press: Oxford.

Breier A, Charney DS, and Nelson JC (1984). Seizures induced by abrupt discontinuation of alprazolam. *Am J Psychiatry*, **141**, 1606–7.

British National Formulary (2002). British Medical Association and Royal Pharmaceutical Society of Great Britain.

Brodie MJ (1990). Established anticonvulsants and treatment of refractory epilepsy. *BMJ*, **336**, 350–4.

Busto U and Sellers E (1991). Anxiolytics and sedatives/hypnotics dependence. *Br J Addict*, **86**, 1647–52.

Busto U, Sellers EM, Naranjo CA, *et al.* (1986). Withdrawal reaction after long-term therapeutic use of benzodiazepines. *New Engl J Med,* **315,** 654–9.

Cantopher T, Olivieri S, Cleave N, *et al.* (1990). Chronic benzodiazepine dependence: a comparative study of abrupt withdrawal under propranolol cover versus gradual withdrawal. *Br J Psychiatry,* **156,** 406–11.

Chaplin (1988). Benzodiazepine prescribing. *Lancet* **1,** 120–1.

Chiu TH and Rosenberg HC (1978). Reduced diazepam binding following chronic benzodiazepine treatment. *Life Sci,* **23,** 1153–8.

Cole JO and Chiarello RJ (1990). The benzodiazepines as drugs of abuse. *J Psychiatry Res,* **24,** 135–44.

Crockford D, White WD, and Campbell B (2001). Gabapentin use in benzodiazepine dependence and detoxification. *Can J Psychiatry,* **46,** 287.

CSM (Committee on Safety of Medicines) (1988). Benzodiazepines, dependence and withdrawal symptoms. *Current Problems,* 21.

Curran HV (1991). Benzodiazepines, memory and mood: a review. *Psychopharmacology* **105,** 1–8.

Curran HV (1992). Memory functions, alertness and mood of long-term benzodiazepine ussers: a preliminary investigation of the effects of normal daily dose. *J Psychopharmacol,* **6,** 69–75.

Di Chiara G and Imperato A (1988). Drugs abused by humans preferentially increase synaptic dopamine concentrations in the mesolimbic system of freely moving rats. *Proc Nat Acad Sci,* **85,** 5274–8.

Drug and Therapeutics Bulletin (1997). Helping patients who misuse drugs. *Drug Ther Bull,* **35,** 18–22.

DuPont RL and Saylor KE (1991). Sedatives, hypnotics and benzodiazepines. In *Clinical Textbook of Addictive Disorders,* RJ Frances and SI Miller (ed.), pp. 69–102. Guilford Press: New York and London.

Edwards JG, Cantopher R, and Olivieri S (1990). Benzodiazepine dependence and the problems of withdrawal. *Postgrad Med J,* **66** (Suppl. 2), S27–35.

Farrell M and Strang J (1988). Misuse of temazepam. *BMJ,* **297,** 1402.

Fyer AJ, Liebowitz MR, Gorman JL, *et al.* (1987). Discontinuation of alprazolam treatment in panic patients. *Am J Psychiatry,* **144,** 303–8.

File S and Baldwin HA (1989). Changes in anxiety in rats tolerant to, and withdrawn from, benzodiazepines: behavioural and biochemical studies. In *Psychopharmacology of Anxiety,* P Tyrer (ed.), pp. 28–51. Oxford University Press: Oxford.

Gallager DW, Heninger K, and Heninger G (1986). Periodic benzodiazepine antagonist administration prevents benzodiazepine withdrawal symptoms in primates. *Eur J Pharmacol,* **5,** 57–61.

Gerra G, Giucasto G, Zaimovic A, *et al.* (1996). Intravenous flumazenil following prolonged exposure to lormetazepam in humans: lack of precipitated withdrawal. *Int Clin Psychopharmacol,* **11,** 81–8.

Gerra G, Zaimovic A, Giusti F, *et al.* (2002). Intravenous flumazenil versus oxazepam tapering in the treatment of benzodiazepine withdrawal: a randomized, placebo-controlled study. *Addict Biol* **7,** 385–95.

Golombok S, Higgitt A, Fonagy P, *et al.* (1987). A follow-up study of patients treated for benzodiazepine dependence. *Br J Med Psychol,* **60,** 141–9.

Golombok S, Moodley P, and Lader M (1988). Cognitive impairment in long-term benzodiazepine users. *Psychol Med,* **18**, 365–74.

Goodman WK, Charney DS, Price LH, *et al.* (1986). Ineffectiveness of clonidine in the treatment of the benzodiazepine withdrawal syndrome: report of three cases. *Am J Psychiatry,* **143**, 900–3.

Gorenstein C, Bernik MA, Pompeia S, *et al.* (1995). Impairment of performance associated with long-term use of benzodiazepines. *J Psychopharmacol,* **9**, 313–18.

Griffiths RR, Evans SM, Guarino JJ, *et al.* (1993). Intravenous flumazenil following acute and repeated exposure to lorazepam in healthy volunteers: antagonism and precipitated withdrawal. *J Pharmacol Exp Therap,* **265**, 1163–74.

Griffiths RR and Weerts EM (1997). Benzopdiazepine self-administration in humans and laboratory animals – implications for problems of long-term use and abuse. *Psychopharmacology,* **134**, 1–37.

Haddad P, Lejoyeux M, and Young A (1998). Antidepressant discontinuation reactions. *BMJ,* **316**, 1105–6.

Haefley W, Pieri L, Pole P, *et al.* (1981). General pharmacology and neuropharmacology of benzodiazepine derivatives. In *Handbook of Experimental Pharmacology,* vol. 55, H Hoffmeister and G Stille (ed.), pp. 13–262. Springer-Verlag: Berlin.

Hallstrom C and Lader MH (1981). Benzodiazepine withdrawal phenomena. *Int Pharmacopsychiatry,* **16**, 235–44.

Heather N, Bowie A, Ashton H, *et al.* (2004). Randomised controlled trial of two brief interventions against long-term benzodiazepine use: outcome of intervention. *Addiction Research and Theory,* (in press).

Hitchcott PK, File SE, Ekwuru M, *et al.* (1990). Chronic diazepam treatment in rats causes long-lasting changes in central [^{3}H]-5-hydroxytryptamine and [^{14}C]-g-aminobutyric acid release. *Br J Pharmacol,* **99**, 11–12.

Hollister LE, Muller-Oerlinghausen B, Rickels K, *et al.* (1993). Clinical uses of benzodiazepines. *J Clin Psychopharmacol,* **13**, 6 (Suppl. 1), 1S–169S.

Kales A, Scharf MB, and Kales JD (1978). Rebound insomnia: a new clinical syndrome. *Science,* **201**, 1039–41.

Kales A, Soldatos CR, Bixler EO, *et al.* (1988). Diazepam: effects on sleep and withdrawal phenomena. *J Clin Psychopharmacol,* **8**, 340–6.

Keshaven MS and Crammer JL (1985). Clonidine in benzodiazepine withdrawal. *Lancet,* **1**, 1325–6.

Klein E, Uhde TW, and Post RM (1986). Preliminary evidence for the utility of carba-mazepine in alprazolam withdrawal. *Am J Psychiatry,* **143**, 235–6.

Koob GF (1992). Drugs of abuse: anatomy, pharmacology and function of reward path-ways. *Trends Pharmacol Sci,* **13**, 177–84.

Lader M (1988). The psychopharmacology of addiction – benzodiazepine tolerance and dependence. In *The Psychopharmacology of Addiction,* M Lader (ed.), pp. 1–14. Oxford Medical Publications: Oxford.

Lader M (1991). Avoiding long-term use of benzodiazepine drugs. *Prescriber,* March, 79–93.

Lader M (1992). Benzos and memory loss: more than just 'old age'. *Prescriber* **3**, 13.

Lader M (1993). Historical development of the concept of tranquillizer dependence. In *Benzodiazepine Dependence,* C Hallsrom (ed.), pp. 46–57, Oxford University Press: Oxford.

ADVERSE SYNDROMES AND PSYCHIATRIC DRUGS: A CLINICAL GUIDE is tagged below.

Lader M and Higgitt AC (1986). Management of benzodiazepine dependence – Update 1986, *Br J Addict*, **81**, 7–9.

Lader MH and Morton SV (1992). A pilot study of the effects of flumazenil on symptoms persisting after benzodiazepine withdrawal. *J Psychopharmacol*, **6**, 19–28.

Lancet, Leading Article (1987). Treatment of benzodiazepine dependence. *Lancet*, **1**, 78–9.

Levy AB (1984). Delirium and seizures due to abrupt alprazolam withdrawal: case report. *J Clin Psychiatry*, **45**, 38–9.

Livingston MG (1991). Benzodiazepine dependence: avoidance, detection and management. *Prescr J*, **31**, 149–56.

Lucki I and Rickels K (1988). The effect of anxiolytic drugs on memory in anxious subjects. In *Benzodiazepine Receptor Ligands, Memory and Information Processing – Psychometric, Psychopharmacological and Clinical Issues*, I Hindmarch and H Ott (ed.), pp. 128–39. Springer: Berlin.

Maletzky BM and Klotter J (1976). Addiction to diazepam. *Int J Addict*, **11**, 95–115.

Malizia AL and Nutt DJ (1995). The effects of flumazenil in neuropsycyhiatric disorders. *Clin Neuropharmacol*, **18**, 215–32.

Medawar C (1997). The antidepressant web. *Int J Risk Saf Med*, **10**, 75–126.

Mintzer MZ, Stoller KB, and Griffiths RR (1999). A controlled study of flumazenil-precipitated withdrawal in chronic low-dose benzodiazepine users. *Psychopharmacology*, **147**, 200–9.

Murphy SM and Tyrer P (1988). The essence of benzodiazepine dependence. In *The Psychopharmacology of Addiction*, M Lader (ed.), pp. 157–67. Oxford University Press: Oxford.

Murphy SM and Tyrer P (1991). A double-blind comparison of the effects of gradual withdrawal of lorazepam, diazepam and bromazepam in benzodiazepine dependence. *Br J Psychiatry*, **158**, 511–16.

Murphy SM, Owen RT, and Tyrer PJ (1984). Withdrawal symptoms after six weeks treatment with diazepam. *Lancet* **2**, 1389.

Noyes R, Perry PJ, Crowe RR, *et al.* (1986). Seizures following the withdrawal of alprazolam. *J Nerv Ment Disorders*, **174**, 50–2.

Nutt DJ (1986). Benzodiazepine dependence in the clinic: a cause for anxiety? *Trends Pharmacol Sci*, **7**, 457–60.

Nutt DJ (1990). Pharmacological mechanisms of benzodiazepine withdrawal. *J Psychiatr Res*, **24**, 105–10.

Nutt DJ (1996). Brain mechanisms and their treatment implications. *Lancet*, **347**, 31–6.

Olajide D and Lader M (1984). Depression following withdrawal from long-term benzodiazepine use: a report of four cases. *Psychol Med*, **14**, 937–40.

Olajide D and Lader M (1987). A comparative study of the efficacy of buspirone in relieving benzodiazepine withdrawal symptoms. *J Clin Psychopharmacol*, **7**, 11–15.

Oswald I, French C, Adam K, *et al.* (1982). Benzodiazepine hypnotics remain effective for 24 weeks. *BMJ*, **2**, 860–3.

Owen RT and Tyrer P (1983). Benzodiazepine dependence: a review of the evidence. *Drugs*, **25**, 385–98.

Pande AC, Davidson JRT, Jefferson JW, *et al.* (1999). Treatment of social phobia with gabapentin: a placebo-controlled study. *J Clin Psychopharmacol*, **19**, 341–8.

Petursson H and Lader MH (1981). Withdrawal from long-term benzodiazepine treatment. *BMJ*, **283**, 634–5.

Petursson H and Lader MH (1984). Benzodiazepine dependence. *B J Addict*, **76**, 133–45.

Podhorna J (2002). The experimental pharmacotherapy of benzodiazepine withdrawal. *Curr Pharmaceut Design*, **8**, 23–43.

Preziosa PJ and Neale JH (1983). Benzodiazepine receptor binding by membranes from brain cell cultures following chronic treatment with diazepam. *Brain Res*, **288**, 354–8.

Rastogi RB, Lapierre YD, and Singhal RL (1976). Evidence for the role of brain norepinephrine and dopamine in 'rebound' phenomenon seen during withdrawal after repeated exposure to benzodiazepines. *J Psychiatry Res*, **13**, 65–75.

Ries RK, Roy-Byrne PP, Ward NG, *et al.* (1989). Carbamazepine treatment for benzodiazepine withdrawal. *Am J Psychiatry*, **146**, 536–7.

Robertson JR and Ronald PJM (1992). Prescribing benzodiazepines to drug misusers. *Lancet*, **339**, 1169–70.

Rosenberg HC and Chiu TH (1979). Decreased ^{3}H-diazepam binding is a specific response to chronic benzodiazepine treatment. *Life Sci*, **24**, 803–8.

Royal College of Psychiatrists (1988). Benzodiazepines and dependence: a College statement. *Bull R Coll Psychiatr*, **12**, 107–8.

Royal College of Psychiatrists (2002). CR59. Benzodiazepines: risks, benefits and dependence. A re-evaluation.

Ruben SM and Morrison CL (1992). Temazepam misuse in a group of injecting drug users. *Br J Addict*, **87**, 1387–92.

Rudolph U, Crestani F, and Mohler H (2001). GABA$_A$ receptor subtypes: dissecting their pharmacological functions. *Trends Pharmacol Sci*, **22**, 188–94.

Savic I, Widen L, and Stone-Elander S (1991). Feasibility of reversing benzodiazepine tolerance with flumazenil. *Lancet*, **337**, 133–7.

Salzman C, Fisher J, Nobel K, *et al.* (1992). Cognitive improvement following benzodiazepine discontinuation in elderly nursing home residents. *Int J Gen Psychiatry*, **7**, 89–93.

Saxon L, Hjemdahl P, Hiltunen AJ, *et al.* (1997). Effects of flumazenil in the treatment of benzodiazepine withdrawal – a double-blind pilot study. *Psychopharmacology* **131**, 153–60.

Schweizer E and Rickels K (1986). Failure of buspirone to manage benzodiazepine withdrawal. *Am J Psychiatry*, **143**, 1590–2.

Schweizer E, Rickels K, Case WG, *et al.* (1991). Carbamazepine treatment in patients discontinuing long-term benzodiazepine therapy. Effects on withdrawal severity and outcome. *Arch Gen Psychiatry*, **48**, 448–52.

Schweizer E, Rickels K, Weiss S, *et al.* (1993). Maintenance drug treatment of panic disorder. I. Results of a prospective, placebo-controlled comparison of alprazolam and imipramine. *Arch Gen Psychiatry*, **50**, 51–60.

Scott RTA (1990). The prevention of convulsions during benzodiazepine withdrawal. *Br J Gen Pract*, **40**, 261.

Seivewright N (1998). Theory and practice in managing benzodiazepine dependence and misuse. *J Subst Misuse*, **3**, 170–7.

Seivewright N and Dougal W (1993). Withdrawal symptoms from high dose benzodi-azepines in polydrug users. *Drug Alcohol Depen*, **32**, 15–23.

Seivewright N, Donmall M, and Daly C (1993). Benzodiazepines in the illicit drugs scene: The picture and some treatment dilemmas. *Int J Drug Pol*, **4**, 42–8.

Shaw M, Brabbins C, and Ruben S (1994). Misuse of benzodiazepines. *BMJ*, **308**, 1709.

Stahl SM (2002). Don't ask, don't tell, but benzodiazepines are still the leading treatments for anxiety disorder. *J Clin Psychiatry*, **63**, 756–7.

Stark DE, Sykes R, and Mullen P (1987). Temazepam abuse. *Lancet* **2**, 802–3.

Strang J, Seivewright N, and Farrell M (1993). Oral and intravenous abuse of benzodi-azepines. In *Benzodiazepine Dependence*, C Hallstrom (ed.), pp. 128–42. Oxford University Press: Oxford.

Strang J, Griffiths P, Abbey J, *et al.* (1994). Survey of use of injected benzodiazepines among drug users in Britain. *BMJ*, **308**, 1082.

Tata PR, Rollings J, Collins M, *et al.* (1994). Lack of cognitive recovery following withdrawal from long-term benzodiazepine use. *Psychol Med*, **24**, 203–13.

Taylor D (1987). Current usage of benzodiazepines in Britain. In *The Benzodiazepines in Current Clinical Practice*, H Freeman and Y Rue (ed.), pp. 13–18. Royal Society of Medicine Services: London.

Tonne U, Hiltunen AJ, Vikander B, *et al.* (1995). Neuropsychological changes during steady-state drug use, withdrawal and abstinence in primary benzodiazepine-dependent patients. *Acta Psychiatr Scand*, **91**, 299–304.

Tyrer P (1987). Benefits and risks of benzodiazepines. In *The Benzodiazepines in Current Clinical Practice*, H Freeman and Y Rue (ed.), pp. 3–12. Royal Society of Medicine Services: London.

Tyrer P (1989*a*). Risks of dependence on benzodiazepine drugs: the importance of patient selection. *BMJ*, **298**, 102–5.

Tyrer P (1989*b*). Choice of treatment in anxiety. In *Psychopharmacology of Anxiety*, P Tyrer (ed.), pp. 255–82. Oxford University Press: Oxford.

Tyrer P (1991). The benzodiazepine post-withdrawal syndrome. *Stress Medicine*, **7**, 1–2.

Tyrer P, Rutherford D, and Higgitt T (1981). Benzodiazepine withdrawal symptoms and propranolol. *Lancet*, **1**, 520–2.

Tyrer P, Owen R, and Dawling S (1983). Gradual withdrawal of diazepam after long-term therapy. *Lancet*, **1**, 1402–6.

Tyrer P, Murphy S, and Riley P (1990). The benzodiazepine withdrawal symptom questionnaire. *J Affect Disorders*, **19**, 53–61.

Tyrer P, Ferguson B, Hallstrom C, *et al.* (1996). A controlled trial of dothiepin and placebo in treating benzodiazepine withdrawal symptoms. *Br J Psychiatry*, **168**, 457–61.

Vinogradov S, Reiss AL, and Csernansky JG (1986). Clonidine therapy in withdrawal from high-dose alprazolam treatment. *Am J Psychiatry*, **143**, 1188.

Warburton DM (1988). The puzzle of nicotine use. In *The Psychopharmacol of Addiction*, M Lader (ed.), pp. 27–49. Oxford University Press: Oxford.

Wells F (1993). Benzodiazepines and the pharmaceutical industry. In *Benzodiazepine Dependence*, C Hallstrom (ed.), pp. 338–49. Oxford University Press: Oxford.

Wise RA and Bozarth MA (1987). A psychomotor stimulant theory of addiction. *Psychol Rev*, **94**, 469–92.

Woods JH, Katz JL, and Winger G (1992). Benzodiazepines: use, abuse and consequences. *Pharmacol Rev,* **44**, 151–338.

Woods JH, Katz JL, and Winger G (1998). Use and abuse of benzodiazepines: issues relevant to prescribing. *J Am Med Assoc,* **260**, 3476–80.

Young A and Haddad P (2000). Discontinuation symptoms and psychotropic drugs. *Lancet,* **355**, 1184.

Zitman FG and Couvee JE (2001). Chronic benzodiazepine use in general practice patients with depression: an evaluation of controlled treatment and taper-off. *Br J Psychiatry,* **178**, 317–24.

Chapter 14

Syndrome of inappropriate antidiuretic hormone secretion

Paul Strickland

Introduction

Water homeostasis involves physiological monitoring of both osmolality and arterial blood pressure. Plasma osmolality is principally determined by sodium ion concentration and is normally maintained between 280–300 mOsmol/L and 135–145 mmol/L respectively. Osmoreceptors in the hypothalamus respond to changes in extracellular osmolality and arterial baroreceptors detect changes in blood pressure and hence circulating blood volume. These receptors influence water balance by altering water and salt excretion in the kidney and by modulating thirst. Therefore, under normal circumstances, when extracellular osmolality increases and/or blood pressure drops, these receptors stimulate the secretion of antidiuretic hormone (ADH) from the posterior pituitary gland and induce thirst, both directly and indirectly via angiotensin II. ADH acts at the nephron to increase water reabsorption thereby concentrating urine (low volume, high sodium concentration). Plasma ADH concentrations are usually low or undetectable when plasma osmolality falls below 280 mOsmol/L.

In SIADH, in the presence of hyponatraemia (plasma sodium <125 mmol/L) and reduced plasma osmolality (<280 mOsmol/L), ADH continues to be secreted, resulting in urine production with high osmolality and high salt concentration (urine, Na >20 mmol/L, osmolality >100 mOsmol/L). Therefore, water is retained and salt lost causing further hyponatraemia. The patient is unable to excrete diluted urine.

SIADH was first described by Schwartz *et al.* (1957) and later further characterized by Bartter and Schwartz (1967). They defined the syndrome of hyponatraemia with renal salt loss, unrelated to adrenal or renal disease, originally in patients with bronchogenic carcinoma. Since then many other causes have been identified and this includes a wide range of drugs (see Table 14.1). There are also reports of SIADH and drugs of abuse, for example ecstasy (MDMA) (Gomez-Balaguer *et al.* 2000).

Table 14.1 Causes of the syndrome of inappropriate secretion of anti-diuretic hormone (SIADH), (after Spigset and Hedenmalm 1995; Kovacs and Robertson 1992)

1 ADH-producing tumours
- Carcinomas: bronchogenic; pancreatic; prostatic; duodenal
- Thymoma
- Lymphoma
- Mesothelioma
- Ewing's sarcoma

2 Pulmonary disease
- Asthma
- Pneumonia (viral, bacterial or fungal)
- Tuberculosis
- Empyema
- Pneumothorax
- Acute respiratory failure

3 CNS disorders
- Meningitis
- Encephalitis
- Brain abscess
- Cerebrovascular accident
- Subarachnoid haemorrhage
- Subdural haemorrhage
- Hydrocephalus
- Head trauma
- Delirium tremens
- Aplasia of corpus callosum
- Acute intermittent porphyria
- Neonatal hypoxia
- Guillain-Barré syndrome

4 General surgery

5 Psychiatric drugs
- Anticholinergic drugs
- Antidepressants (all classes)
- Antipsychotics (all classes)
- Benzodiazepines
- Carbamazepine (and oxcarbamazepine)

6 Other drugs
- Amiloride
- Clofibrate
- Cyclophosphamide
- Desmopressin
- Oxytocin
- Thiazide diuretics
- Vasopressin
- Vinca alkaloids

Some of the earliest descriptions of SIADH involved conventional antipsychotic drugs (Spigset and Hedenmalm 1995) but the syndrome may also occur with atypical antipsychotics (Collins and Anderson 2000; Whitten and Ruehter 1997). All classes of antidepressants have been implicated in causation including tricyclic antidepressants, monoamine oxidase inhibitors, selective serotonin reuptake inhibitors and serotonin-noradrenalin reuptake inhibitors (Spigset and Hedenmalm 1997; Meynaar *et al.* 1997; Kirby and Ames 2001). SIADH occurs with both carbamazepine and oxcarbamazepine usage (Van Amelsvoort *et al.* 1994). Benzodiazepines have also been implicated (Engel and Grau 1988).

Clinical features

Typically SIADH develops in the early weeks of treatment with antidepressants and later with antipsychotic drugs. The clinical presentations of SIADH are due to water retention and hyponatraemia. Symptoms do not usually occur until plasma sodium is <130 mmol/L. However, approximately 50 per cent of patients with plasma sodium concentrations <125 mmol/L may be asymptopmatic (Kirby and Ames 2001). Furthermore, symptoms are more severe if hyponatraemia develops acutely, rather than chronically. Common symptoms of hyponatraemia are weakness, lethargy, weight gain without oedema, muscle cramps, headache, vomiting and anorexia. As hyponatraemia progresses, or develops acutely, the patient may develop confusion, convulsions and ultimately coma followed by death (Sandifer 1983). Table 14.2 summarises common signs and symptoms of hyponatraemia. Because many patients with chronic hyponatraemia may be asymptomatic, or have non-specific and vague symptoms, a common presentation of SIADH is as a chance finding from a routine blood electrolyte assay.

Incidence

The incidence of SIADH caused by psychotropic drugs is not known, as there are no systematic studies, only spontaneous reports of adverse reactions.

Table 14.2 Symptoms and signs of SIADH

1 Often absent
2 Early/mild/chronic: a. weakness; lethargy; weight gain without oedema; muscle cramps   b. headache; vomiting; anorexia
3 Late/severe/acute: confusion; convulsions; coma; death

The drugs most commonly implicated are antidepressants, including tricyclics, selective serotonin reuptake inhibitors (SSRIs) and selective serotonin and noradrenaline reuptake inhibitors (SNRIs), antipsychotic medications and carbamazepine/oxcarbamazepine. It has been suggested that serotonergic antidepressants are more likely to cause the syndrome than other antidepressants (Movig *et al.* 2002*a,b*) but this has been disputed (Kirby and Ames 2001). Hyponatraemia occurring with carbamazepine has been reported to be as high as 22 per cent in patients treated for epilepsy or trigeminal neuralgia (Van Amelsvoort *et al.* 1994) and there have also been case reports involving carbamazepine used in affective disorders (Palladino 1986).

Pharmacological basis

The mechanism whereby psychotropic drugs cause SIADH is not fully understood. It is proposed that serotonin (via 5-HT_2 or 5-HT_{1C} receptors) and noradrenalin (via alpha_1 receptors) stimulate ADH secretion, and that dopamine may inhibit or stimulate ADH secretion dependant on receptor subtype. Furthermore, monoamine systems are involved in thirst regulation. Finally anticholinergic drugs may induce thirst through reduced salivation and consequent dry mouth (Spigset and Hedenmalm 1995).

Differential diagnosis

The assessment of patients presenting with hyponatraemia is first to determine whether they are hyper/hypo or eu-volaemic and to exclude other medical conditions which may cause hyponatraemia, for example, loop diuretic use, nephritis, hypothyroidism, adrenal insufficiency, oedema, self induced water intoxication (SIWI), or severe hyperglycaemia (see Table 13.1). In SIADH the patient is hyper or eu-volaemic, but without oedema.

Self-induced water intoxication (SIWA) or compulsive water drinking has long been recognized in psychiatric patients, most commonly with schizophrenia, for example, Riggs *et al.* (1991). However, this differs from SIADH in that patients with SIWA drink large volumes of water, up to and above 25 L per day, and produce high volume dilute urine (low sodium, low osmolality). Although in SIWA hyponatraemia may be present, ADH levels are low. This contrasts with SIADH where the patient is unable to excrete dilute urine, thereby retaining water and losing salt.

Suggested initial investigation of patients with suspected SIADH is shown in Table 14.3. As described, the first step is to exclude other medical causes of hyponatraemia and then to confirm SIADH. Severe hyponatraemia is a medical emergency (plasma sodium <120 mmol/L), especially if acute, and requires urgent medical attention.

Table 14.3 Investigation of suspected SIADH

1	**Blood** Plasma urea and electrolytes, full blood count, ESR, glucose, liver function tests, plasma osmolality, thyroid function tests, morning cortisol
2	**Urine** Sodium, glucose, osmolality, specific gravity
3	**Other** Chest X-ray
4	**Consider** referral to nephrologist for further assessment, and advice-management of severe hyponatraemia and/or possible water loading tests and drug re-challenge.

Management

Treatment of hyponatraemia once it is detected depends on the severity and identifying the cause. Withdrawal of the suspected drug, followed by water loading and re-challenge with the agent will clarify the aetiology: however, this is not often done.

If the SIADH is believed to be caused by a psychotropic drug, the initial step is to consider whether the patient continues to require this agent. In some cases the clinician will be able to stop the drug without starting a replacement compound but in other cases switching to an alternative drug will be preferred. Since each class of psychotropics tends to have similar modes of action it is often preferable to try switching between classes. For example if an SSRI is causing SIADH it may be worth switching to a noradrenergic antidepressant or a tricyclic antidepressant.

Although treatment of the underlying cause is preferable, there may be cases of mild hyponatraemia where it is felt necessary to continue with the drug suspected of causing SIADH. In such cases it will be necessary to correct the hyponatraemia. Attempts at rapid correction of hyponatraemia are hazardous and potentially fatal. Rapid changes in extracelluar sodium concentration may cause central pontine myelinosis. Spigset and Hedenmalm (1995) suggest that if the hyponatraemia is mild and asymptomatic (plasma Na >125 mmol/L), the treatment of choice is fluid restriction (as low as 250 ml per day) and/or change in suspected drug. However, if the hyponatraemia is more severe (plasma sodium concentration <125 mmol/L) and symptoms are present, especially with acute onset, the suspected drug should be withdrawn, the preliminary investigations performed as described above and the advice of a nephrologist sought. Again the mainstay of treatment is water restriction, and it is beyond the usual clinical competencies of a psychiatrist to engage in administering intravenous saline and diuretics.

In some cases of SIADH resistant to fluid restriction, sodium chloride tablets with or without frusemide, urea, demeclocycline and lithium have all been used (Illowsky and Kirsch 1988; Riggs *et al.* 1991; Siegel *et al.* 1998). Once again, this should only be considered with the support and advice of a nephrologist.

Table 14.4 Risk factors for SIADH (Spigset and Hedenmalm 1995, 1997)

Older age (especially >60 years)
Female sex
Low body weight
Smoking
Past/current history of polydypsia
Treatment in summer months
Existing renal disease
Medical comorbidity (e.g. hypothyroidism, head injury, CVA, various cancers)
Other concurrent medication, for example, diuretics

Risk factors and prevention

Risk factors have been identified in predisposing to SIADH. These are summarized in Table 14.4 (Spigset and Hedenmalm 1995, 1997). Clearly prevention of severe hyponatraemia is the ideal. This can partly be achieved by identifying vulnerable patients and ensuring that plasma urea and electrolytes are assessed prior to their commencing psychotropic medication and are then monitored regularly during treatment.

Conclusion

Many psychotropic drugs can cause SIADH. If mild and chronic it is often asymptomatic; however, as hyponatraemia worsens if can become life threatening. High-risk groups have been identified and these patients require electrolyte monitoring before and during treatment. Following diagnosis the treatment of choice is to switch medication, however if this not possible water restriction and advice from a nephrologist are usually effective. Rapid intravenous administration of saline may be fatal through too rapid correction of sodium ion concentration and central pontine myelinosis.

Summary: Syndrome of inappropriate ADH secretion

Definition	In the presence of hyponatraemia (plasma sodium <125 mmol/L) and reduced plasma osmolality (<280 mOsmol/L), ADH continues to be secreted, resulting in concentrated urine production (urine, Na >20 mmol/L, osmolality >100 mOsmol/L). Water is retained and salt lost causing further hyponatraemia. The patient is unable excrete diluted urine.

	The onset is typically early on in treatment with the causal drug.
Incidence	Variable depending on drug, patient sex, age and general health. Up to 22% with carbamazepine (Van Amelsvoort et al. 1994). Largely unknown.
Drugs causing syndrome	Carbamazepine and oxcarbamazepine are the most common drugs implicated.
	Occurs with all antidepressants (unclear if serotonergic drugs are associated with high risk). Recognized with conventional and atypical antipsychotics and occasionally with benzodiazepines. For non-psychiatric drugs see Table 14.1.
Key symptoms	Often absent. Early features include weakness, lethargy, weight gain without oedema and muscle cramps, followed by headache, vomiting and anorexia.
	Late and severe symptoms are confusion, convulsions, coma and death.
Pharmacological mechanism	Unknown; ?Serotonin (via 5-HT$_2$ or 5-HT$_{1C}$ receptors) and noradrenalin (via alpha1 receptors) stimulate ADH secretion, and dopamine may inhibit or stimulate ADH secretion dependant on receptor sub-type. Monoamine systems are involved in thirst regulation. Anticholinergic drugs may induce thirst through reduced salivation and consequent dry mouth (Spigset and Hedenmalm 1995).
Investigations to confirm diagnosis	History will detect symptoms. Blood and urine sodium and osmolality measurement are central to diagnosis. Chest X-ray, morning cortisol and thyroid function tests are important in differentiation from other syndromes.
Management	Depends on the severity of hyponatraemia and identifying the cause.
	Withdrawal of the suspected drug, followed water loading and re-challenge with the agent will clarify the aetiology.
	Seek advice from physician or nephrologists.
	If the SIADH is believed to be caused by a psychotropic drug, the initial step if to consider whether the patient continues to require this agent.
	It is extremely hazardous to attempt rapid correction of hyponatraemia.
Further reading	Spigset O and Hedenmalm K (1995). Hyponatraemia and the syndrome of inappropriate antidiuretic hormone secretion (SIADH) induced by psychotropic drugs. Drug Saf, **12**, 209–25.

Spigset O and Hedenmalm K (1997). Hyponatraemia related to treatment with antidepressants: A survey of reports in the World Health Organization data base for spontaneous reporting of adverse drug reactions. *Pharmacotherapy*, **17**, 348–52.

Kirby D and Ames D (2001). Hyponatraemia and selective serotonin re-uptake inhibitors in elderly patients. *International Journal of Geriatric Psychiatry*, **16**, 484–93.

Acknowledgement

I would like to thank Dr David Lewis, consultant nephrologist at Hull Royal Infirmary, for his advice on this text.

References

Bartter FC and Schwartz WB (1967). The syndrome of inappropriate secretion of antidiuretic hormone. *Am J Med*, **42**, 790–806.

Blass DM and Pearson VE (2000). SIADH with multiple antidepressants in a geriatric patient. *J Clin Psychiatry*, **61**, 448–9.

Collins A and Anderson J (2000). SIADH induced by two atypical antipsychotics.[erratum appears in *Int J Geriatr Psychiatry* 2000 Jul, 15 (7), 667] *Int J Geriatr Psychiatry*, **15**, 282–3.

Engel WR and Grau A (1988). Inappropriate secretion of antidiuretic hormone associated with lorazepam. *BMJ*, **297** (6652), 858.

Gomez-Balaguer M, Pena H, Morillas C, *et al.* (2000). Syndrome of inappropriate antidiuretic hormone secretion and 'designer drugs' (ecstasy). *J Pediatr Endocrinol Metab*, **13**, 437–8.

Illowsky BP and Kirch DG (1988). Polydipsia and hyponatremia in psychiatric patients. *Am J Psychiatry*, **145**, 675–83.

Kirby D and Ames D (2001). Hyponatraemia and selective serotonin re-uptake inhibitors in elderly patients. *Int J Geriatr Psychiatry*, **16**, 484–93.

Kovacs L and Robertson GL (1992). Syndrome of inappropriate antidiuresis. *Endocrinol Metab Clin North Am*, **21**, 859–75.

Meynaar IA, Peeters AJ, Mulder AH, *et al.* (1997). Syndrome of inappropriate ADH secretion attributed to the serotonin re-uptake inhibitors, venlafaxine and paroxetine. *Neth J Med*, **50**, 243–5.

Movig KL, Leufkens HGM, Lenderink AW, *et al.* (2002*a*). Serotonergic antidepressants associated with an increased risk for hyponatraemia in the elderly. *Eur J Clin Pharmacol*, **58**, 143–8.

Movig KL, Leufkens HGM, Lenderink AW, *et al.* (2002*b*). Association between antidepressant drug use and hyponatraemia: a case-control study. *Br J Clin Pharmacol*, **53**, 363–9.

Palladino A (1986). Hyponatremia associated with carbamazepine therapy. *Am J Psychiatry*, **143**, 1190.

Riggs AT, Dysken MW, Kim SW, *et al.* (1991). A review of disorders of water homeostasis in psychiatric patients. *Psychosomatics*, **32**, 133–48.

Sandifer MG (1983). Hyponatremia due to psychotropic drugs. *J Clin Psychiatry*, **44**, 301–3.

Schwartz WB, Bennett W, Curelop S, *et al.* (1957). A syndrome of renal sodium loss and hyponatremia probably resulting from inappropriate secretion of antidiuretic hormone. *Am J Med*, **23**, 529–42.

Siegel AJ, Baldessarini RJ, Klepser MB, *et al.* (1998). Primary and drug-induced disorders of water homeostasis in psychiatric patients: principles of diagnosis and management. *Harv Rev Psychiatry*, **6**, 190–200.

Spigset O and Hedenmalm K (1995). Hyponatraemia and the syndrome of inappropriate antidiuretic hormone secretion (SIADH) induced by psychotropic drugs. *Drug Saf*, **12**, 209–25.

Spigset O and Hedenmalm K (1997). Hyponatraemia related to treatment with antidepressants: A survey of reports in the World Health Organization data base for spontaneous reporting of adverse drug reactions. *Pharmacotherapy*, **17**, 348–52.

Van Amelsvoort T, Bakshi R, Devaux CB, *et al.* (1994). Hyponatremia associated with carbamazepine and oxcarbazepine therapy: a review. *Epilepsia*, **35**, 181–8.

Whitten JR and Ruehter VL (1997). Risperidone and hyponatremia: a case report. *Ann Clin Psychiatry*, **9**, 181–3.

Chapter 15

Dermatological syndromes

R Hamish McAllister-Williams and
Suzy N Leech

Introduction

Dermatological syndromes are fairly common consequences of psychotropic drug treatment, occurring in up to 5 per cent of patients exposed (Srebrnik *et al.* 1991). It is not possible in this short chapter to cover every dermatological syndrome that has been reported to be associated with psychotropic medication. As a result we will concentrate on two broad groupings of syndromes: those related to hypersensitivity reactions (Stevens–Johnson syndrome, toxic epidermal necrolysis, hypersensitivity syndrome associated with eosinophilia and vasculitis) and pigmentation changes often induced or exacerbated by light exposure (hyperpigmentation and photosensitivity). This differentiation is not absolute since photosensitivity may also trigger or exacerbate Stevens–Johnson syndrome (Suarez Moro *et al.* 2000) and photosensitivity can result from an allergic reaction to photoproducts of medication. Other miscellaneous syndromes will only be mentioned briefly.

Stevens–Johnson syndrome and toxic epidermal necrolysis

These entities are immune complex-mediated hypersensitivity syndromes believed to form part of a continuum of dermatological conditions of increasing severity ranging from erythema multiforme minor (EMM), Stevens–Johnson syndrome (SJS; also known as erythema multiforme major) and at the worst end of the spectrum, toxic epidermal necrolysis (TEN) with the syndromes being related pathophysiologically (Ghislain and Roujeau 2002). These disorders tend to be recurrent with increasing severity if subjects are re-exposed to potential aetiological agents in the future. They are associated with significant mortality rates and are the most serious dermatological syndromes known to be associated with psychotropic drug use.

Clinical features

EMM is a self-limiting disease characterized by symmetrically and often acrally distributed erythematous plaques classically occurring as 'target lesions' (Fig. 15.1) and regarded as pathognomonic for this condition. Target lesions are composed of three colour zones: a central area of dusky erythema surrounded by a paler ring and an outer erythematous ring. The central area may blister. The oral mucosa can sometimes be affected to a mild degree. However, as the name suggests a variety of lesions may be seen clinically. It is commonly a reaction to herpes simplex infection or other viral illnesses as well as a reaction to drugs.

In SJS, the syndrome typically begins with non-specific upper respiratory tract symptoms of fever, sore throat, headache, arthralgia and malaise. This lasts from anything between one and 14 days before mucocutaneous lesions develop, which occur abruptly and last for two to four weeks. Oral and mucous membrane lesions are more prominent than in EMM and may be severe enough to prevent patients eating or drinking, or cause epistaxis and involvement of the lower respiratory tract and gastrointestinal tract which can lead to gastrointestinal bleeding and pneumonia. Conjunctivitis is common. Genitourinary involvement can cause dysuria or an inability to void. Examination of the skin reveals a rash beginning as macular erythematous

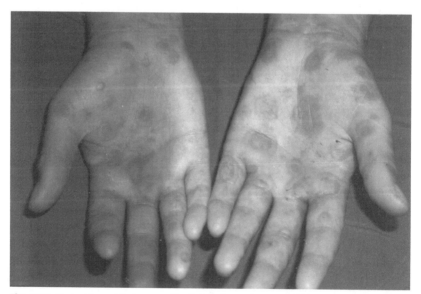

Fig. 15.1 Typical target lesions on the hands in erythema multiforme minor (EMM). The targets have a central erythematous area surrounded by a paler ring and another erythematous ring (see Plate 1 of the plate section at the centre of this book).

lesions which subsequently develop into papules, vesicles, bullae, urticated plaques or confluent erythema (Figs 15.2 and 15.3). Target lesions may be present. Lesions are generally non-pruritic but may be painful. Distribution may be widespread but the palms, soles, dorsum of the hands and the extensor surfaces are most commonly affected. SJS is diagnosed when mucosal lesions

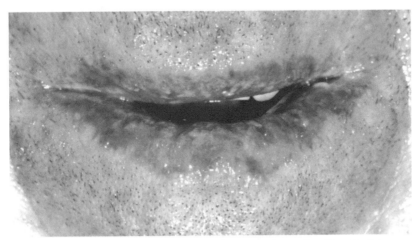

Fig. 15.2 Mucosal involvement in Stevens–Johnson syndrome (see Plate 2 of the plate section at the centre of this book).

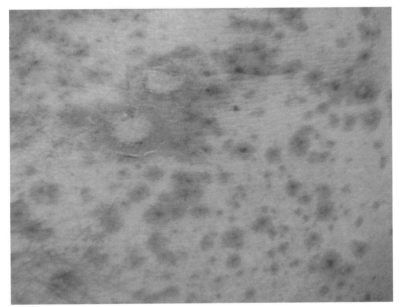

Fig. 15.3 Extensive erythema with some epidermal attachment and target lesions becoming confluent on the trunk (see Plate 3 of the plate section at the centre of this book).

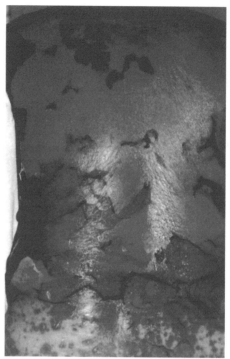

Fig. 15.4 Toxic epidermal necrolysis due to carbamazepine treated successfully with IVIG (see Plate 4 of the plate section at the centre of this book).

are present and epidermal detachment is less than 10 per cent of the surface area (Ghislain and Roujeau 2002).

In TEN, cutaneous lesions are more extensive (Fig. 15.4) and the diagnosis is made when more than 30 per cent of the epidermis is detached (Ghislain and Roujeau 2002). The skin becomes diffusely erythematous and painful with areas of necrotic epidermis and occasionally flaccid blistering. Nikolsky's sign is positive – where apparently intact-looking epidermis is readily separated at the basal layer by friction e.g. pressure applied in a sliding motion with the finger to the surface of the skin. Mucous membranes may be extensively involved. Systemic signs include fever, myalgia, arthritis, orthostasis, tachycardia and hypotension. Severe illness can be associated with alterations in consciousness, seizures and coma.

Several complications of SJS/TEN can occur. The most frequent are those associated with scarring including keratitis and uveitis, occasionally resulting in permanent visual impairment. Vaginal stenosis and penile scarring have been reported. Epidermal detachment may be extensive leading to a number of management problems. These include fluid loss leading to electrolyte imbalances, secondary infections, thermoregulatory impairment, excessive energy expenditure, alterations of immunological functions and haematological abnormalities. Pneumonia has been noted in up to 30 per cent of SJS patients. However it is not clear if this is a complication or a component of the aetiology of the condition. There are rare case reports of hepatic damage, renal insufficiency, haematological complications, orchitis and thyroiditis (Knowles *et al.* 1999; Schlienger and Shear 1998). Mortality ranges from around 5 per cent with SJS to 30–35 per cent with TEN (Roujeau *et al.* 1995). Prognostic factors include age, percentage of denuded skin, neutropenia, serum urea nitrogen level and visceral involvement (Ghislain and Roujeau 2002).

Pharmacological basis

The pathology in all cases of SJS and TEN is probably a cell-mediated hypersensitivity basis (Fritsch and Sidoroff 2000). The mechanism is currently thought to be related to Fas ligand mediated cell death (Wehrli *et al.* 2000). It is suggested that drugs are aetiologically important in almost all cases of TEN and 40–50 per cent of cases of SJS (Sane and Bhatt 2000). Non-drug causes include infections (especially herpes simplex, influenza, mumps, histoplasmosis and mycoplasma) and malignancies. Drug causes include both psychotropic and non-psychotropic medication, particularly sulfonamide antibiotics, allopurinol, non-steroidal anti-inflammatories, penicillins (Roujeau *et al.* 1995). The most important group of psychotropics aetiologically related to SJS and TEN are anticonvulsants. Phenytoin, phenobarbitol, carbamazepine (Rzany *et al.* 1999), lamotrigine (Calabrese *et al.* 2002) and possibly valproic acid (Rzany *et al.* 1999; Tsai and Chen 1998) are all implicated. While gabapentin is often considered a safe agent for patients with a previous history of drug allergies, there is a report of SJS in a patient with a previous history of drug reactions with phenytoin and carbamazepine (DeToledo *et al.* 1999). There have also been case reports of SJS following treatment with sertraline (Jan *et al.* 1999) and cocaine usage (Hofbauer *et al.* 2000). The period of risk with medication appears to be largely confined to the first eight weeks of treatment (Rzany *et al.* 1999).

Differential diagnosis

Other than differentiation between SJS, EMM and TEN, the differential diagnosis is from other conditions associated with erythematous skin lesions including burns, exfoliative dermatitis, staphylococcal scalded skin syndrome and autoimmune blistering disorders such as bullous pemphigoid and pemphigus. The presence of target lesions in SJS is thought to be pathognomonic. A definitive diagnosis of SJS or TEN can be established by skin biopsy.

Management

Prompt diagnosis and early withdrawal of all suspected drugs is essential. Morbidity and mortality is increased if the causative drug is withdrawn late and if the drug has a long half-life (Garcia-Doval *et al.* 2000). Supportive care is the mainstay of treatment for SJS. Referral to a dermatologist is essential and the advice of an opthalmologist may also be required. Speedy transfer to a specialist unit is associated with a decreased mortality rate (McGee and Munster 1998). The general principles of management of TEN are similar to those of burns patients and if extensive lesions are present, patients should be managed on ITU or a burns unit.

With regard to topical management, it has been suggested that areas with a positive Nikolsky sign heal faster when the epidermis is left *in situ* than if it is removed (Ghislain and Roujeau 2002). Otherwise protective dressings and topical antibiotics can be used as necessary. Prevention of ocular sequelae require daily examination by an ophthalmologist, with physiological saline or antibiotics administered as frequently as necessary.

With regard to systemic treatment, the use of corticosteroids is controversial (Sane and Bhatt 2000) with no randomized controlled trials. Some case series have suggested benefit (Tegelberg-Stassen *et al.*1990) and others no effect (Engelhardt *et al.* 1997). It has also been argued that corticosteroids may provoke prolonged wound healing, increased risk of infection and mask early signs of sepsis or severe gastrointestinal bleeding. This is supported by a retrospective study suggesting that corticosteroid treatment is an independent risk factor for increased mortality (Kelemen *et al.* 1995). As a result the current view is that corticosteroids are of unproven value in mild cases but may be deleterious in advanced forms of SJS and TEN (Ghislain and Roujeau 2002). More recently intravenous immunoglobulin, (IVIG), has been advocated for the treatment of TEN. There are no randomized controlled trials but a retrospective study of 48 patients showed a rapid reduction in new lesions and a survival rate of 88 per cent (Prins *et al.* 2003) though a prospective study of 34 patients suggested no benefit (Bachot *et al.* 2003). This treatment should only be considered in severe cases.

Sun exposure should be avoided for several months because ultraviolet light can worsen hyperpigmentation sequelae. In this regard sun blocks are recommended. Ophthalmological follow up is essential given the propensity for ocular complications. Glycaemia must be followed up because diabetes may develop after SJS and TEN (Ghislain and Roujeau 2002).

Risk factors and prevention

Observational studies suggest that the incidence of SJS is between one and six per million people per year and between 0.5 and 1.5 per million per year for TEN (Chan *et al.* 1990; Roujeau *et al.* 1990). Increased liability to SJS and TEN is present in patients with human immunodeficiency virus or systemic lupus erythematosus (Roujeau *et al.* 1995; Saiag *et al.* 1992).

The clinical use of drugs can influence the risk of SJS and TEN. For example, the risk of SJS with lamotrigine appears higher in children under 12 (Messenheimer 1998), when used concurrently with valproate (Yalcin and Karaduman 2000) or when the dose is rapidly increased (Wong *et al.* 1999). This led to a change in the manufacturer's dosage recommendations for lamotrigine in 1994. In Germany this was associated with a drop in the incidence of SJS secondary to lamotrigine treatment from 4.2 per cent to 0.02 per cent (Mockenhaupt *et al.* 2000). How these rates compare to rates reported for other drugs in different studies is difficult to ascertain. However, it has been reported that the risk from carbamazepine is about twice that of phenobarbitone and phenytoin, and four times the risk for valproate. To put this into a wider context, the risk associated with carbamazepine is around half that of sulphonamides (Roujeau *et al.* 1995).

With regard to prevention the most important factor is that survivors should not be re-exposed to the drug that led to the syndrome, or related compounds. Cross-reactions have been reported between different anticonvulsants. However if the underlying psychiatric illness requires treatment then it is safest to use alternate drugs that are structurally the most different from the causative agent. Because genetic factors are suspected in these conditions, it is recommended that the suspect drug should not be used in first degree relatives of the patient (Roujeau 1999).

Hypersensitivity syndrome associated with eosinophilia

A variety of hypersensitivity responses are responsible for most cutaneous reactions to drugs. The term 'hypersensitivity syndrome' usually refers to a specific, severe, idiosyncratic reaction also referred to as 'drug reaction with eosinophilia and systemic symptoms' or DRESS (Callot *et al.* 1996).

Clinical features

The skin manifestation of DRESS include a widespread and long-lasting morbilliform erythematous skin eruption often progressing to exfoliative dermatitis. Facial oedema occurs with a periorbital prominence. Vesicles and pustules may also be seen. Signs usually begin two to six weeks after starting the causal drug. Systemic symptoms include fever, lymphadenopathy and more rarely hepatitis, pneumonitis, myocarditis, periarditis and nephritis (Sullivan and Shear 2001). Blood abnormalities include an eosinophilia (by definition) but also mononucleosis in about 40 per cent of cases (Callot *et al.* 1996). Rash and hepatitis may last for several weeks following drug discontinuation though recovery is usually total. However there is an estimated mortality rate early in the illness of around 10 per cent (Ghislain and Roujeau 2002).

Pharmacological basis

DRESS has been associated with the anticonvulsants phenytoin, carbamazepine and phenobarbital with an estimated incidence of 1 per 5,000 to 10,000 exposures (Tennis and Stern 1997). Sulfonamides, allopurinol, nevirapine, minocycline and gold salts have also been implicated (Ghislain and Roujeau 2002).

Differential diagnosis

This is from other erythematous skin reactions to drugs. This would include EMM, SJS, TEN, toxic erythema and viral exanthems. Clinically, EMM/SJS can be distinguished by the presence of target lesions and TEN by denuded areas of skin and a positive Nikolsky sign. Viral exanthems would not occur with an eosinophilia. A skin biopsy may help in differentiation.

Management

Prompt recognition and withdrawal of the offending drug is the most important management issue. In the acute period, systemic steroids (0.5 to 1 mg/kg hydrocortisone) can be used. This leads to alleviation of symptoms and improved blood measures but its effect on the long term course is not known. However, since corticosteroids may exacerbate viral co-infections, it has been recommended that steroids be reserved for patients with life-threatening visceral manifestations (Ghislain and Roujeau 2002). In milder cases, topical steroids might be preferred.

Risk factors and prevention

It has been suggested that DRESS results from a defect of detoxification processes, such as slow acetylation (Ghislain and Roujeau 2002). This implies that patients with first degree relatives who have had DRESS may be at increased risk. A role of viral co-infection is also suspected, specifically with the herpes virus HHV6 (Suzuki *et al.* 1998).

Identification of the causative agent is important with regard to preventing further episodes. Cross-reactions are frequent between aromatic anticonvulsants (phenytoin, carbamazepine and Phenobarbital) and so all must be avoided if one has been causative.

Vasculitis

This is essentially inflammation and damage to blood vessel walls. It is an immune complex-mediated disease with many causes including infection

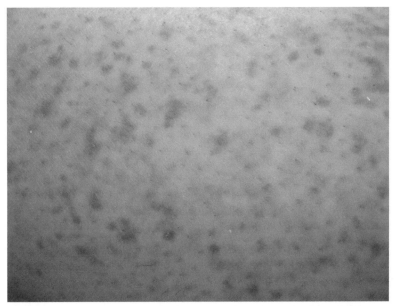

Fig. 15.5 Typical non blanching palpable purpuric papules on the lower leg in vasculitis (see Plate 5 of the plate section at the centre of this book).

(e.g. streptococcal), autoimmune diseases (e.g. rheumatoid arthritis) and an adverse reaction to drugs.

Clinical features

Vasculitis commonly occurs on the lower legs and arms but may be widespread. The onset is usually sudden. Clinical features may be variable but usually presents as palpable, non blanching, purpuric papules (Fig. 15.5). Pustular lesions, blisters, urticarial lesions and necrotizing ulcers can also occur. A prodrome of headache, general malaise, fever and arthralgia frequently occur before onset. Lesions usually subside within 2–3 weeks. Systemic involvement occurs with renal involvement seen most frequently in up to 60 per cent of patients (Ramsay and Fry 1969). The joints, gastrointestinal tract, CNS and lungs may also be affected.

Pharmacological basis

In drug-induced vasculitis, the vessels involved are usually small and are thought to become damaged due to immune complex deposition within the vessel wall. This is regarded as a type III hypersensitivity reaction mediated by antibodies directed against drug-related haptens. This usually occurs within a few weeks of starting a drug but may occur within days if a patient has previously received the drug and become sensitized to it. Phenytoin is the most commonly reported anticonvulsant causing vasculitis with sodium valproate and carbamazepine also being recognized. Less frequently, antidepressant and antipsychotic drugs have also been implicated (ten Holder *et al.* 2002). Non-psychiatric drugs that can cause vasculitis include angiotensin-converting enzyme inhibitors (ACE inhibitors), non-steroidal anti-inflammatory drugs (NSAIDs) and penicillins.

Differential diagnosis

This includes other causes of purpura including sepsis, (disseminated intravenous coagulopathy), thrombocytopenia, clotting abnormalities, vitamin C deficiency, steroid-induced purpura, and capillaropathy. A skin biopsy is usually diagnostic showing fibrinoid necrosis and leucocyte infiltration of the vessel wall in vasculitis.

Management

Identification and withdrawal of the offending drug is essential. Other causes of vasculitis need to be excluded with an infection screen, Antistreptolysin O Titre (ASOT), autoantibody screen, chest X-ray etc. Patients should be monitored closely for renal involvement with daily urine analysis and regular electrolytes check. Bed rest and leg elevation is usually adequate as treatment but if there is ulceration intervention with oral steroids or dapsone may be considered. If renal involvement occurs referral to a renal physician is necessary as aggressive immunosuppressive therapy may be warranted.

Risk factors and prevention

Stasis changes and oedema of the legs, other precipitants of vasculitis such as malignancy, autoimmune disease or infection, may increase the risk of development. Avoidance of the offending drug (and/or related drugs) is necessary for future prevention.

Photosensitivity

Two mechanisms exist for photosensitivity though both depend on the action of light, altering the molecular structure of the drug to produce a new photoproduct. Dermatological reactions result from either a toxic effect of these new molecules or, less commonly (Epstein and Wintroub 1985), an allergic reaction. Both will be considered together.

Clinical features

Photosensitivity may present with a wide morphological spectrum ranging from sunburn to eczematous, lichenoid and even bullous lesions occurring in light exposed areas of the skin. Phototoxic reactions are generally confined to the exposed areas and resemble sunburn, whereas photo-allergic reactions may become more generalized. Photo-allergic reactions, as opposed to photo-toxic effects, may present with a wheal and flare soon after exposure to light. A long-term consequence of photosensitivity is hyperpigmentation of the involved skin (see Fig. 15.6).

Photosensitivity can be accompanied by systemic complications, presumably caused by the presence in the body of phototoxic molecules. Neuropathy (Roelcke *et al.* 1992) and hepatitis (Ljunggren and Bojs 1991) have both been reported.

Pharmacological basis

Exposure of certain drugs to ultraviolet-A (UVA) and ultraviolet-B (UVB) light can lead to the generation of various photoproducts. These can be toxic and/or lead to allergic reactions. For example exposure of chlorpromazine to UVA produces a number of photoproducts including a promazinyl radical which has been shown to be toxic *in vivo* and *in vitro* (Chignell *et al.* 1985). It is possible to test for potential phototoxic effects of drugs *in vitro* by incubating erythrocytes with particular drugs together with exposure to UVA and UVB light. Toxicity is demonstrated by haemolysis. Such testing demonstrates the well known phototoxic effects of several phenothiazines and thioxanthenes, with the former being the most potent (Eberlein-Konig *et al.* 1997*a*).

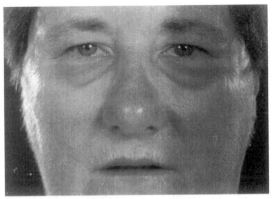

Fig.15.6 A patient with chlorpromazine induced pigmentation in sun exposed areas (see Plate 6 of the plate section at the centre of this book).

Clinically photosensitivity has been reported with many antipsychotics and antidepressants, the most common being chlorpromazine. However other typical antipsychotics can also cause these problems as well as atypicals including risperidone (Almond *et al.* 1998) and clozapine (Howanitz *et al.* 1995). Likewise antidepressants reported to be associated with photosensitivity include first generation drugs such as amitriptyline (Taniguchi and Hamada 1996) and phenelzine (Case *et al.* 1988), as well as newer ones such as fluoxetine (Gaufberg and Ellison 1995) and fluvoxamine (Gillet-Terver *et al.* 1996). Photosensitivity has also been reported as one of the most common side effects of hypericum (St John's Wort) with one case per 300,000 treated patients (Schulz 2001). Photosensitivity has also been reported with other psychotropic medication including alprazolam (Watanabe *et al.* 1999) and carbamazepine (Ljunggren and Bojs 1991) as well as non-psychiatric drugs, for exmaple amiodarone, quinine and thiazide diuretics.

Differential diagnosis

The diagnosis of photosensitivity can be complicated since, at the mild end of the severity spectrum, the syndrome needs to be differentiated from 'normal' sunburn. More severe reactions may resemble porphyria cutanea tarda (Harth and Rapoport 1996). The latter may be excluded by a porphyria screen. For a definitive diagnosis, photoprovocation tests can be conducted.

Management

Once the diagnosis is confirmed it may be necessary for the patient to discontinue treatment with the offending drug. However if the photosensitivity is mild and the need for the drug great, then the situation may be managed with sun block that reduces UVA and UVB absorption by the skin.

Risk factors and prevention

The absolute numbers of patients experiencing photosensitivity with psychotropic drugs is unknown. It is likely that patients treated with chlorinated phenothiazines (such as chlorpromazine, prochlorpromazine and perphenazine) and tricyclic antidepressants with a nitrogen and/or a sulphur molecule in their structure (such as amitriptyline and clomipramine), thioxanthenes and carbamazepine are at greatest risk. Photosensitivity occurs in patients of all ethnic backgrounds irrespective of skin pigmentation (Pazzagli *et al.* 1998). Patients who have had a photosensitive reaction to one drug may be more prone to developing one to other medication.

Given the risks of photosensitivity it is important to advise patients treated with higher risk drugs to use sun block if they have a high degree of exposure to sun light. It is important to remember that exposure to UVA and UVB occurs even in cloudy weather. There has been a report suggesting that oral vitamin C and E combined may protect against photosensitivity (Eberlein-Konig *et al.* 1997*b*).

Hyperpigmentation

Clinical features

Hyperpigmentation secondary to medication typically has a photo-distribution. Pigmentation is seen on the face, dorsum of the hands and extensor aspects of the forearms but skin folds and mucous membranes tend to be spared. The pigmentation typically has a blue or slate grey colouration, which is non-pruritic (Fig. 15.6). This dermatological syndrome is usually seen only after several years of treatment with the causative agent.

Lenticular and corneal pigmentary deposits also occur in patients with hyperpigmentation. Retinitis pigmentosa, characterized by black pigment deposited around the fundus together with a loss of night vision, is associated with antipsychotic treatment, particularly with thioridazine. However the mechanism behind this syndrome may be different to that underlying other ocular deposits (Fornaro *et al.* 2002; see below).

Pharmacological basis

Hyperpigmentation has most commonly been reported following long term imipramine treatment (Angel *et al.* 2002; Atkin and Fitzpatrick 2000) but has also been reported following treatment with other tricyclic antidepressants (Milionis *et al.* 2000) and phenothiazines (Kass and Hsu 2001). There are also case reports of hyperpigmentation associated with citalopram (Inaloz *et al.* 2001) and oxprenolol administration (Harrower and Strong 1977). Non-psychiatric drugs associated with skin hyperpigmentation include hydroxy-chloroquine and minocycline (Mehrany *et al.* 2003). The characteristic pathological features have been suggested to result from the development of drug-melanosome complexes caused by chronic photoactivation (Sicari *et al.* 1999).

Retinitis pigmentosa, particularly associate with antipsychotic usage, may have a different pharmacological basis. It has been suggested that dopamine D_4 receptor blockade by antipsychotics disrupts the normal control of melatonin sysnthesis which increases photoreceptor susceptibility to light (Fornaro *et al.* 2002). This may explain the lack of an association between this condition and atypical antipsychotics.

Differential diagnosis

Other causes of pigmentation within the skin need to be excluded, such as Addison's disease, haemochromatosis, hyperthyroidism, post inflammatory pigmentation, chloasma etc. Diagnosis of drug-induced pigmentation can be confirmed by skin biopsy. Yellow-brown deposits in macrophages are found in the upper and mid dermis. These stain for melatonin with a Fontana–Masson stain, but do not stain for iron (Angel *et al.* 2002; Sicari *et al.* 1999).

Management

Few treatments exist for hyperpigmentation. Withdrawal of the drug may be associated with a slow gradual improvement in skin pigmentation over months to years, though ocular deposits may persist for much longer (Lal *et al.* 1993). Laser treatment may be successful (Atkin and Fitzpatrick 2000) but this is not in routine use.

Risk factors and prevention

This syndrome appears to be entirely idiosyncratic with no risk factors reported but may be related to length of time on the drug.

Miscellaneous dermatological syndromes

Many other drug reactions that are less serious are reported with drugs used by psychiatrists. These will not be covered here, but they include the exacerbation of pre-existing psoriasis and possible induction of psoriasis by lithium carbonate. Other reactions attributed to lithium include acneiform eruptions, lupus like eruptions and alopecia (Abel *et al.* 1986). Lupus-like reactions have also been reported with chlorpromazine (Fabius and Gaulhofer 1971). Other drug reactions to psychotropic medications include exfoliative dermatitis, lichenoid drug eruptions, fixed drug eruptions and seborrheic rashes (Kimyai-Asadi *et al.* 1999). Other idiosyncratic reactions include curly hair with valproate therapy (Jeavons *et al.* 1977).

Summary: Stevens–Johnson syndrome and toxic epidermal necrolysis

Definition	Widespread erythema and blistering with systemic illness.
Incidence	Unclear and varies between drugs. Probably less than 0.1% of patients prescribed at risk drugs.
Drugs causing syndrome	Carbamazepine, lamotrigine, phenobarbital, phenytoin, valproate. Low risk with gabapentin, sertraline and cocaine. Can occur with non-psychiatric drugs

	e.g. sulfonamide antibiotics, allopurinol, non-steroidal anti-inflammatories, penicillins.
Key symptoms	Target lesions and positive Nikolsky's sign. Mucosal membrane involvement.
	Frequent eye involvement. Systemic illness. Onset within eight weeks of start of drug.
Pharmacological mechanism	Hypersensitivity reaction. Genetic and infective factors increase risk.
Investigations to confirm diagnosis	Skin biopsy.
Management	Discontinuation of drug treatment. Referral to specialist services: dermatology, ophthalmology and burns unit or intensive care for severe illness. Supportive therapy.
Further reading	Ghislain PD and Roujeau JC (2002) Treatment of severe drug reactions: Stevens–Johnson syndrome, toxic epidermal necrolysis and hypersensitivity syndrome. *Dermatology Online Journal*, **8**, 5.
	Fritsch PO and Sidoroff A (2000) Drug-induced Stevens–Johnson syndrome/toxic epidermal necrolysis. *American Journal of Clinical Dermatology*, **1**, 349–60.
	Calabrese JR, Sullivan JR, Bowden CL, *et al.* (2002) Rash in multicenter trials of lamotrigine in mood disorders: clinical relevance and management. *Journal of Clinical Psychiatry*, **63**, 1012–19.

Summary: Hypersensitivity syndrome with eosinophilia (DRESS)

Definition	Skin eruption with eosinophilia and systemic symptoms
Incidence	One per 5,000–10,000 exposures.
Drugs causing syndrome	Carbamazepine, phenytoin and phenobarbitol. Non-psychiatric drugs causing
	DRESS include sulfonamides, allopurinol, nevirapine, minocycline and gold salts.
Key symptoms	Maculopapular erythematous skin rash arising two to six weeks after drug commencement. Fever, lymphadenopathy and hepatitis.
Pharmacological mechanism	Hypersensitivity reaction. Genetic and infective risk factors. Reduction in metabolism of drug.
Investigations to confirm diagnosis	Eosinophil count, liver function tests.

Management	Discontinuation of causative agent. Specialist advice. Topical steroids. Systemic steroids in acute phase for patients with life threatening visceral manifestations.
Further reading	Callot V, Roujeau JC, Bagot M, et al. (1996) Drug-induced pseudolymphoma and hypersensitivity syndrome. Two different clinical entities. Archives of Dermatology, **132**, 1315–21.
	Ghislain PD and Roujeau JC (2002) Treatment of severe drug reactions: Stevens–Johnson syndrome, toxic epidermal necrolysis and hypersensitivity syndrome. Dermatology Online Journal, **8**, 5.
	Sullivan JR and Shear NH (2001) The drug hypersensitivity syndrome: what is the pathogenesis? Archives of Dermatology, **137**, 357–64.

Summary: Vasculitis

Definition	Vessel wall damage due to immune complex deposition
Incidence	Varies between drugs. Probably less than 0.1% of patients prescribed at risk drugs.
Drugs causing syndrome	Fluoxetine, carbamazepine, phenytoin and sodium valproate. Can occur with non-psychiatric drugs including ACE inhibitors, NSAIDs and penicillins.
Key symptoms	Palpable painful purpuric (non blanching) lesions over legs and arms.
Pharmacological mechanism	Presumed type III hypersensitivity reaction.
Investigations to confirm diagnosis	Skin biopsy, vasculitis screen, monitor for renal and other systemic involvement (gastrointestinal system, respiratory system, CNS).
Management	Discontinuation of drug treatment. Bed rest. Referral to specialist dermatological services plus renal if evidence of kidney involvement. May need systemic immunosuppression.
Further reading	Kimyai-Asadi A, Harris JC, and Nousari HC (1999) Critical overview: adverse cutaneous reactions to psychotropic medications. Journal of Clinical Psychiatry, **60**, 714–25.
	ten Holder SM, Joy MS, and Falk RJ (2002) Cutaneous and systemic manifestations of drug-induced vasculitis. The Annals of Pharmacotherapy, **36**, 130–47.

Roujeau JC and Stern RS (1994) Severe adverse cutaneous reactions to drugs. *New England Journal of Medicine*, **331**, 1272–85.

Summary: Skin photosensitivity

Definition	Erythema/pigmentation of sun exposed skin.
Incidence	Unknown – rare.
Drugs causing syndrome	Phenothiazines and more rarely thioxanthenes. Also reported with atypical antipsychotics (risperidone, clozapine) antidepressants (amitriptyline, phenelzine, fluoxetine, fluvoxamine), St John's Wort, alprazolam and carbamazepine. Can occur with non-psychiatric drugs e.g. amiodarone, quinine and thiazide diuretics.
Key symptoms	Erythema +/− blistering or increased pigmentation in sun-exposed sites.
Pharmacological mechanism	Development of photo toxic products or haptens after ultraviolet light exposure, abnormal accumulation of drug within skin.
Investigations to confirm diagnosis	Photochallenge testing, skin biopsy.
Management	Withdrawal of drug, topical steroids for acute inflammation.
Further reading	Allen JE (1993) Drug-induced photosensitivity. *Clinical Pharmacology*, **12**, 580–7.
	Harth Y and Rapoport M (1996) Photosensitivity associated with antipsychotics, antidepressants and anxiolytics. *Drug Safety*, **14**, 252–9.

Summary: Skin hyperpigmentation

Definition	Pigmentation following long-term drug treatment.
Incidence	Rare.
Drugs causing syndrome	Tricyclic antidepressants (especially imipramine) and phenothiazines (especially chlorpromazine). Can occur with non-psychiatric drugs e.g. minocycline and hydroxychloroquine.
Key symptoms	Blue or slate-grey coloured pigmentation in skin areas exposed to the light.
	Occurs after several years treatment.
Pharmacological mechanism	Photoactivation leading to drug-melanosome complexes that are phagocytosed by macrophages in the dermis.

Investigations to confirm diagnosis	Skin biopsy.
Management	Withdrawal of drug. Sun-block.
Further reading	Bloom D, Krishnan B, Thavundayil JX, *et al.* (1993) Resolution of chlorpromazine-induced cutaneous pigmentation following substitution with levomepromazine or other neuroleptics. *Acta Psychiatrica Scandinavica*, **87**, 223–4.
	Lal S, Bloom D, Silver B, *et al.* (1993) Replacement of chlorpromazine with other neuroleptics: effect on abnormal skin pigmentation and ocular changes. *J. Psychiatr. Neurosci.*, **18**, 173–7.
	Satanove A (1965) Pigmentation due to phenothiazines in high and prolonged dosage. *JAMA*, **191**, 263–8.

References

Abel EA, DiCicco LM, Orenberg EK, *et al.* (1986). Drugs in exacerbation of psoriasis. *J Am Acad Dermatol*, **15**, 1007–22.

Allen JE (1993). Drug-induced photosensitivity. *Clin Pharmacol*, **12**, 580–7.

Almond DS, Rhodes LE, and Pirmohamed M (1998). Risperidone-induced photosensitivity. *Postgrad Med J*, **74**, 252–3.

Angel TA, Stalkup JR, and Hsu S (2002). Photodistributed blue-gray pigmentation of the skin associated with long-term imipramine use. *Int J Dermatol*, **41**, 327–9.

Atkin DH and Fitzpatrick RE (2000). Laser treatment of imipramine-induced hyperpigmentation. *J Am Acad Dermatol*, **43**, 77–80.

Bachot N, Revuz J, and Roujeau JC (2003). Intravenous immunoglobulin treatment for Stevens–Johnson syndrome and toxic epidermal necrolysis: a prospective noncomparative study showing no benefit on mortality or progression. *Arch Dermatol*, **139**, 33–6.

Bloom D, Krishnan B, Thavundayil JX, *et al.* (1993). Resolution of chlorpromazine-induced cutaneous pigmentation following substitution with levomepromazine or other neuroleptics. *Acta Psychiatr Scand*, **87**, 223–4.

Calabrese JR, Sullivan JR, Bowden CL, *et al.* (2002). Rash in multicenter trials of lamotrigine in mood disorders: clinical relevance and management. *J Clin Psychiatry*, **63**, 1012–19.

Callot V, Roujeau JC, Bagot M, *et al.* (1996). Drug-induced pseudolymphoma and hypersensitivity syndrome. Two different clinical entities. *Arch Dermatol*, **132**, 1315–21.

Case JD, Yusk JW, and Callen JP (1988). Photosensitive reaction to phenelzine: a case report. *Photodermatology*, **5**, 101–2.

Chan HL, Stern RS, Arndt KA, *et al.* (1990). The incidence of erythema multiforme, Stevens–Johnson syndrome, and toxic epidermal necrolysis. A population-based study with particular reference to reactions caused by drugs among outpatients. *Arch Dermatol*, **126**, 43–7.

Chignell CF, Motten AG, and Buettner GR, (1985). Photoinduced free radicals from chlorpromazine and related phenothiazines: relationship to phenothiazine-induced photosensitization. *Environ Health Perspect*, **64**, 103–10.

DeToledo JC, Minagar A, Lowe MR, *et al.* (1999). Skin eruption with gabapentin in a patient with repeated AED-induced Stevens–Johnson's syndrome. *Ther Drug Monit*, **21**, 137–8.

Eberlein-Konig B, Bindl A, and Przybilla B (1997*a*). Phototoxic properties of neuroleptic drugs. *Dermatol*, **194**, 131–5.

Eberlein-Konig B, Placzek M, and Przybilla B (1997*b*). Phototoxic lysis of erythrocytes from humans is reduced after oral intake of ascorbic acid and d-alpha-tocopherol. *Photodermatol Photoimmunol Photomed*, **13**, 173–7.

Engelhardt SL, Schurr MJ, and Helgerson RB (1997). Toxic epidermal necrolysis: an analysis of referral patterns and steroid usage. *J Burn Care Rehabil*, **18**, 520–4.

Epstein JH and Wintroub BU (1985). Photosensitivity due to drugs. *Drugs*, **30**, 42–57.

Fabius AJ and Gaulhofer WK (1971). Systemic lupus erythematosus induced by psychotropic drugs. *Acta Rheumatol Scand*, **17**, 137–47.

Fornaro P, Calabria G, Corallo G, *et al.* (2002). Pathogenesis of degenerative retinopathies induced by thioridazine and other antipsychotics: a dopamine hypothesis. *Doc Ophthalmol*, **105**, 41–9.

Fritsch PO and Sidoroff A (2000). Drug-induced Stevens–Johnson syndrome/toxic epidermal necrolysis. *Am J Clin Dermatol*, **1**, 349–60.

Garcia-Doval I, LeCleach L, Bocquet H, *et al.* (2000). Toxic epidermal necrolysis and Stevens–Johnson syndrome: does early withdrawal of causative drugs decrease the risk of death? *Arch Dermatol*, **136**, 323–7.

Gaufberg E and Ellison JM (1995). Photosensitivity reaction to fluoxetine. *J Clin Psychiatry*, **56**, 486.

Ghislain PD and Roujeau JC (2002). Treatment of severe drug reactions: Stevens–Johnson syndrome, toxic epidermal necrolysis and hypersensitivity syndrome. *Dermatol Online J*, **8**, 1, 5.

Gillet-Terver MN, Modiano P, Trechot P, *et al.* (1996). Fluvoxamine photosensitivity. *Aus J Dermatol*, **37**, 62.

Harrower AD and Strong JA (1977). Hyperpigmentation associated with oxprenolol administration. *BMJ*, **2**, 6082, 296.

Harth Y and Rapoport M (1996). Photosensitivity associated with antipsychotics, antidepressants and anxiolytics. *Drug Saf*, **14**, 252–9.

Hofbauer GF, Burg G, and Nestle FO (2000). Cocaine-related Stevens–Johnson syndrome. *Dermatol*, **201**, 258–60.

Howanitz E, Pardo M, and Losonczy M (1995). Photosensitivity to clozapine. *J Clin Psychiatry*, **56**, 589.

Inaloz HS, Kirtak N, Herken H, *et al.* (2001). Citalopram-induced photopigmentation. *J Dermatol*, **28**, 742–5.

Jan V, Toledano C, Machet L, *et al.* (1999). Stevens–Johnson syndrome after sertraline. *Acta Derm Venereol*, **79**, 401.

Jeavons PM, Clark JE, and Harding GF (1977). Valproate and curly hair. *Lancet*,1, no. 8007, 359.

Kass J and Hsu S (2001). What is your diagnosis? Hyperpigmentation due to long-term chlorpromazine use. *Cutis*, **68**, 252, 260.

Kelemen JJ, Cioffi WG, McManus WF, *et al.* (1995). Burn center care for patients with toxic epidermal necrolysis. *J Am Coll Surg*, **180**, 273–8.

Kimyai-Asadi A, Harris JC, and Nousari C (1999). Critical overview: adverse cutaneous reactions to psychotropic medications. *J Clin Psychiatry*, **60**, 714–25.

Knowles SR, Shapiro LE, and Shear NH (1999). Anticonvulsant hypersensitivity syndrome: incidence, prevention and management. *Drug Saf*, **21**, 489–501.

Lal S, Bloom D, Silver B, *et al.* (1993). Replacement of chlorpromazine with other neuroleptics: effect on abnormal skin pigmentation and ocular changes. *J Psychiatr Neurosci*, **18**, 173–7.

Ljunggren B and Bojs G (1991). A case of photosensitivity and contact allergy to systemic tricyclic drugs, with unusual features. *Contact Dermatitis*, **24**, 259–65.

McGee T and Munster A (1998). Toxic epidermal necrolysis syndrome: mortality rate reduced with early referral to regional burn center. *Plast Reconstr Surg*, **102**, 1018–22.

Mehrany K, Kist JM, Ahmed DD, *et al.* (2003). Minocycline induced cutaneous pigmentation. *Int J Dermatol*, **42**, 551–2.

Messenheimer JA (1998). Rash in adult and pediatric patients treated with lamotrigine. *Can J Neurolog Sci*, **25**, S14–18.

Milionis HJ, Skopelitou A, and Elisaf MS (2000). Hypersensitivity syndrome caused by amitriptyline administration. *Postgrad Med J*, **76**, 361–3.

Mockenhaupt M, Schlingmann J, and Schroeder W (2000). Antiepileptic therapy and the risk of severe cutaneous reactions (SCAR). *Neurology*, **54** (Suppl. 3), A84.

Pazzagli L, Banfi R, Borselli G, *et al.* (1998). Photosensitivity reaction to fluoxetine and alprazolam. *Pharm World Sci*, **20**, 136.

Prins C, Kerdel FA, Padilla RS, *et al.* (2003). Treatment of toxic epidermal necrolysis with high-dose intravenous immunoglobulins: multicenter retrospective analysis of 48 consecutive cases. *Arch Dermatol*, **139**, 26–32.

Ramsay C and Fry L (1969). Allergic vasculitis: clinical and histological features and incidence of renal involvement. *Br J Dermatol*, **81**, 96–102.

Roelcke U, Hornstein C, Hund E, *et al.* (1992). Acute neuropathy in perazine-treated patients after sun exposure. *Lancet*, **340**, 729–30.

Roujeau JC (1999). Treatment of severe drug eruptions. *J Dermatol*, **26**, 718–22.

Roujeau JC, Guillaume JC, Fabre JP, *et al.* (1990). Toxic epidermal necrolysis (Lyell syndrome). Incidence and drug etiology in France, 1981–1985. *Arch Dermatol*, **126**, 37–42.

Roujeau JC, Kelly JP, Naldi L, *et al.* (1995). Medication use and the risk of Stevens–Johnson syndrome or toxic epidermal necrolysis. *New Engl J Med*, **333**, 1600–7.

Roujeau JC and Stern RS (1994). Severe adverse cutaneous reactions to drugs. *New Engl J Med*, **331**, 1272–85.

Rzany B, Correia O, Kelly JP, *et al*. (1999). Risk of Stevens–Johnson syndrome and toxic epidermal necrolysis during first weeks of antiepileptic therapy: a case-control study. Study Group of the International Case Control Study on Severe Cutaneous Adverse Reactions. *Lancet*, **353**, 2190–4.

Saiag P, Caumes E, Chosidow O, *et al*. (1992). Drug-induced toxic epidermal necrolysis (Lyell syndrome) in patients infected with the human immunodeficiency virus. *J Am Acad Dermatol*, **26**, 567–74.

Sane SP and Bhatt AD (2000). Stevens–Johnson syndrome and toxic epidermal necrolysis-challenges of recognition and management. *J Assoc Physician*, **48**, 999–1003.

Satanove A (1965). Pigmentation due to phenothiazines in high and prolonged dosage. *JAMA*, **191**, 263–8.

Schlienger RG and Shear NH (1998). Antiepileptic drug hypersensitivity syndrome. *Epilepsia*, **39** (Suppl. 7), S3–7.

Schulz V (2001). Incidence and clinical relevance of the interactions and side effects of Hypericum preparations. *Phytomedicin*, **8**, 152–60.

Sicari MC, Lebwohl M, Baral J, *et al*. (1999). Photoinduced dermal pigmentation in patients taking tricyclic antidepressants: histology, electron microscopy, and energy dispersive spectroscopy. *J Am Acad Dermatol*, **40**, 2, Pt 2, 290–3.

Srebrnik A, Hes JP and Brenner S (1991). Adverse cutaneous reactions to psychotropic drugs. *Acta Derm Venereol Suppl (Stockholm)*, **158**, 1–12.

Suarez Moro R, Trapiella Martinez L, Avanzas Gonzalez E, *et al*. (2000). Stevens–Johnson syndrome secondary to carbamazepine mediated by photosensitivity. *An Med Interna*, **17**, 105–6.

Sullivan JR and Shear NH (2001). The drug hypersensitivity syndrome: what is the pathogenesis? *Arch Dermatol*, **137**, 357–64.

Suzuki Y, Inagi R, Aono T, *et al*. (1998). Human herpesvirus 6 infection as a risk factor for the development of severe drug-induced hypersensitivity syndrome. *Arch Dermatol*, **134**, 1108–12.

Taniguchi S and Hamada T (1996). Photosensitivity and thrombocytopenia due to amitriptyline. *Am J Hematol*, **53**, 49–50.

Tegelberg-Stassen MJ, van Vloten WA, and Baart dlF (1990). Management of nonstaphylococcal toxic epidermal necrolysis: follow-up study of 16 case histories. *Dermatologica*, **180**, 124–9.

ten Holder SM, Joy MS, and Falk RJ (2002). Cutaneous and systemic manifestations of drug-induced vasculitis. *Ann Pharmacother*, **36**, 130–47.

Tennis P and Stern RS (1997). Risk of serious cutaneous disorders after initiation of use of phenytoin, carbamazepine, or sodium valproate: a record linkage study. *Neurology*, **49**, 542–6.

Tsai SJ and Chen YS (1998). Valproic acid-induced Stevens–Johnson syndrome. *J Clin Psychopharmacol*, **18**, 420.

Watanabe Y, Kawada A, Ohnishi Y, *et al*. (1999). Photosensitivity due to alprazolam with positive oral photochallenge test after 17 days administration. *J Am Acad Dermatol*, **40**, 5, Pt 2, 832–3.

Wehrli P, Viard I, Bullani R, *et al.* (2000). Death receptors in cutaneous biology and disease. *J Invest Dermatol*, **115**, 141–8.

Wong IC, Mawer GE, and Sander JW (1999). Factors influencing the incidence of lamotrigine-related skin rash. *Ann Pharmacother*, **33**, 1037–42.

Yalcin B and Karaduman A (2000). Stevens–Johnson syndrome associated with concomitant use of lamotrigine and valproic acid. *J Am Acad Dermatol*, **43**, 898–9.

Chapter 16

Miscellaneous syndromes: anticholinergic toxicity, clozapine toxicity, and hypertensive crisis with MAOIs

Trevor I Prior and Glen B Baker

Introduction

Many medications have pharmacological properties which extend beyond their intended targets in therapy and result in adverse effects. In many cases, the range of symptoms produced is broad and multisystemic, resulting in a syndrome rather than a single clinical complaint. This chapter deals with three such syndromes: anticholinergic toxicity, clozapine toxicity and hypertensive crisis.

Anticholinergic toxicity can be produced by individual psychotropic drugs but is often the result of the additive effects of the anticholinergic properties of a number of medications. Clozapine toxicity can be caused by an increase in serum levels of clozapine as a result of either inhibition of catabolic enzymes involved in its degradation by concomitantly prescribed drugs or reversal of the induction of these enzymes. Hypertensive crisis, as described in this chapter, results from an interaction between monoamine oxidase inhibitors (MAOIs) and certain foodstuffs and medications leading to an increased release of noradrenaline (norepinephrine).

In their own way, these syndromes also serve to remind the clinician of the need to be aware of pharmacodynamic and pharmacokinetic properties of the medications being taken by their patients. This information aids not only in diagnosing the cause of the syndromes, but also provides knowledge to avoid these side effects in the first place.

Anticholinergic toxicity

Clinical features

The symptoms of anticholinergic toxicity are diverse (see Table 16.1) and can involve the central nervous system, cardiovascular system, gastrointestinal

Table 16.1 Symptoms of anticholinergic toxicity

Central nervous system:
– sedation
– stuttering
– restlessness and irritability
– confusion
– hallucinations
– seizures
– coma
Eye:
– blurred vision
– dry eyes
– dilated pupils
– photophobia
– exacerbation of narrow angle glaucoma
Cardiovascular:
– sinus tachycardia
– flushed facies
Gastrointestinal:
– dry mouth
– constipation
– decreased bowel sounds
Genitourinary:
– urinary retention
Sweat glands:
– decreased sweating
– increased temperature

system and genitourinary system as well as the eyes and sweat glands (Meltzer and Fatemi 1998). Isolated symptoms of anticholinergic toxicity are very common, but are often seen as being a part of the disease process, an unavoidable consequence of treatment, or as a normal part of life processes such as ageing. They may be merely uncomfortable in a younger individual of good physical health, but may have significant impact upon the quality of life of the physically ill or the elderly. The full syndrome often emerges gradually and is potentially life-threatening.

Early features include dry mouth, blurred vision, dilated pupils, tachycardia and difficulty passing urine. As the syndrome progresses there may be difficulty swallowing, restlessness and fatigue, and the skin becomes hot, dry and red. Changes in mental state usually occur later than the physical symptoms and include agitation, delirium, auditory and visual hallucinations and eventually coma. Death can occur via hyperpyrexia or injury sustained while delirious.

Pharmacological basis

The clinical features are primarily the effect of blockade of muscarinic receptors (Brown and Taylor 1996). Thus the syndrome is more correctly termed antimuscarinic toxicity rather than anticholinergic toxicity. Medications with anticholinergic properties come from a range of classes, including antidepressants (tricyclics, paroxetine), antihistamines, antipsychotics (conventional agents, olanzapine, clozapine), antispasmodics, mydriatics and anticholinergic drugs. The latter are often prescribed to treat antipsychotic-induced parkinsonism. Anticholinergic toxicity is normally a result of the additive effects of these agents, although monotherapy may cause symptoms. The syndrome can also result from intentional overdose of a drug with a significant antimuscarinic effect and also from ingestion of some plants, including deadly nightshade, red sage, Jerusalem cherry, burdock root and certain mushrooms (gyromitra toxin).

The visual effects of anticholinergic agents occur via three main mechanisms. First, muscarinic blockade inhibits pupillary constrictor muscles, resulting in unopposed dilation. In susceptible individuals this can result in exacerbation of narrow angle glaucoma. Similarly, ciliary muscle function is impaired, resulting in a loss of ocular accommodation, particularly in near vision. Finally, lacrimation can be impaired, resulting in dry eyes or a 'sandy' feeling in the eyes.

Sinus tachycardia caused by anticholinergic agents is the result of blockade of vagal nerve stimulation. The mechanism by which these agents cause peripheral cutaneous vasodilation, resulting in the blush reaction, is unclear.

Inhibition of salivary secretions results in a dry oral mucosa. In addition, anticholinergic activity causes relaxation of the smooth muscles of the intestine with a subsequent decrease in both tone and propulsion. The result is a lengthening of intestinal transit time and constipation. In extreme cases, the gastric musculature can be completely paralysed resulting in an ileus. In a similar fashion, inhibition of the contraction of the smooth muscle of the bladder can cause urinary retention.

Sweat glands are innervated by cholinergic fibres. Thus, blockade by anticholinergic agents results in a decrease in secretion. This can manifest in decreased sweating and a disruption in thermoregulation, resulting in an elevated temperature and an increased risk of heat stroke.

Differential diagnosis

As with any medical syndrome which can cause a variety of symptoms in a diverse range of body systems, the list of differential diagnoses is extensive. Therefore, it is imperative that the clinician be able to recognize the multi-system pattern of symptoms. It is extremely unlikely that anticholinergic toxicity states will cause only one or two symptoms. Broadly, the differential diagnoses include hyperthyroidism, hypoglycaemia, meningitis, neuroleptic malignant syndrome (NMS) and exacerbation of schizophrenia.

Both anticholingeric toxicity and NMS are characterized by pyrexia, fluctuating levels of consciousness and tachycardia. One of the most useful distinguishing features is that the skin is dry in anticholinergic toxicity but sweaty in NMS. Also rigidity is a key feature of NMS but is absent in anticholinergic toxicity.

Management

Since anticholinergic toxicity is often the direct result of the additive effects of the anticholinergic activity of a number of pharmaceutical agents, the mainstay of treating this syndrome is to reduce the dose and number of medications taken.

In extreme cases of anticholinergic intoxication, characterized by delirium, coma, seizures, hallucinations and tachycardia (in addition to the usual peripheral symptoms), treatment should begin with the immediate discontinuation of all medications with anticholinergic activity. In these cases, physostigmine (a cholinesterase inhibitor) can be administered both to confirm the diagnosis and to treat the toxic state. It should only be used when cardiac monitoring and life support services are available since this medication can cause profound bradycardia, severe hypotension and bronchospasm. Physostigmine is given 1 to 2 mg IV over 2–3 minutes (repeated every 30 to 60 minutes) and should be repeated in 15 to 20 minutes if no improvement is seen (*Drug Facts and Comparisons* 2001). Benzodiazapines can be given to control agitation.

Complaints of eye pain may indicate the presence of acute ocular hypertension caused by exacerbation of narrow angle glaucoma. An urgent ophthalmic examination is required.

Constipation can be lessened by maintaining adequate hydration or by regular administration of a stool softener or bulk laxative.

Risk factors and prevention

The development of anticholinergic toxicity is usually the result of concomitant therapy with medications that have anticholinergic activity. Thus, minimizing the number and dosage of these agents is an effective tool in preventing this syndrome.

Individuals with organic brain dysfunction are at greater risk of developing central nervous system symptoms.

The elderly are more likely to receive multiple medications, and are also at increased risk of developing the cognitive and peripheral symptoms of anticholinergic toxicity (Tune 2001).

Individuals with pre-existing medical problems may present with a more limited symptom profile. For example, an individual with pre-existing narrow angle glaucoma may complain of eye pain (due to an acute increase in ocular pressure). Similarly, an individual with ischaemic heart disease may complain of an increase in angina-related pain due to increased heart rate. Being cognizant of the other symptoms related to anticholinergic toxicity will alert the clinician to the cause of these more severe conditions.

Clozapine toxicity

Clinical features

Clozapine toxicity reflects high plasma levels of clozapine and/or its metabolites. Symptoms include drowsiness, delirium, hypotension, hypersalivation, tachycardia, respiratory depression, myoclonic jerks, seizures and coma (Le Blaye *et al.* 1992). The syndrome may result from an excessive dose of clozapine being prescribed or from deliberate overdose. However in this chapter we focus on it occurring as a result of pharmacokinetic interactions between clozapine and concomitant medication.

Pharmacological basis

The liver is the primary site of the metabolism of clozapine. Clozapine is oxidized by a family of enzymes called the cytochrome P450 (CYP) system. Specifically, clozapine is metabolized primarily by CYP1A2, with additional contributions by CYP2C19, CYP2D6 and CYP3A4. Like most CYP enzymes, the activity of CYP1A2 can be affected by other consumed medications. A drug, or its metabolites, may be a substrate for, an inhibitor of, or an inducer of a CYP enzyme. Thus, concomitantly prescribed medications which affect these CYPs can alter serum levels of clozapine and its metabolites (reviewed in Prior and Baker 2003).

As stated, clozapine is primarily metabolized by the enzyme CP1A2. Several other medications are known to inhibit or increase the activity of CYP1A2 (Table 16.2). The inhibition of clozapine metabolism has been shown to have clinical consequences. For example, concomitant treatment with the selective serotonin reuptake inhibitor (SSRI) antidepressant fluvoxamine, an inhibitor of CYP1A2, causes an increase in serum clozapine levels and can have adverse effects, including seizures (Wetzel *et al.* 1998). Individuals vary in their susceptibility to pharmacokinetic interactions and one cannot predict, on an individual basis, the extent to which a patient's plasma level of clozapine will change following such co-prescribing. Thus vigilance is required if such drug combinations are used. In a prospective study, the addition of fluvoxamine 50 mg per day increased the mean trough concentration of serum clozapine,

Table 16.2 Representative inhibitors and inducers of CYP1A2

Inhibitors	Inducers
cimetidine	carbamazepine
ciprofloxacin	cigarette smoke
erythromycin	rifampin
fluvoxamine	
grapefruit juice	
norfloxacin	
fluroquinoline	

at steady state, by three-fold compared to baseline (Wetzel *et al.* 1998). However, in some patients clozapine levels can rise up to nine-fold with the addition of fluvoxamine 100 to 200 mg per day (Dequardo and Roberts 1996; Armstrong and Stephans 1997).

Reversal of CYP1A2 induction also can have clinical consequences. For example, cigarette smoking is known to induce CYP1A2 activity. Therefore, cessation of smoking causes a decrease in CYP1A2 activity resulting in an increase in serum clozapine levels. In one study smoking cessation was followed by a mean 72 per cent increase in clozapine levels (Meyer 2001). Clozapine-induced seizures have been reported to occur after patients stopped smoking (Skogh *et al.* 1999).

Inhibition of other CYP enzymes involved in the metabolism of clozapine appears to be less problematic. Inhibition of CYP2D6 can cause an increase in serum clozapine levels, but clinical features have not been reported. Inhibition of CYP3A4 has been reported to cause symptoms of clozapine toxicity, but seizures have not been reported (Prior and Baker 2003 for review).

Differential diagnosis

The differential diagnosis of clozapine toxicity include anticholinergic toxicity, diabetic ketoacidosis, hyperglycemia, infection (secondary to agranulocytosis), neuroleptic malignant syndrome and other CNS pathology. The possibility that the syndrome could reflect a deliberate overdose of clozapine also needs to be considered.

Management

The immediate management of patients is dictated by the severity of the presenting symptoms. With less severe symptoms, patients can be managed with supportive measures. If a known inhibitor of a CYP enzyme acting on clozapine has been introduced recently, consideration should be given to discontinuing this medication. Alternatively, the dose of clozapine can be reduced. In the latter case, the clozapine dose will need to be readjusted once treatment with the CYP inhibitor or inducer is discontinued. Clozapine levels can be measured, but are not routinely available in acute settings.

In the case of severe symptoms, such as delirium, alterations in mental status or seizures, management should include immediate cessation of clozapine, appropriate supportive measures, and investigations to rule out other pathologies. Seizures can be controlled using standard methods. If clozapine is required for management of the patient's psychiatric illness, it can be reintroduced after appropriate anticonvulsant prophylaxis (carbamazepine is not recommended given the increased risk of agranulocytosis) (Meltzer and Fatemi 1998).

Risk factors and prevention

Clozapine toxicity caused by inhibition of CYP enzymes is easily preventable by avoiding the use of medications which inhibit these enzymes, especially CYP1A2 (Table 16.2). Where concomitant therapy is unavoidable, serum clozapine levels can be measured and, if necessary, clozapine dose adjusted for the duration of treatment. Clozapine toxicity caused by reversal of CYP induction, such as by quitting smoking, can be prevented by close monitoring of the patient during this period (Greenwood-Smith *et al.* 2003).

Individual CYP enzymes may be present in different amounts or forms in different people as a result of genetic polymorphisms. Information about such genetic polymorphism would be useful, but in most clinical situations routine phenotyping or genotyping is not done.

Hypertensive crisis with MAOIs

Introduction

A hypertensive crisis is a medical emergency involving an acute, severe blood pressure elevation that can result in impairment of organ systems (e.g. central nervous system, renal, cardiovascular). In these conditions, the blood pressure must be lowered over minutes to hours. Phenelzine, tranylcypromine and isocarboxazid are the common monoamine oxidase inhibitors (MAOIs) associated with hypertensive crisis. All three drugs cause irreversible inhibition of MAO. In contrast, moclobemide, a reversible inhibitor of MAO-A, is less likely to cause hypertensive crisis.

Clinical features

As with most syndromes, the clinical signs and symptoms are individually non-specific. It is the combination of symptoms, along with a history of

Table 16.3 Clinical features of hypertensive crisis

Central nervous system:
– headache (often occipital)
– new-onset blurred vision
– dilated pupils
– photophobia
– neck stiffness
– confusion
– change in mental state
– loss of consciousness
– stroke
Cardiovascular:
– elevated blood pressure
– palpitations
Gastrointestinal:
– abdominal pain
– nausea and vomiting
Miscellaneous:
– weakness and fatigue
– sweating
– motor agitation

MAOI use, that should alert the clinician and assist with diagnosis (Krishnan 1998). The severity of a MAOI hypertensive crisis varies. Symptoms usually begin suddenly within a few minutes to a few hours after the ingestion of another drug or a foodstuff that has the potential to interact with the MAOI. The symptoms that can occur are summarized in Table 16.3.

A pounding headache, often occipital, is often the first feature. It may lessen after an hour or so to leave a dull ache. Other symptoms can include flushing, palpitations, nausea and vomiting, dilatation of the pupils, photophobia, neck stiffness, sweating and restlessness. The systolic blood pressure may range from 150 to 220 mmHg and the diastolic from 100 to 130 mmHg. In severe cases convulsions and cerebral haemorrhage can occur. It has been estimated that 1 in every 8000 hypertensive reactions is fatal and that this equates to about 1 per 100 000 patients treated with tranylcypromine (Davidson 1992).

Pharmacological basis

The biological action of MAOIs is to increase the concentration of centrally acting monoamine neurotransmitters, such as 5-hydroxytryptamine (5-HT, serotonin), noradrenaline and dopamine, by inhibiting their degradation by MAO.

Two types of MAO enzymes have been identified, MAO-A and MAO-B. Both are located in the cerebral cortex, liver, stomach and intestine. MAO-A is selectively located in adrenergic and serotonergic nerve terminals in the CNS and peripheral sympathetic terminals. The platelets contain only MAO-B. Serotonin and noradrenaline are metabolized almost exclusively by MAO-A. 2-Phenylethylamine is metabolized by MAO-B. Dopamine and tyramine are substrates for both forms of MAO. Only MAO-A inhibition is thought to be relevant to the treatment of depression.

A hypertensive crisis can result from the interaction of MAOIs with foods and drinks (the so-called 'cheese reaction') as well as with other drugs. The dietary interaction occurs with foods that are rich in indirect-sympathomimetic amines such as tyramine and 2-phenylethylamine. These amines are normally metabolized by MAO-A and MAO-B in the gut and liver. However in patients treated with an MAOI, inhibition of intestinal and liver MAO allows increased amounts of the dietary amines to enter the systemic circulation. Inhibition of neuronal MAO-A results in increased storage of norepinephrine in pre-synaptic storage vesicles. Consequently tyramine and other indirect-sympathomimetic amines can cause an abnormal release of noradrenaline from the neuronal vesicles into synapses leading to stimulation of post-ganglionic sympathetic adrenergic neurones and hypertension. Food and drinks that are high in tyramine and/or other sympathomimetic amines (e.g. 2-phenylethylamine) or precursors of bioactive amines (e.g. DOPA) and should be avoided by patients are listed in Table 16.4. Most of the reported interactions between MAOIs and foodstuffs, and nearly all the deaths, have involved cheese (McCabe 1986).

Moclobemide is a reversible inhibitor of MAO-A, in contrast to tranyl-cypromine and phenelzine which are non-reversible inhibitors. Moclobemide is far less likely to be involved in a hypertensive reaction because excess tyramine can displace moclobemide from its binding site on MAO-A and so be metabolized by the enzyme.

A number of medications can also interact with MAOIs and precipitate a hypertensive crisis (Table 16.5). These include certain antihypertensives (e.g. guanethidine), precursors of biogenic amines (e.g. L-tryptophan, L-dopa) and indirect-acting sympathomimetics (e.g. methylphenidate, amphetamine, ephedrine, pseudoephedrine). Many over-the-counter cough and cold remedies contain ephedrine or pseudoephedrine and so also need to be avoided. Concomitant treatment with MAOIs and noradrenergic antidepressants can potentially cause a hypertensive reaction. The combination of a serotonergic antidepressant with an MAOI can cause serotonin syndrome, which is discussed in Chapter 3 of this book.

Table 16.4 Representative foodstuffs with high concentrations of tyramine or other sympathomimetic amines (or their precursors)

Beverages
– Chianti wine
– Beer (especially unfiltered)
Fruits and vegetables
– Broad and fava beans
– Canned figs and raisins
– Over-ripe fruits and vegetables
– Orange pulp
– Sauerkraut
Meat and Fish
– Beef and chicken liver
– Fermented sausages
– Cured meats
– Caviar
– Herring
– Dried fish, shrimp paste
Other
– Yeast extracts
– Packaged soups
– Aged cheese

Table 16.5 Representative medications that can interact with MAOIs

Antiasthmatics (beta-agonists)
Antidepressants (selective serotonin reuptake inhibitors, clomipramine, venlafaxine, buproprion)
Antihypertensives (alpha-methyldopa, guanethidine, pargyline, reserpine)
L-Tryptophan
Narcotics (especially meperidine)
Over-the-counter cold, hayfever and sinus medications containing phenylpropanolamine, pseudoephedrine, ephedrine, or dextromethorphan
Sympathomimetics (amphetamine, cocaine, methylphenidate, dopamine, epinephrine, norepinephrine, isoproterenol)

Differential diagnosis

Differential diagnosis includes:

 • acute coronary syndromes (aneurysms)

 • acute glomerulonephritis

- acute anxiety, panic attack
- delirium tremens
- encephalitis
- headaches (cluster, migraine, tension)
- hyperthyroidism (including thyroid storm, Graves' disease)
- myocardial infarction
- pheochromocytoma
- pregnancy (eclampsia, pre-eclampsia)
- serotonin syndrome
- stroke
- subarachnoid hemorrhage
- systemic lupus erythematosus
- use of over-the-counter or recreational sympathomimetic drugs.

Management

Hypertensive crisis is a medical emergency and should be treated in an appropriate setting. The MAOI should be immediately discontinued as should any contributory medications e.g. those that contain sympathomimetic amines. Clinical evaluation and investigations, including the following, are required to rule out other causes of hypertensive crisis:

Laboratory:

- serum electrolytes, urea, creatinine
- full blood count
- urinalysis (for evidence of haematuria or proteinuria)
- toxicology screen
- endocrine testing (TSH, T_4, T_3).

Imaging:

- chest x-ray
- head CT.

Other:

- ECG.

The α-adrenergic receptor blocker, phentolamine (5 mg intramuscularly or intravenously) is the recommended treatment for an MAOI-induced hypertensive crisis (Tueth *et al.* 1998). This drug has a rapid onset of action (usually within 5 minutes), and a single dose is generally effective. A diuretic such as frusemide (furosemide) may be given intravenously to avoid fluid retention, and, if necessary, a beta-blocker such as propranolol may be given to control tachycardia. Additional doses of phentolamine, if required, can be given over several hours. A recent alternative treatment is nifedipine (10 mg, bite and swallow or sublingual, with a repeat dose after 20 minutes if required). The onset of action with nifedipine usually occurs within 5 minutes (Schenk and Remick 1989; Tueth *et al.* 1998).

It is essential that the patient be monitored in case the hypertensive state returns or they become dangerously hypotensive.

Risk factors and prevention

Patient education is the mainstay of prevention. All patients receiving an MAOI should receive a list of food, beverages, and medications to be avoided. These medications and food restrictions should remain in place for 10 to 14 days after an MAOI is discontinued and an appropriate washout period of other medications (such as SSRIs) observed prior to initiating treatment with an MAOI. Patients can be given a card explaining they are on an MAOI and advised to carry it with them at all times. Patients may benefit from wearing a medical bracelet if long-term therapy is likely.

Summary: Anticholinergic Toxicity

Definition	A characteristic group of both central and peripheral symptoms caused by medications with anticholinergic activity.
Incidence	Unknown, but common. Increased risk in the elderly, patients with organic brain dysfunction or those taking more than one medication.
Drugs causing the syndrome	Tricyclic antidepressants
	Antipsychotic agents (both conventional and atypical agents)
	Anticholinergic drugs
Key symptoms	Altered mental status, blurred vision, elevated temperature, tachycardia, constipation, dry mouth, dry flushed skin, urinary retention
Pharmacological mechanism	Blockade of muscarinic receptors
Relevant investigations to confirm diagnosis	Physostigmine test
Management	Reduce or discontinue medications
	Supportive therapy
	Physostigmine (in acute intoxication)

Further reading	Beaver KM and Gavin JJ (1998). Treatment of acute anticholinergic poisoning with physostigmine. *American Journal of Emergency Medicine*, **16**, 505–7.
	Teoh R, Page AV, and Hardern R (2001). Physostigmine as treatment for severe CNS anticholinergic toxicity. *Emergency Medical Journal*, **18**, 412.
	Tune LE (2001). Anticholinergic effects of medication in elderly patients. *Journal of Clinical Psychiatry*, **62**, Suppl 21, 11–14.

Summary: Clozapine Toxicity

Definition	Symptoms due to an elevation in serum clozapine levels. This may be caused by concomitant treatment with medications that block the enzymes responsible for clozapine metabolism (particularly CYP1A2) or conversely by stopping medications that have previously induced these enzymes. Stopping smoking can have the same effect.
Incidence	Unknown
Drugs causing syndrome	Concomitant treatment with clozapine and medications which inhibit CYP1A2 e.g. fluvoxamine
Key symptoms	Sedation, hypotension, hypersalivation, tachycardia, myoclonic jerks, seizures
Pharmacological mechanism	Inhibition or reversal of induction of CYP enzymes involved in clozapine metabolism
Investigations to confirm diagnosis	History of prescribing change, consistent with above mechanism, shortly before symptom onset. Serum clozapine levels
Management	Stop concomitant medication, reduce or discontinue clozapine, control seizure if necessary
Further reading	Greenwood-Smith C, Lubmann DI, and Castle DJ (2003). Serum clozapine levels: a review of their clinical utility. *Journal of Psycholopharmacology*, **17**, 234–8.
	Prior TI and Baker GB (2003). Interactions between the cytochrome P450 system and the second-generation antipsychotics. *Journal of Psychiatry & Neuroscience*, **28**, 99–112.
	Wetzel H, Anghelescu I, and Szegedi A, *et al*. (1998). Pharmacokinetic interactions of clozapine with selective serotonin reuptake inhibitors: differential effects of fluvoxamine and paroxetine in a prospective study. *Journal of Clinical Psychopharmacology*, **18**, 2–9.

Summary: Hypertensive Crisis

Definition	A sudden, severe rise in blood pressure
Incidence	Unknown with psychotropics. Of patients with hypertension, approximately 1–2% can develop a hypertensive emergency with end-organ damage.
Drugs causing syndrome	Combination of MAOIs and certain foods rich in indirectly-acting sympathomimetics.
	Concomitant use of MAOIs with certain antihypertensives, sympathomimetics (may be present in over-the-counter cough and cold remedies), antidepressants*, narcotics and L-tryptophan,
Key symptoms	Headache, blurred vision, nausea, vomiting, neck stiffness, sweating, palpitations, change in mental status, stroke, sudden death
Pharmacological mechanism	Dietary interactions reflect blockade of intestinal and liver MAO allowing increased levels of biogenic amines to enter systemic circulation. These have an indirect-sympathomimetic action. This is enhanced by inhibition of neuronal MAO leading to increased intracellular stores of monoamines. The latter mechanism accounts for many of the drug interactions.
Investigations to confirm diagnosis	History may confirm combination of an MAOI and a contraindicated drug or foodstuff. Examination will show characteristic mental state and physical signs including elevation of blood pressure. Investigations can help exclude other causes of hypertensive crisis e.g. TFTs.
Management	Stop MAOI and causal agents, begin supportive treatment, correct blood pressure (nifedipine or phentolamine)
Further reading	Janicak PG, Davis JM, Preskorn SH *et al.* (2001). *Principles and Practice of Psychopharmacotherapy*, pp. 300–1. Lippincott Williams & Wilkins, PA.
	Kennedy SH, McKenna KF, and Baker GB (2001). Monoamine Oxidase Inhibitors. In: BJ Sadock and VA Sadock (ed.) *Kaplan & Sadock's Comprehensive Textbook of Psychiatry*, 7th edn, pp. 2397–406. Lippincott Williams & Wilkins, PA.
	Krishnan KRR (1998). Monoamine oxidase inhibitors. In: AF Schatzberg and CB Nemeroff (ed.) *The American Psychiatric Press Textbook of Psychopharmacology*, 2nd edn, pp. 239–249. American Psychiatric Press, Inc. Washington, DC.

* *Combined use of a noradrenergic antidepressant and a MAOI can potentially cause a hypertensive crisis. The combination of a serotonergic antidepressant and a MAOI is a well recognized cause of serotonin syndrome.*

References

Armstrong SC and Stephans JR (1997) Blood clozapine levels elevated by fluvoxamine: potential for side effects and lower clozapine dosage. *J Clin Psychiatry*, **58**, 499.

Beaver KM and Gavin JJ (1998). Treatment of acute anticholinergic poisoning with physostigmine. *Am J Emerg Med*, **16**, 505–7.

Brown JH and Taylor P (1996). Muscarinic receptor agonists and antagonists. In Goodman and Gilman's *The Pharmacological Basis of Therapeutics*, 9th edn, JG Hardman and LE Limbird (ed.), pp. 141–60. McGraw-Hill: New York, NY.

Davidson J (1992). Monoamine oxidase inhibitors. In *Handbook of Affective Disorders*. ES Paykel (ed.) Churchill Livingstone: Edinburgh.

Dequardo JR and Roberts M (1996). Elevated clozapine levels after fluvoxamine initiation. *Am J Psychiatry*, **153**, 840–1.

Drug Facts and Comparisons Burnham TH (ed.) (2001). 55th edn, pp. 393–4. Wolter Kluwer: St Louis, MO.

Greenwood-Smith C, Lubmann DI, and Castle DJ (2003). Serum clozapine levels: a review of their clinical utility. *J Psychopharmacol*, **17**, 234–8.

Janicak, PG, Davis JM, Preskorn SH, *et al.* (2001). *Principles and Practice of Psychopharmacotherapy*, pp. 300–1. Lippincott Williams and Wilkins: Philadelphia.

Kennedy SH, McKenna KF, and Baker GB (2001). Monoamine Oxidase Inhibitors. In *Kaplan and Sadock's Comprehensive Textbook of Psychiatry*, 7th edn, BJ Sadock and VA Sadock (ed.), pp. 2397–406. Lippincott Williams and Wilkins: Philadelphia.

Krishnan KRR (1998). Monoamine oxidase inhibitors. In *The American Psychiatric Press Textbook of Psychopharmacology*, 2nd edn, AF Schatzberg and CB Nemeroff (ed.), pp. 239–49. American Psychiatric Press, Inc.: Washington, DC.

Le Blaye I, Donatini B, Hall M, *et al.* (1992). Acute overdosage with clozapine: a review of available clinical experience. *Pharmaceut Med*, **6**, 169–78.

McCabe BJ (1986). Dietary tyramine and other pressor-amines in MAOI regimens: a review. *J Am Diet Assoc*, **86**, 1059–64.

Meltzer HY and Fatemi SH (1998). Treatment of schizophrenia. In *The American Psychiatric Press Textbook of Psychopharmacology*, 2nd edn, AF Schatzberg and CB Nemeroff (ed.), pp. 747–74. American Psychiatric Press Inc.: Washington, DC.

Meyer JM (2001). Individual changes in clozapine levels after smoking cessation: results and a predictive model. *J Clin Psychopharmacol*, **21**, 569–74.

Prior TI and Baker GB (2003). Interactions between the cytochrome P450 system and the second-generation antipsychotics. *J Psychiatry Neurosci*, **28**, 99–112.

Schenk CH and Remick RA (1989). Sublingual nifedipine in the treatment of hypertensive crisis associate with monoamine oxidase inhibitors. *Ann Emerg Med*, **18**, 114–15.

Skogh E, Bengtsson F, and Nordin C (1999). Could discontinuing smoking be hazardous for patients administered clozapine medication? A case report. *Ther Drug Monit*, **21**, 580–2.

Teoh R, Page AV, and Hardern R (2001). Physostigmine as treatment for severe CNS anticholinergic toxicity. *Emerg Med J*, **18**, 412.

Tueth MJ, DeVane CL, and Evans DL (1998). Treatment of psychiatric emergencies. In *The American Psychiatric Press Textbook of Psychopharmacology*, 2nd edn,

AF Schatzberg and CB Nemeroff (ed.), pp. 917–29. American Psychiatric Press Inc.: Washington, DC.

Tune LE (2001). Anticholinergic effects of medication in elderly patients. *J Clin Psychiatry*, **62** (Suppl. 21), 11–14 (review).

Wetzel H, Anghelescu I, Szegedi A, *et al.* (1998). Pharmacokinetic interactions of clozapine with selective serotonin reuptake inhibitors: differential effects of fluvoxamine and paroxetine in a prospective study. *J Clin Psychopharmacol*, **18**, 2–9.

Index

NB: summaries and tables are indicated in **bold**.